Essentials in Ophthalmology

Series Editor
Arun D. Singh
Cleveland Clinic Foundation
Cole Eye Institute
Cleveland, OH, USA

More information about this series at http://www.springer.com/series/5332

Narsing A. Rao • Julie Schallhorn
Damien C. Rodger
Editors

Posterior Uveitis

Advances in Imaging and Treatment

Springer

Editors
Narsing A. Rao
Ophthalmology
USC Roski Eye Institute Ophthalmology
Los Angeles, CA
USA

Julie Schallhorn
Department of Ophthalmology
and Francis I. Proctor Foundation
University of California, San Francisco
San Francisco, CA
USA

Damien C. Rodger
Department of Ophthalmology
Kaiser Permanente Los Angeles
Medical Center
Los Angeles, CA
USA

ISSN 1612-3212 ISSN 2196-890X (electronic)
Essentials in Ophthalmology
ISBN 978-3-030-03139-8 ISBN 978-3-030-03140-4 (eBook)
https://doi.org/10.1007/978-3-030-03140-4

Library of Congress Control Number: 2019930846

This Springer imprint is published by the registered company Springer Nature Switzerland AG
The registered company address is: Gewerbestrasse 11, 6330 Cham, Switzerland

Preface

We have the great fortune of practicing medicine at a time of rapid discovery and advancement. Every coming year brings new diagnostics, new therapeutics, and an evolving insight into the genesis of uveitis and related intraocular inflammatory diseases. We have collected here an in-depth examination of the diseases, imaging techniques, and treatments that are being reshaped by the advances in our field.

The first section will tour a multitude of infectious and noninfectious uveitidies and explore how advances are aiding our diagnosis and treatment. The second section will delve into established and emerging therapeutics, including advances in drug delivery. We are aided in this journey by a panoply of experts from around the world, bringing a truly international view to this subject.

We hope that readers find *Advances in Intraocular Inflammation Imaging and Treatment* useful as they navigate and incorporate the changes in the field in diagnosis and management of intraocular inflammation and prepare for what is to come.

Los Angeles, CA, USA — Narsing A. Rao
San Francisco, CA, USA — Julie Schallhorn
Los Angeles, CA, USA — Damien C. Rodger

Contents

Contributors

Nisha Acharya, MD, MS F.I. Proctor Foundation, University of California, San Francisco, San Francisco, CA, USA

Thomas A. Albini, MD Bascom Palmer Eye Institute, University of Miami Miller School, Department of Ophthalmology, Miami, FL, USA

Soumyava Basu, MS Retina and Uveitis Service, L V Prasad Eye Institute, Bhubaneswar, India

Jesse L. Berry, MD USC Roski Eye Institute, Keck School of Medicine of the University of Southern California, Department of Ophthalmology, Los Angeles, CA, USA

Children's Hospital Los Angeles, Keck School of Medicine of the University of Southern California, Los Angeles, CA, USA

Sujay Chauhan, DO Narayana Nethralaya, Department of Uveitis and Ocular Immunology, Bangalore, India

Dana Yousef Darwish, BS Illinois Eye and Ear Infirmary, University of Illinois at Chicago, Department of Ophthalmology and Visual Sciences, Chicago, IL, USA

Brian K. Do, MD USC Roski Eye Institute, Keck School of Medicine of the University of Southern California, Department of Ophthalmology, Los Angeles, CA, USA

John A. Gonzales, MD F.I. Proctor Foundation, University of California, San Francisco, San Francisco, CA, USA

Ankush Kawali, DNB Narayana Nethralaya, Department of Uveitis and Ocular Immunology, Bangalore, India

Phuc V. Le, MD, PhD UCLA Department of Ophthalmology, Doheny Eye Institute, Pasadena, CA, USA

Ashleigh Laurin Levison, MD Colorado Retina Associates, Denver, CO, USA

Ann-Marie Lobo, MD Illinois Eye and Ear Infirmary, University of Illinois at Chicago, Department of Ophthalmology and Visual Sciences, Chicago, IL, USA

Padmamalini Mahendradas, DO, DNB Narayana Nethralaya, Department of Uveitis and Ocular Immunology, Bangalore, India

Hossein Nazari Khanamiri, MD University of Texas medical Branch, Department of Ophthalmology and Visual Sciences, Galveston, TX, USA

Francesco Pichi, MD Eye Institute, Cleveland Clinic Abu Dhabi, Abu Dhabi, UAE

Cleveland Clinic Lerner College of Medicine, Case Western Reserve University, Cleveland, OH, USA

Narsing A. Rao, MD Ophthalmology, USC Roski Eye Institute Ophthalmology, Los Angeles, CA, USA

Damien C. Rodger, MD, PhD Department of Ophthalmology, Kaiser Permanente Los Angeles Medical Center, Los Angeles, CA, USA

Julie Schallhorn, MD, MS Department of Ophthalmology and Francis I. Proctor Foundation, University of California, San Francisco, San Francisco, CA, USA

Jeffrey J. Tan, MD USC Roski Eye Institute, Department of Ophthalmology, Los Angeles, CA, USA

Daniel Vitor Vasconcelos-Santos, MD, PhD Universidade Federal de Minas Gerais, Faculdade de Medicina, Belo Horizonte, Brazil

Mei Zhou, MD Illinois Eye and Ear Infirmary, University of Illinois at Chicago, Department of Ophthalmology and Visual Sciences, Chicago, IL, USA

Part I

Introduction

Posterior Uveitis: Role of Imaging Modalities

Phuc V. Le

Introduction

Clinical judgment is key to the diagnosis and management of intraocular inflammation. However, with the development of new imaging technologies and modalities, clinicians have more clinically relevant information available to them. This makes understanding the different imaging modalities an important adjunct to the clinical exam. The goal of this chapter is to review the principles underlying these imaging technologies and help the clinician understand how to utilize them appropriately. Several reviews of imaging in ocular inflammation have previously been published [1–3]. Thus, we will briefly discuss traditional photography and angiography, but the emphasis of this chapter will be on newer technologies. These include ultra-widefield imaging, autofluorescence, optical coherence tomography (OCT), and advanced OCT applications such as en face imaging and OCT-angiography (OCT-A).

Two technological developments have occurred which are relevant to several of the imaging modalities discussed in this chapter. The first is that imaging systems are now digital. This can be as simple as replacing a film-based capturing unit with a digital SLR camera. Digitization has many benefits, including electronic storage and computerized manipulation of images. The second development is the capability to capture noncontact ultra-widefield images with up to 200° field of view, such as seen in Fig. 1. This improves our ability to assess the retinal periphery and can be especially useful in evaluating peripheral retinal vasculitis [4, 5]. Widefield imaging will be discussed in detail later on in this chapter.

P. V. Le (✉)
UCLA Department of Ophthalmology, Doheny Eye Institute, Pasadena, CA, USA
e-mail: ple@doheny.org

N. A. Rao et al. (eds.), *Posterior Uveitis*, Essentials in Ophthalmology,
https://doi.org/10.1007/978-3-030-03140-4_1

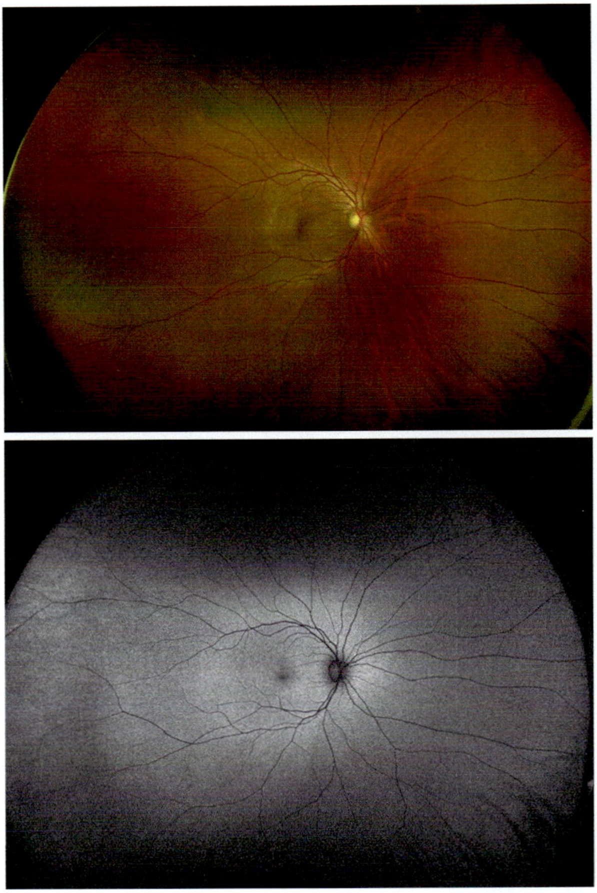

Fig. 1 Ultra-widefield pseudocolor and green-light autofluorescence image, normal eye. Top panel shows pseudocolor (combination of red and green channel signal) image. Bottom panel shows green-light autofluorescence image

Color Photography

Traditional anterior segment and fundus photography still plays an important role in the diagnosis and management of intraocular inflammation. Photographs capture the clinical appearance of the area of interest, allowing the clinician to share clinical findings as well as assess changes over time. Some conditions can be diagnosed solely on the basis of a single fundus photograph. In addition to standard color or black and white photography, filters can be utilized to help accentuate certain aspects of the image. One example is the use of so-called red-free filters to help detect retinal hemorrhage.

Intravenous Angiography

Traditional fluorescein angiography (FA) and indocyanine green angiography (ICGA) are performed by injecting a fluorescent dye into a peripheral vein and capturing time-stamped images of the posterior pole with a flash photography system.

The imaging system utilizes filters matched to the excitation and emission spectra of the fluorescent dye, approximately 480/520 nm for fluorescein and 790–800/820 nm for indocyanine green [6].

Several modifications to the traditional imaging technique have been developed. One is the replacement of the excitation light source and filter by a laser tuned to the specific wavelength of the fluorescent dye. Some devices have two laser light sources, allowing for simultaneous FA and ICGA at one sitting [6, 7]. Another improvement is the use of confocal technology to block out light that is not in the focal plane, thus reducing noise [8]. As previously discussed, digitization of the images allows for immediate review and image adjustment for optimal interpretation, while the combination of angiography and widefield imaging allows clinicians to better evaluate peripheral pathology.

Fluorescein Angiography

Fluorescein angiography is a primary tool in the assessment of ocular blood flow. Fluorescein sodium has a molecular weight of 376 daltons and in the intravascular space is incompletely bound to albumin. Because of the presence of unbound or "free" fluorescein sodium, it easily leaks out of even minimally damaged or inflamed retinal vessels. Examples of application of fluorescein angiography to ocular inflammation include the detection of cystoid macular edema, vasculitis, vein occlusion, and secondary choroidal neovascularization [1]. Less commonly, FA can be utilized for the anterior segment to assess for iris nonperfusion or leakage from inflamed vessels.

Areas of brightness, or hyperfluorescence, can be caused by leaking, pooling, staining, or so-called "window defect." The first three represent accumulation of fluorescein dye, whereas the latter represents increased visibility of the fluorescein in the choroidal circulation due to loss of overlying retinal pigment epithelium. In some forms of choroidal inflammation, such as serpiginous choroiditis, loss of the choroidal vasculature can lead to overlying retinal pigment epithelium (RPE) atrophy [9]. In these areas, there may be very little hyperfluorescent "window defect" effect because of the loss of the underlying choriocapillaris.

Areas of darkness, or hypofluorescence, can be caused by either blockage of fluorescence by overlying material, such as hemorrhage, or lack of fluorescein dye due to nonperfusion.

Indocyanine Green Angiography

The mechanics of capturing ICGA images are similar to that of FA. However, the differences between the indocyanine green (ICG) molecule and fluorescein sodium molecule lead to several important differences between the two imaging modalities. The ICG molecule is of higher molecular weight (775 daltons vs. 376 daltons) and has a higher binding affinity to serum proteins than fluorescein sodium [10]. Thus, while fluorescein readily leaks out of even minimally damaged retinal vessels, ICG typically remains bound to serum proteins and therefore tends to stay within the

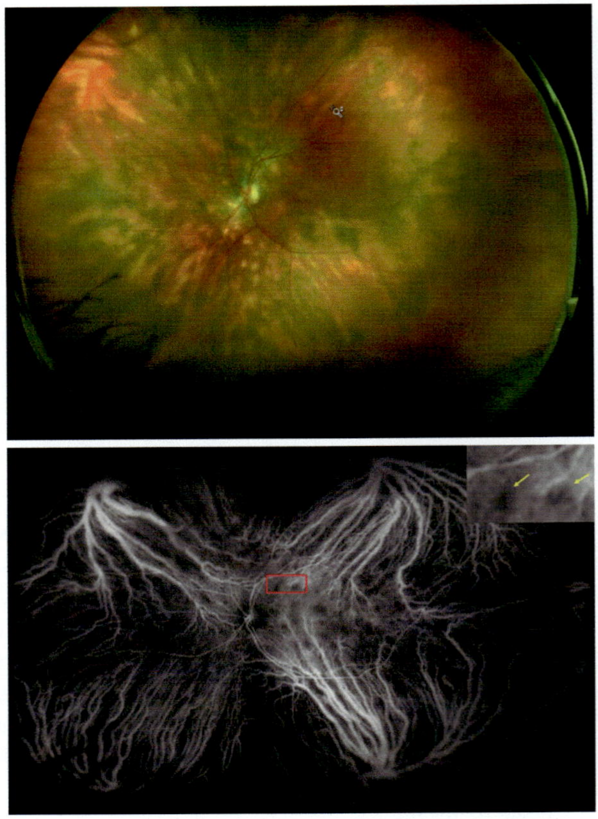

Fig. 2 Ultra-widefield pseudocolor and indocyanine green angiography (ICGA) image of patient with birdshot chorioretinopathy. Top panel: Pseudocolor image demonstrating multiple hypopigmented lesions scattered throughout the posterior pole. Bottom panel: ICG angiography image, demonstrating multiple areas of hypofluorescence due to nonperfusion. Inset shows two areas of nonperfusion (arrows). (Courtesy of Rao NA)

intravascular space. In an ICGA image, areas of increased brightness are typically referred to as either hyperfluorescent or hypercyanescent, while areas of decreased brightness can be called hypofluorescent or hypocyanescent.

Because of its longer excitation/emission spectra, ICG angiography is better able to penetrate the RPE and thin layers of hemorrhage than FA. Thus, ICG angiography can better image choroidal vascular pathology such as choroidal hemangiomas and polypoidal choroidal vasculopathy. In ocular inflammation, ICG angiography can be utilized to detect choroidal inflammation and nonperfusion such as seen in birdshot chorioretinopathy (BCR), MEWDS, APMPPE, and serpiginous [9, 11]. An image of a patient with BCR is shown in Fig. 2.

Autofluorescence and Infrared Reflectance

Autofluorescence (AF) imaging is a relatively new, non-invasive imaging modality that captures the distribution of fluorophores within the retina. This allows the detection of areas of pathological fluorophore accumulation, as well as areas of RPE and retinal atrophy in which there is decreased or absent autofluorescence signal. A review of autofluorescence imaging was recently published [12], as well as a review of autofluorescence imaging in uveitis [13].

The primary fluorophore in the retina is lipofuscin, which is composed of incompletely digested photoreceptor outer segments. Lipofuscin accumulates within RPE cells with age and accumulates more rapidly in conditions of abnormal vitamin A recycling such as Stargardt's disease [14]. One important component of lipofuscin is the bis-retinoid N-retinylidene-N-retinylethanolamine (A2E).

The accumulation of A2E and other products of vitamin A recycling that make up lipofuscin can be both an indicator and a cause of RPE cell dysfunction and death. This is because dysfunctional RPE cells may be unable to process photoreceptor outer segments efficiently, leading to the accumulation of lipofuscin and the idea that hyperautofluorescence is a marker of "sick or dying" RPE. Lipofuscin within the cell may be directly toxic to cells due to its detergent effect and the increased formation of free radicals. Thus, there is a potential for a vicious cycle of lipofuscin accumulation in dysfunctional RPE cells, causing toxicity and worsening RPE dysfunction and increased levels of lipofuscin accumulation.

Image Capture

Related to its initial detection as part of fluorescein angiography imaging, the early autofluorescence imaging systems were flash photography systems with excitation and emission filter wavelengths matched to that of fluorescein sodium. These flash photography systems are still in use today, but new, optimized filter sets have been developed. These filter sets use an excitation bandwidth shifted into the wavelength of green light. These images are therefore often called green-light autofluorescence images. The ultra-widefield imaging systems also generate green-light autofluorescence images but are not flash-based.

The other commonly used system used to capture autofluorescence images is based on the confocal scanning laser ophthalmoscope (Spectralis, Heidelberg Engineering, Heidelberg Germany). In this system, the excitation system consists of a low-power blue laser which is scanned across the area in a raster pattern. The emitted light passes through a confocal pinhole onto a detector. This technique allows multiple signals to be averaged, and the confocal optics prevent light that is out of focus from contributing to the signal. These images are sometimes referred to as blue-light autofluorescence images. Because the system utilizes confocal imaging, it is more sensitive to inaccuracies in the focus of the camera.

Interpretation

In a fundus autofluorescence image, the pixel brightness represents the intensity of the autofluorescence signal. Bright regions are called hyperautofluorescent, and these represent areas of increased lipofuscin from subretinal deposits such as drusen, vitelliform lesions, or accumulation within dysfunctional RPE cells.

Hyperautofluorescence can also occur due to so-called unmasking. This occurs when dysfunctional photoreceptors do not absorb the autofluorescence signal from the underlying RPE. This can occur due to temporary photobleaching, such as when the eye has just recently been imaged with another modality or due to a disease process that causes loss of photoreceptors without loss of the underlying RPE.

Dark regions on AF images are described as hypoautofluorescent. Hypoautofluorescence can occur due to blockage of either the excitation or emission by overlying heme or fluid or due to lack of autofluorescence signal due to RPE atrophy. It is important to note that in blue-light autofluorescence, the fovea and juxtafoveal region are normally hypoautofluorescent due to blockage of the autofluorescence signal from luteal pigments such as lutein and zeaxanthin. Thus, true decreased autofluorescence is difficult to assess adjacent to the fovea, and complementary modalities such as infrared reflectance and OCT are often utilized. The optic disc and retinal vasculature typically have no autofluorescent signal and therefore can be used as a comparator for the level of "black" to expect in the fundus image from a particular eye at a specific setting. The optic disc, blood vessels, and fovea are typically much more hypoautofluorescent on blue-light autofluorescence than green-light autofluorescence images.

A normal fundus autofluorescence image is shown in Fig. 1. The optic nerve and blood vessels appear black or hypoautofluorescent, due to lack of lipofuscin. There is a general low level of background autofluorescence that increases slightly in the parafoveal area but then decreases quickly in the fovea, again due to blockage by luteal pigments within the photoreceptors.

In general, AF imaging in inflammation demonstrates focal areas of abnormal autofluorescence. Abnormalities in autofluorescence are often more numerous than the lesions that are seen on color fundus photography or clinical biomicroscopy. These areas may be hypo or hyperautofluorescent in the acute phase, and hyperautofluorescent lesions can become hypoautofluorescent over time. Examples of conditions with hyperautofluorescence in the acute stage include multiple evanescent white dot syndrome (MEWDS) and serpiginous choroiditis [15]. Hyperautofluorescence may be due to increased lipofuscin accumulation from RPE dysfunction or unmasking due to overlying photoreceptor dysfunction. These regions of hyperautofluorescence tend to fade as the inflammation subsides. If the inflammation results in RPE atrophy, the lesion will become hypoautofluorescent. If the tissue recovers, the area will may return to its normal autofluorescence (iso-autofluorescent). Other conditions appear to have lesions which are solely hypoautofluorescent, such as seen in birdshot chorioretinopathy [16]. Areas of hypoautofluorescence from RPE atrophy are analogous to areas of geographic atrophy in age-related macular degeneration.

(Near) IR Reflectance

Near-infrared reflectance (IR) imaging is commonly utilized with blue-light autofluorescence imaging. This imaging modality utilizes excitation in the wavelength of approximately 820–830 nm. Because it is a longer wavelength than blue light, infrared reflectance penetrates deeper into the tissue and is less affected by media opacity or hemorrhage.

On IR imaging, areas of RPE atrophy appear bright. This modality can be used to detect atrophy in the perifoveal region, since perifoveal hypoautofluorescence is a normal finding. Infrared imaging can also be used to follow choroidal nevi. Since it penetrates heme, hemorrhage is often poorly visible on IR reflectance images. An example of FAF and IR imaging is shown in Fig. 3.

Ultra-widefield Imaging

Noncontact ultra-widefield imaging systems with the capability to image 150–200° of the fundus are currently available. Such systems typically capture in multiple modalities, including color photography, fluorescein and/or indocyanine green angiography, and autofluorescence. The color image is typically a pseudocolor image generated by combining the signal from individual green, red, and sometimes blue channels.

The obvious benefit of ultra-widefield imaging is the ability to detect peripheral pathology. When coupled with FA, this includes the ability to detect peripheral retinal vasculitis such as seen in Fig. 4. Several reports have now demonstrated peripheral leakage in patients with uveitis that were thought to be quiescent on clinical exam or standard macular angiography [5].

Optical Coherence Tomography

The development of optical coherence tomography (OCT) by Huang and colleagues has revolutionized ophthalmology [16]. Using OCT, clinicians are now able to obtain micron level structural information, improving both our understanding of pathophysiology and our diagnostic ability. Further developments in OCT-related technology, such as enhanced depth imaging, swept-source OCT, and OCT-angiography, provide even more information. The plethora of imaging options available once again emphasizes the importance of understanding the basis of each technique.

Technology

In the original description of OCT, called time-domain OCT, a low-coherence light beam is split between a reference arm and a sample arm [16]. The light traveling down the sample arm reflects or backscatters at each interface it encounters. The light traveling down the reference arm encounters a reference mirror, which is scanned (moved) in the Z-direction. The reflected light from both arms is combined, and the interference pattern is used to calculate a reflectance at each position along the path of the beam through the sample. This is analogous to an axial ultrasound

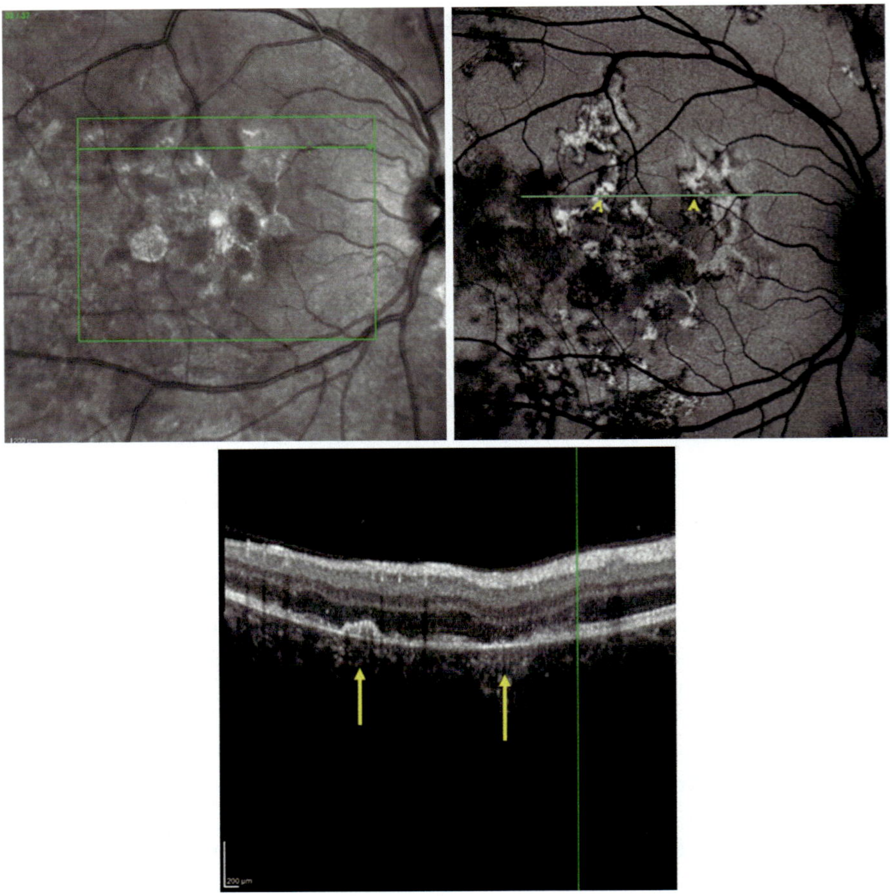

Fig. 3 Infrared reflectance, blue-light autofluorescence, and optical coherence tomography (OCT) B-scan of patient with tuberculous choroiditis. Top left panel: Infrared reflectance image. Top right panel: Blue-light autofluorescence image. There are areas of hyper- and hypoautofluoresence. The hyperautofluorescent areas can represent lipofuscin accumulation in a subretinal pigment epithelium (RPE) deposit (left arrowhead) or active choroiditis causing dysfunctional or degenerating RPE and lipofuscin accumulation. The hypoautofluorescent areas (right arrowhead) typically represent areas of RPE atrophy and therefore absent lipofuscin. The arrowheads correspond to arrows on the OCT B-scan. Bottom panel – OCT B-scan through the region marked by the green line in panels A and B. The right arrow indicates an area of RPE degeneration with overlying photoreceptor loss. There is no external limiting membrane visible in that area, and the region dips downward due to inner and outer segment atrophy. The outer nuclear layer is still present. The left arrow demonstrates a sub-RPE deposit that corresponds to the hyperautofluorescent area in panel B. (Courtesy of Rao NA)

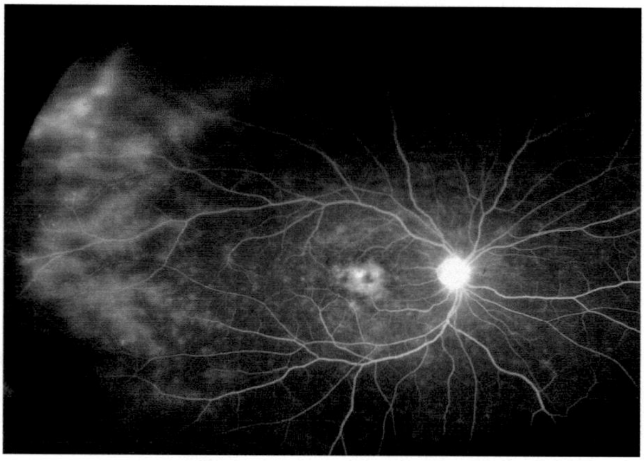

Fig. 4 Ultra-widefield fluorescein angiogram of patient with ANCA-positive granulomatosis polyangiitis (Wegener's granulomatosis). There is cystoid macular edema, seen as hyperfluorescence in the macula, and leakage in the periphery. (Courtesy of Rao NA)

beam, and the terminology is the same. The reflectance along a single beam is called an A-scan or amplitude scan because the magnitude of the reflectance along the axial scan was originally plotted as the amplitude on a two-dimensional graph. Multiple parallel A-scans can be displayed by converting the amplitude at each axial position into a brightness, thus creating a cross-sectional B-scan (brightness scan).

Fourier domain or spectral domain OCT (SD-OCT) utilizes a broadband light source and spectrometer [17]. The reference mirror is fixed instead of moving, and the interference pattern measured by the spectrometer undergoes a Fourier transform to provide a scan profile that is similar to a time-domain A-scan but without the physical movement of the reference mirror. These SD-OCT devices have improved both speed and resolution, with current mass-produced models capable of capturing approximately 20,000–50,000 A-scans per second with resolution in the range of a few microns. This has enabled the capture of three-dimensional volume scans within seconds.

Interpretation

The OCT signal represents the backscatter at a specific location or depth within the tissue. Increased backscatter is represented by a brighter pixel intensity and is called hyperreflective. Decreased backscatter is represented by a dark pixel intensity and is called hyporeflective. For instance, the RPE layer is normally hyperreflective, while fluid and vitreous are hyporeflective.

A normal retinal B-scan has alternating hyper- and hyporeflective layers. The nerve fiber layer and RPE are highly hyperreflective. The ganglion cell and plexiform layers are hyperreflective but less so than the nerve fiber layer, and the nuclear layers are hyporeflective.

There are many applications of OCT imaging in ocular inflammation. In the anterior segment, OCT imaging can be utilized to quantify (inflammatory) cells and document peripheral anterior synechiae and posterior synechiae [18, 19]. It has also been used to quantify vitreous haze [20].

Today, OCT is a routine tool for assessing retinal pathology. It can detect vitreomacular interface disease such as epiretinal membranes and macular pucker. Fluid within the retina, such as cystoid edema and subretinal fluid, is seen as a hyporeflective space. There is high agreement between FA and OCT in evaluating uveitic macular edema [21]. Atrophy of the RPE appears as a triad of thinning of the RPE/Bruch's complex, hypertransmission into the choroid and sclera, and photoreceptor thinning (Fig. 3 panel C). Optical coherence tomography is also a primary modality to detect signs of choroidal neovascularization, a possible sequelae of ocular inflammation.

Advanced OCT Applications

En Face Imaging

Just as multiple parallel one-dimensional A-scans can be used to create a two-dimensional B-scan, multiple B-scans can be combined to form a three-dimensional volume scan. A traditional horizontal B-scan would represent a transverse or axial section of the volume scan. An image that represents a coronal section of the volume scan is called a "C-scan" or en face image [22]. It attempts to mimic the view one would have if they were looking directly at a particular depth within the fundus.

Due to the curvature of the fundus, a single C-scan at a fixed depth within the cube scan would cut through different layers of the retina. A more useful view may be one that is based on the curvature of the fundus. Therefore, a commonly utilized modification of en face imaging utilizes automated segmentation of the retinal layers and allows the user to display a C-scan "slice" that is not at a fixed depth relative to the camera system but instead is relative to a particular retinal layer. The retinal layers commonly utilized as reference layers include the RPE and internal limiting membrane, since these layers are easier to detect automatically. The software is capable of displaying different thicknesses within the volume scan, from "slices" as thin as a few pixels to thicker "slabs" representing tens or hundreds of microns of thickness. For instance, one can select the so-called ellipsoid zone of the retina by selecting a slab positioned immediately above the RPE with a thickness of approximately 20 microns. An example en face image and the OCT B-scan source is shown in Fig. 5.

Because it combines the signal from multiple B-scans, en face imaging is very sensitive to motion artifact. Image registration and eye tracking are some of the techniques used by the device manufacturers to minimize these artifacts [23, 24].

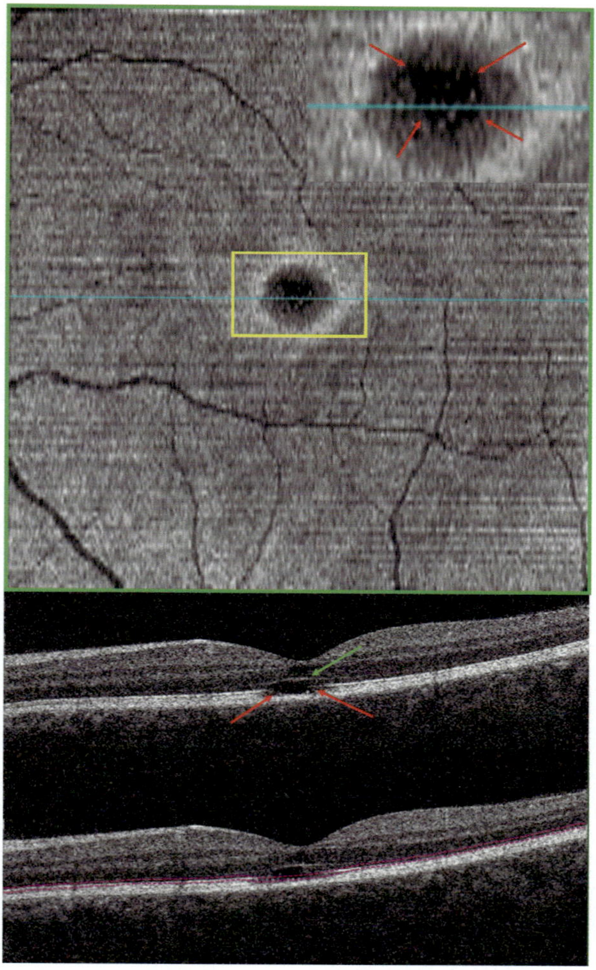

Fig. 5 En face solar retinopathy. En face image of photoreceptor damage from solar retinopathy (sungazing). Top panel: en face slab of the so-called ellipsoid zone (EZ)-band, generated from the macular cube scan. Inset shows the absent signal in the fovea, indicating loss of the EZ-band (red arrows). Middle panel – OCT B-scan through the fovea. The foveal external limiting membrane is intact (higher green arrow), but there is a hyporeflective space where the inner and outer segments should be (lower red arrows). Bottom panel – OCT B-scan through the fovea. Dotted purple lines immediately anterior to the retinal pigment epithelium show the upper and lower boundaries of the slab used to generate the en face image in the top panel

Enhanced Depth Imaging Optical Coherence Tomography (EDI-OCT)

In a conventional SD-OCT B-scan, the point of maximal signal, called the zero delay line, is placed near the interface between the posterior vitreous and the retina. This allows improved visualization of vitreomacular interface disease such as epiretinal membranes and vitreomacular traction. Unfortunately, sensitivity decreases with depth (called sensitivity roll-off). Thus, imaging of the choroid and sclera is hampered by both distance from the zero delay line as well as the presence of overlying light-absorbing structures such as photoreceptors and RPE. By placing the subject closer to the device, an inverted image (which is normally suppressed) is obtained with the choroid much closer to the zero delay line. This technique, called enhanced depth imaging or EDI-OCT, significantly improves the ability to image the deeper structures such as the choroid and sclera [25].

The development of EDI-OCT has allowed improved measurements of choroidal thickness, as well as the ability to detect abnormal reflectivity within the choroid itself [26]. These changes in reflectivity may indicate choroidal inflammation, such as in BCR [27].

Swept Source OCT

A recent development in OCT technology is swept-source OCT (SS-OCT) [28]. In SS-OCT, both the excitation and detection aspects of the OCT device have been modified. While conventional SD-OCT systems typically use a superluminescent diode laser centered in the 820–870 nm range, the SS-OCT uses a tunable laser centered at a wavelength of approximately 1000 nm. "Tunable" means that the wavelength of the laser is changed, or "tuned," to span a spectrum of wavelengths. The detector in the SS-OCT is also different. The SS-OCT utilizes photodetectors instead of a combination of charge coupled device (CCD) camera and spectrometer. With these modifications, the SS-OCT has increased penetration, less signal noise ratio drop-off, and increased speed. Typical SS-OCT devices are able to obtain approximately 100,000 A-scans/second, which is about twice the speed of conventional SD-OCT systems. Higher A-scan speeds can be utilized to scan larger areas, perform multiple scans of the same location, and/or decrease the time required to obtain a single volume scan. Swept-source OCT can also be utilized with en face imaging and OCT-angiography.

Optical Coherence Tomography Angiography

Optical coherence tomography angiography (OCT-A) is based on the premise that variations in the reflectance at a single location in repeated OCT B-scans must be due to blood flow or noise. Thus, by obtaining multiple B-scans of the same position and then detecting differences in the amplitude and phase of the reflectance signal, OCT-A generates images of blood flow and presumably blood vessels. Once a volume scan is created, "slabs" of retina are selected, and the blood vessels within the slab boundaries are displayed as a two-dimensional en face image. An OCT-A image from a normal eye is shown in Fig. 6. Similar to the standard en face imaging technique, implementation of OCT-A can utilize image registration and eye tracking in order to increase the likelihood that the same location is sampled. A review of OCT-A applied to intraocular inflammation was recently published [29]. An OCT-A image from an eye with cystoid macular edema before and after treatment is shown in Fig. 7.

Compared to traditional angiography, OCT-A has several advantages. First, it is non-invasive and fast. Since there is no intravenous dye, the risk of triggering a severe allergic reaction is eliminated. The scan takes just slightly longer than a traditional OCT macular cube scan. The actual scan volume parameters such as the scan dimensions and number of repeated B-scans vary by device and can be adjusted for each individual patient. Unlike in dye-based angiography, there is no leakage that can obscure the imaging of adjacent areas. The exact depth of the flow within the volume scan is known and can be individually highlighted. For instance, the vessels within the superficial retinal layer can be isolated and viewed separately from the deep retinal layer. In addition, OCT-A can be used to image both the retina and choroid simultaneously.

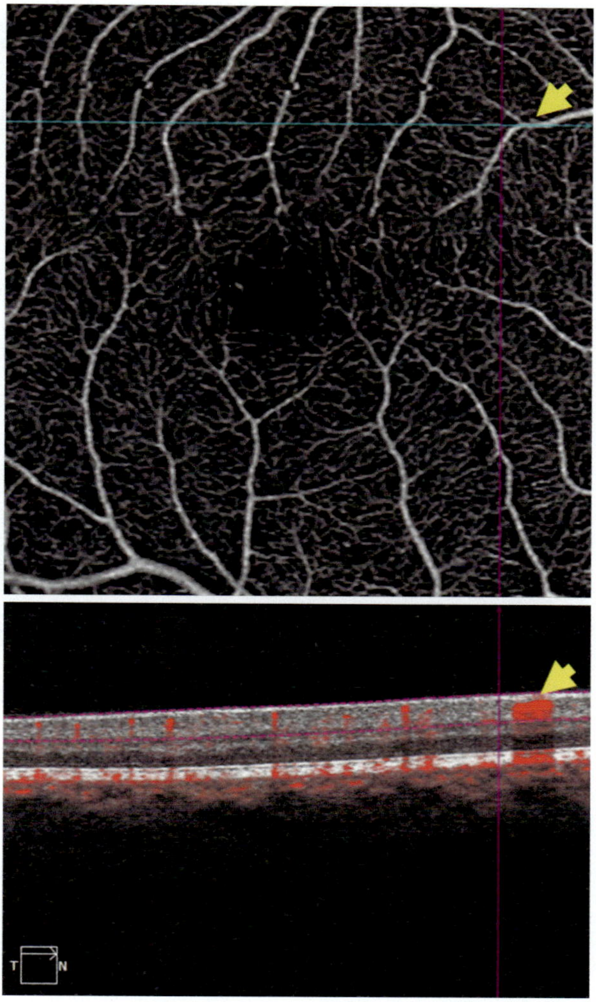

Fig. 6 Optical coherence tomography angiography image, normal eye. Top panel: En face optical coherence tomography (OCT-A) image of the superficial retinal layer. Bottom panel: One of the OCT B-scans used to generate the OCT-A image. The dotted purple lines show the upper and lower boundaries of the slab that represents the superficial retinal layer. The red color indicates the magnitude of the angiography signal (variation between repeated B-scans of the same location). Arrowhead shows corresponding location of a retinal vessel traveling parallel to the OCT B-scan for a short distance

The OCT-A technology has limitations. Importantly, since there is no dye, OCT-A imaging cannot detect leakage from inflamed vessels. It may be possible to measure parameters such as vascular index and dilation/width of retinal vessels to detect vasculitis, but these may be nonspecific, or the "normal" range may vary so much that few patients with intraocular inflammation fall outside the normal range. Second, OCT-A images can suffer from several different types of artifacts. As stated previously, the technology depends on the ability of the device to scan the same location repeatedly. Thus it may be difficult or impossible to image patients with poor fixation. There is also significant projection artifact from superficial blood vessels into en face images of the deeper retina and choroid. The removal of these projection artifacts is an active area of research [30]. This technology is also sensitive to low signal strength due to media opacity or hemorrhage.

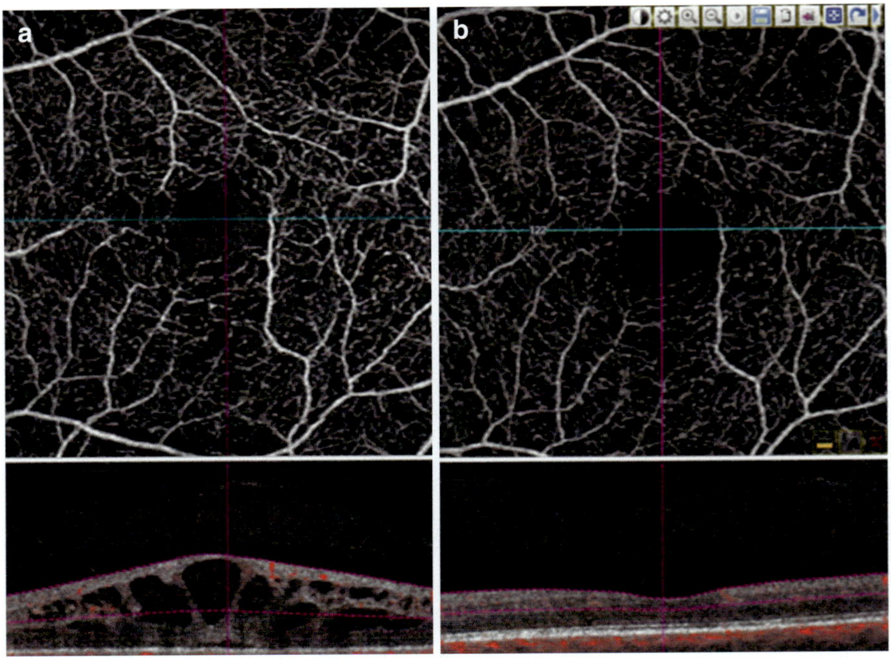

Fig. 7 OCT-A CME. Optical coherence tomography angiography (OCT-A) of the superficial retinal layer in a patient with severe cystoid macular edema, before and after treatment. The two images are essentially identical and demonstrate the robustness of current automated segmentation algorithms in the presence of structural distortion. (**a**) Before treatment. Top panel shows OCT-A image of the superficial retinal layer. Bottom panel shows one of the OCT B-scans used to generate the OCT-A image. There is severe cystoid macular edema. Purple lines show the upper and lower boundaries of the slab used to generate the OCT-A image. (**b**) After treatment with intravitreal steroid injection. Top panel shows OCT-A image of the superficial retinal layer. The image is virtually identical to the one generated prior to treatment (panel A). Bottom panel demonstrates that the macular edema has resolved. The purple dotted lines show the upper and lower boundaries of the slab used to generate the OCT-A image

Summary

The availability of multiple imaging modalities has expanded the ability of clinicians to diagnose and monitor ocular disease. This chapter has focused on recent imaging techniques such as autofluorescence, widefield imaging, and OCT. Understanding the contents of this chapter should aid the reader in interpreting the images in this book and elsewhere. More importantly, understanding the principles, advantages, and limitations of each technology can help to maximize patient outcomes.

Compliance with Ethical Requirements Phuc V. Le declares no conflict of interest. All procedures followed were in accordance with the ethical standards of the responsible committee on human experimentation (institutional and national) and with the Helsinki Declaration of 1975, as revised in 2000. Informed consent was obtained from all patients for being included in the study. No animal studies were carried out by the authors for this article.

References

1. De Laey JJ. Fluorescein angiography in posterior uveitis. Int Ophthalmol Clin. 1995;35:33–58.
2. Ciardella AP, Prall FR, Borodoker N, Cunningham ET. Imaging techniques for posterior uveitis. Curr Opin Ophthalmol. 2004;15:519–30.
3. Gupta V, Al-Dhibi HA, Arevalo JF. Retinal imaging in uveitis. Saudi J Ophthalmol. 2014;28:95–103. https://doi.org/10.1016/j.sjopt.2014.02.008.
4. Manivannan A, Plskova J, Farrow A, et al. Ultra-wide-field fluorescein angiography of the ocular fundus. Am J Ophthalmol. 2005;140:525–7. https://doi.org/10.1016/j.ajo.2005.02.055.
5. Leder HA, Campbell JP, Sepah YJ, et al. Ultra-wide-field retinal imaging in the management of non-infectious retinal vasculitis. J Ophthalmic Inflamm Infect. 2013;3:30. https://doi.org/10.1186/1869-5760-3-30.
6. Jorzik JJ, Bindewald A, Dithmar S, Holz FG. Digital simultaneous fluorescein and indocyanine green angiography, autofluorescence, and red-free imaging with a solid-state laser-based confocal scanning laser ophthalmoscope. Retina. 2005;25:405–16.
7. Bischoff PM, Niederberger HJ, Török B, Speiser P. Simultaneous indocyanine green and fluorescein angiography. Retina. 1995;15:91–9.
8. Bartsch DU, Weinreb RN, Zinser G, Freeman WR. Confocal scanning infrared laser ophthalmoscopy for indocyanine green angiography. Am J Ophthalmol. 1995;120:642–51.
9. Herbort CP. Fluorescein and indocyanine green angiography for uveitis. Middle East Afr J Ophthalmol. 2009;16:168–87. https://doi.org/10.4103/0974-9233.58419.
10. Yannuzzi LA. Indocyanine green angiography: a perspective on use in the clinical setting. Am J Ophthalmol. 2011;151:745–51.e1. https://doi.org/10.1016/j.ajo.2011.01.043.
11. Fardeau C, Herbort CP, Kullmann N, et al. Indocyanine green angiography in birdshot chorioretinopathy. Ophthalmology. 1999;106:1928–34. https://doi.org/10.1016/S0161-6420(99)90403-7.
12. Yung M, Klufas MA, Sarraf D. Clinical applications of fundus autofluorescence in retinal disease. Int J Retina Vitr. 2016;2:12. https://doi.org/10.1186/s40942-016-0035-x.
13. Durrani K, Foster CS. Fundus autofluorescence imaging in posterior uveitis. Semin Ophthalmol. 2012;27:228–35. https://doi.org/10.3109/08820538.2012.711414.
14. Cideciyan AV, Aleman TS, Swider M, et al. Mutations in ABCA4 result in accumulation of lipofuscin before slowing of the retinoid cycle: a reappraisal of the human disease sequence. Hum Mol Genet. 2004;13:525–34. https://doi.org/10.1093/hmg/ddh048.
15. Knickelbein JE, Sen HN. Multimodal imaging of the white dot syndromes and related diseases. J Clin Exp Ophthalmol. 2016;7(3):570.
16. Huang D, Swanson EA, Lin CP, et al. Optical coherence tomography. Science. 1991;254:1178–81.
17. Wojtkowski M, Bajraszewski T, Gorczyńska I, et al. Ophthalmic imaging by spectral optical coherence tomography. Am J Ophthalmol. 2004;138:412–9. https://doi.org/10.1016/j.ajo.2004.04.049.
18. Li Y, Lowder C, Zhang X, Huang D. Anterior chamber cell grading by optical coherence tomography. Invest Ophthalmol Vis Sci. 2013;54:258–65. https://doi.org/10.1167/iovs.12-10477.
19. Sharma S, Lowder CY, Vasanji A, et al. Automated analysis of anterior chamber inflammation by spectral-domain optical coherence tomography. Ophthalmology. 2015;122:1464–70. https://doi.org/10.1016/j.ophtha.2015.02.032.
20. Keane PA, Karampelas M, Sim DA, et al. Objective measurement of vitreous inflammation using optical coherence tomography. Ophthalmology. 2014;121:1706–14. https://doi.org/10.1016/j.ophtha.2014.03.006.
21. Tran THC, de Smet MD, Bodaghi B, et al. Uveitic macular oedema: correlation between optical coherence tomography patterns with visual acuity and fluorescein angiography. Br J Ophthalmol. 2008;92:922–7. https://doi.org/10.1136/bjo.2007.136846.
22. van Velthoven MEJ, Verbraak FD, Yannuzzi LA, et al. Imaging the retina by en face optical coherence tomography. Retina. 2006;26:129–36.

23. Kraus MF, Liu JJ, Schottenhamml J, et al. Quantitative 3D-OCT motion correction with tilt and illumination correction, robust similarity measure and regularization. Biomed Opt Express. 2014;5:2591–613. https://doi.org/10.1364/BOE.5.002591.
24. Zhang Q, Huang Y, Zhang T, et al. Wide-field imaging of retinal vasculature using optical coherence tomography-based microangiography provided by motion tracking. J Biomed Opt. 2015;20:066008. https://doi.org/10.1117/1.JBO.20.6.066008.
25. Spaide RF, Koizumi H, Pozzoni MC, Pozonni MC. Enhanced depth imaging spectral-domain optical coherence tomography. Am J Ophthalmol. 2008;146:496–500. https://doi.org/10.1016/j.ajo.2008.05.032.
26. Baltmr A, Lightman S, Tomkins-Netzer O. Examining the choroid in ocular inflammation: a focus on enhanced depth imaging. J Ophthalmol. 2014;2014:459136. https://doi.org/10.1155/2014/459136.
27. Böni C, Thorne JE, Spaide RF, et al. Choroidal findings in eyes with birdshot chorioretinitis using enhanced-depth optical coherence tomography. Invest Ophthalmol Vis Sci. 2016;57:OCT591–9. https://doi.org/10.1167/iovs.15-18832.
28. Z hang J, Rao B, Chen Z. Swept source based Fourier domain functional optical coherence tomography. Conf Proc Annu Int Conf IEEE Eng Med Biol Soc IEEE Eng Med Biol Soc Annu Conf. 2005;7:7230–3. https://doi.org/10.1109/IEMBS.2005.1616179.
29. Pichi F, Sarraf D, Arepalli S, et al. The application of optical coherence tomography angiography in uveitis and inflammatory eye diseases. Prog Retin Eye Res. 2017;59:178–201. https://doi.org/10.1016/j.preteyeres.2017.04.005.
30. Jia Y, Bailey ST, Wilson DJ, et al. Quantitative optical coherence tomography angiography of choroidal neovascularization in age-related macular degeneration. Ophthalmology. 2014;121:1435–44. https://doi.org/10.1016/j.ophtha.2014.01.034.

Part II

Non-Infectious Posterior or Pan Uveitis

Ocular Sarcoidosis

Padmamalini Mahendradas, Ankush Kawali, and Sujay Chauhan

Introduction

Sarcoidosis is an idiopathic multisystem granulomatous inflammatory disorder characterized by formation of noncaseating epithelioid cell granulomas. It affects people of all ages throughout the world, with highest incidence seen in the age group of 20–40 years. Women are more often affected than men. African Americans are about three times more likely to have sarcoidosis than Caucasian Americans [1].

Etiopathogenesis

The exact etiology of sarcoidosis is still unknown. Interplay of environmental and genetic predisposition has been proposed as the likely mechanism.

Environmental Factors

An increased risk of sarcoidosis has been observed in people with exposure to insecticides, industrial organic dust, and agricultural or moldy environments [2]. *Mycobacterium tuberculosis* infection has also been often associated with sarcoidosis.

Genetic Factors

Genetic factors play a significant role in prevalence, clinical presentations, and severity of sarcoidosis. First-degree relatives of sarcoidosis patients are at a fivefold

P. Mahendradas (✉) · A. Kawali · S. Chauhan
Narayana Nethralaya, Department of Uveitis and Ocular Immunology, Bangalore, India

N. A. Rao et al. (eds.), *Posterior Uveitis*, Essentials in Ophthalmology,
https://doi.org/10.1007/978-3-030-03140-4_2

risk for developing the disease than the general population. HLA-A1, B8, DR3 haplotype, and HLA-DR17 have been associated with an increased risk of developing sarcoidosis in whites and HLA-DR11 in white, African American, and Japanese patients. Recently butyrophilin-like 2 (BTNL2) receptor gene on chromosome 6p has also been linked to sarcoidosis in whites [3, 4].

Immunopathogenesis

Any infectious, organic, or inorganic agents acting as antigen can initiate a cross-reacting immune response to self-antigen. Antigen-presenting cells (APC) lead to secretion of multiple inflammatory mediators like TNF-α, interleukin-12, interleukin-15, and interleukin-18, macrophage inflammatory protein 1 (MIP-1), monocyte chemotactic protein 1 (MCP-1), and granulocyte macrophage colony-stimulating factor (GM-CSF) [5]. A cardinal feature of sarcoidosis is the interaction of CD4+ T cells with APCs causing release of interleukin-2 and interferon-$_{\gamma}$ and formation of granulomas [6]. Sarcoidal granulomas are composed of macrophages and their derivatives, epithelioid cells, giant cells, and T cells and shows "non-caseating" necrosis in histopathological examination. They may persist, resolve, or lead to fibrosis. Activated alveolar macrophages stimulate fibroblast proliferation and collagen production, leading to progressive fibrosis.

Clinical Manifestations

Sarcoidosis can have varied presentation, ranging from an abnormal chest radiograph in an asymptomatic individual to severe multiorgan involvement.

Systemic Disease

Sarcoidosis is a multisystem inflammatory disorder with predominant pulmonary involvement, bilateral hilar lymphadenopathy being the most characteristic finding seen in 50–85% patients [7]. Other organs involved in sarcoidosis include the liver, spleen, lymph nodes, salivary glands, heart, nervous system, muscles, and bones [8]. Systemic disease can manifest with an acute or an insidious onset. Acute disease can present as two distinct syndromes: Löfgren's syndrome and Heerfordt's syndrome. Löfgren's syndrome is characterized by triad of erythema nodosum, bilateral hilar lymphadenopathy on chest radiograph, and arthritis. It has good prognosis with more than 90% resolution by 2 years. Heerfordt's syndrome, also called uveoparotid syndrome, is associated with uveitis, parotid enlargement, and fever with or without facial nerve palsy. Disease with insidious onset, especially with

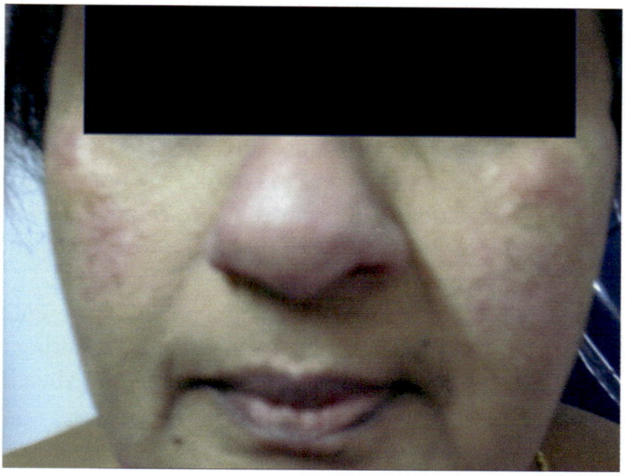

Fig. 1 Face photograph showing lupus pernio in a case of sarcoidosis

multiple extrapulmonary lesions, may result in progressive fibrosis of the lungs and other organs.

I. *Lungs*. Pulmonary fibrosis occurs in 20–25% of patients with sarcoidosis and can lead to respiratory failure [9]. Patients with pulmonary sarcoidosis usually present with complaints of nonproductive cough, dyspnea, and chest pain [10].

II. *Heart*. Cardiac involvement is seen in 2–10% of patients with sarcoidosis and is associated with poor prognosis if untreated [11].

III. *Skin*. Cutaneous lesions are present in up to 25% patients, sometimes as the initial manifestation. Erythema nodosum is the most common cutaneous lesion in sarcoidosis with spontaneous resolution within weeks or months. Lupus pernio (Fig. 1) results in destruction of underlying cartilage and bone causing facial disfigurement.

IV. *Nervous system*. Nervous system involvement occurs in 5–15% of patients with sarcoidosis and can have serious sequelae [12, 13]. Cranial nerve palsies may occur secondary to nerve granulomas, increased intracranial pressure, or granulomatous basal meningitis, Bell's palsy (cranial nerve VII palsy) being the most common. Bilateral dysfunction can occurs, both simultaneously and sequentially.

V. *Liver*. Hepatic granulomas can occur. Liver enzymes can be elevated.

VI. Lymph nodes. Patients may have lymphadenopathy and lymph node biopsy may show multiple non-caseating granulomas consisting of epithelioid cells, Langerhans giant cells, lymphocytes, monocytes, and fibroblasts.

Ocular Disease

Ocular involvement is seen in about 30–50% of patients with sarcoidosis.

I. *Anterior uveitis*. Granulomatous anterior uveitis is the characteristic ocular manifestation and foremost cause of ocular morbidity in sarcoidosis. It is usually unilateral at the onset, but second eye involvement occurs commonly at some point during the course of the disease. Features include mutton-fat keratic precipitates (KPs). Figure 11b, peripheral or angle KPs, placoid peripheral keratic precipitates, and iris nodules (Figure 4, Koeppe and Busacca nodules) are seen. Nodular deposits may occasionally be seen in anterior chamber angle and trabecular meshwork. Tent-like peripheral anterior synechiae (PAS) may also be seen.

II. *Intermediate uveitis*. Intermediate uveitis presents with vitritis and exudative vasculitis. Vitritis is seen as "snowball" or "string of pearls" in vitreous cavity. Retinal perivasculitis is seen as segmental sheathing mostly in equatorial or peripheral retina.

III. *Posterior uveitis*. Multiple orangish-yellow chorioretinal granulomas can be observed in posterior pole and in the mid-periphery. A solitary choroidal granuloma can be confused with tuberculoma. Retinal granulomas poorly responding to steroids are rarely been described in literature [14].

IV. *Retinal vasculitis*. Nodular or segmental periphlebitis appearing as candle wax drippings (or so called "taches de bougie") is classically described for exudative sarcoid vasculitis. Rarely, occlusive periphlebitis may mimic branch retinal vein occlusion. Periphlebitis is occasionally complicated by retinal neovascularization which simulates the peripheral "sea fans" seen in sickle cell retinopathy.

V. *Optic nerve granuloma*. Optic nerve involvement in form of granulomas may occur without systemic involvement [15]. The granulomas are usually unilateral (Fig. 5) but may be bilateral as well in some cases. It can manifest as an acute disease with good response to corticosteroids or as a chronic progressive form that responds poorly to corticosteroids [12, 16, 17].

VI. *Other manifestations* include dacryoadenitis, conjunctival granulomas, nonspecific conjunctivitis, interstitial keratitis, episcleritis, scleritis, and orbital or extraocular muscle granulomas. Conjunctival inflammation occasionally resolves with symblepharon formation. Band keratopathy may occur as a complication of chronic uveitis.

Diagnosis

The diagnosis of sarcoidosis is based on the presence of a compatible clinical picture, supportive laboratory findings, and, in most cases, a confirmatory biopsy.

International Japanese Criteria

International guidelines for systemic sarcoidosis were based on chest radiographic findings. The Ministry of Health, Labour and Welfare in Japan established new criteria for the diagnosis of sarcoidosis in 2006, which divided patients with sarcoidosis into two groups as biopsy-proven and clinically diagnosed subjects (Table 1) [18]. Lymph node biopsy may show multiple non-caseating granulomas

Table 1 Biopsy-proven and clinically diagnosed sarcoidosis

I. *Biopsy-proven group*: Patients have non-caseating granuloma histologically proven and any of i–iii in (II)-1
II. *Clinically diagnosed group*: Patients have two or more of i–vi of investigations shown below and clinical features which strongly indicate sarcoidosis in two organs or more (pulmonary, ocular, cardiovascular, skin, neurological)
1. *Investigation for sarcoidosis*
i. Chest X-ray (Fig. 2) or CT scan to detect bilateral hilar lymphadenopathy (Fig. 3)
ii. Serum angiotensin-converting enzyme (ACE) levels
iii. Skin test for anergy to PPD
iv. Gallium-67 citrate scan
v. Bronchoalveolar lavage (BAL) to detect increase of lymphocytes or CD4/CD8 ratio,
vi. Serum or urine calcium
2. *Ocular clinical features strongly indicating sarcoidosis (two or more items are required)*
I. Granulomatous anterior segment intraocular inflammation, e.g., mutton-fat keratic precipitates or iris nodules (Fig. 4)
II. Gonionodules or peripheral anterior synechiae (PAS)
III. Snowball or beaded vitreous opacities
IV. Retinal perivascular inflammation and sheathing of the retinal vein
V. Multiple candle wax exudates in the choroid and retina or photocoagulation-like retinochoroidal atrophy
VI. Optic nerve granuloma or choroidal granuloma (Fig. 6)
For ocular sarcoidosis, international criteria recommend four levels of certainty for the diagnosis when in patients in whom other possible causes of uveitis are excluded (Table 2) [19]:
I. *Definite ocular sarcoidosis*: Biopsy-supported diagnosis with a compatible uveitis
II. *Presumed ocular sarcoidosis*: Presence of bilateral hilar lymphadenopathy with a compatible uveitis though biopsy has not been performed
III. *Probable ocular sarcoidosis*: Patients where biopsy is not done and in whom the chest X-ray does not show bilateral hilar lymphadenopathy, but there are three suggestive intraocular signs and two supportive investigations positive
IV. *Possible ocular sarcoidosis*: When biopsy is found negative but there are four or more intraocular signs with at least two positive laboratory results

Table 2 International criteria for the diagnosis of ocular sarcoidosis (IWOS) [19]

Clinical signs suggestive of ocular sarcoidosis
1. Mutton-fat KPs (large and small) and/or iris nodules at pupillary margin (Koeppe) or in stroma (Busacca)
2. Trabecular meshwork (TM) nodules and/or tent-shaped peripheral anterior synechiae (PAS)
3. Snowballs/string-of-pearl vitreous opacities
4. Multiple chorioretinal peripheral lesions (active and atrophic)
5. Nodular and/or segmental periphlebitis (± candle-wax drippings) and/or macroaneurysm in an inflammed eye
6. Optic disc nodule(s)/granuloma(s) and/or solitary choroidal nodule
7. Bilaterality (assessed by clinical examination or investigational tests showing subclinical inflammation)
Laboratory investigations in suspected ocular sarcoidosis
1. Negative tuberculin test in a BCG-vaccinated patient or having had a positive PPD (or Mantoux) skin test previously
2. Elevated serum angiotensin converting enzyme (ACE) and/or elevated serum lysozyme
3. Chest X-ray; look for bilateral hilar lymphadenopathy (BHL)
4. Abnormal liver enzyme tests (any two of alkaline phosphatase, ASAT, ALAT, LDH, or γ-GT)
5. Chest CT scan in patients with negative chest X-ray

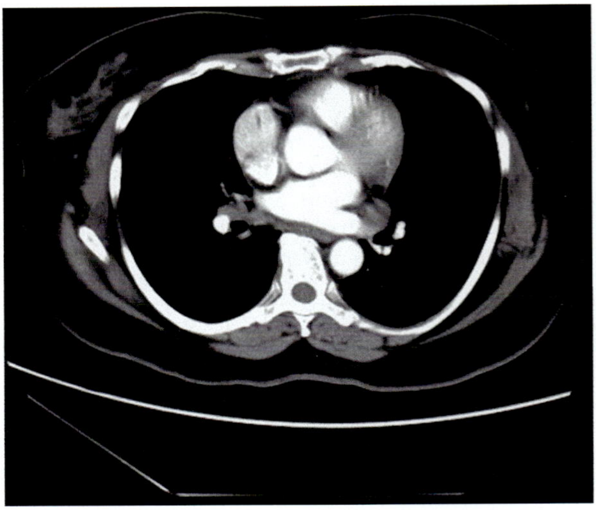

Fig. 2 CT scan of the chest showing enlarged hilar lymph node in a case of granulomatous panuveitis due to sarcoidosis

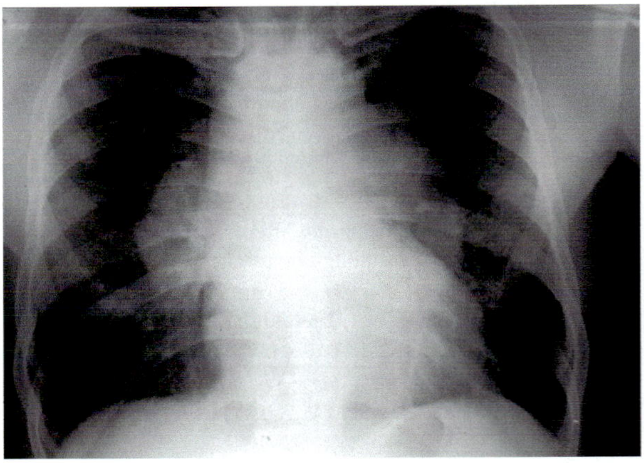

Fig. 3 Chest X-ray PA view shows bilateral hilar lymphadenopathy in a case of bilateral granulomatous panuveitis due to sarcoidosis

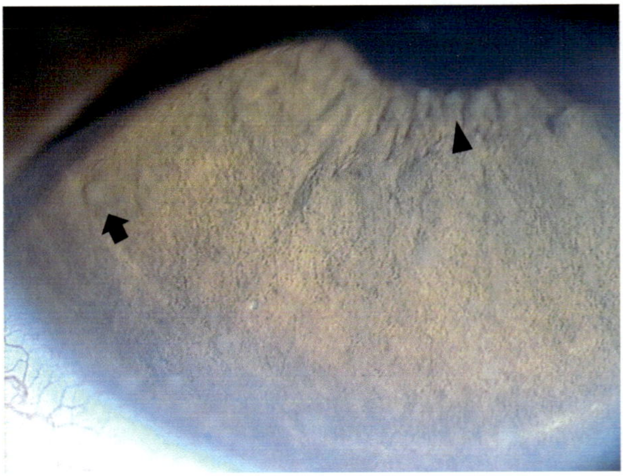

Fig. 4 Diffuse slit lamp biomicroscopic photograph showing the presence of Koeppe's (black arrow head) and Busacca nodules (black arrow) in granulomatous panuveitis

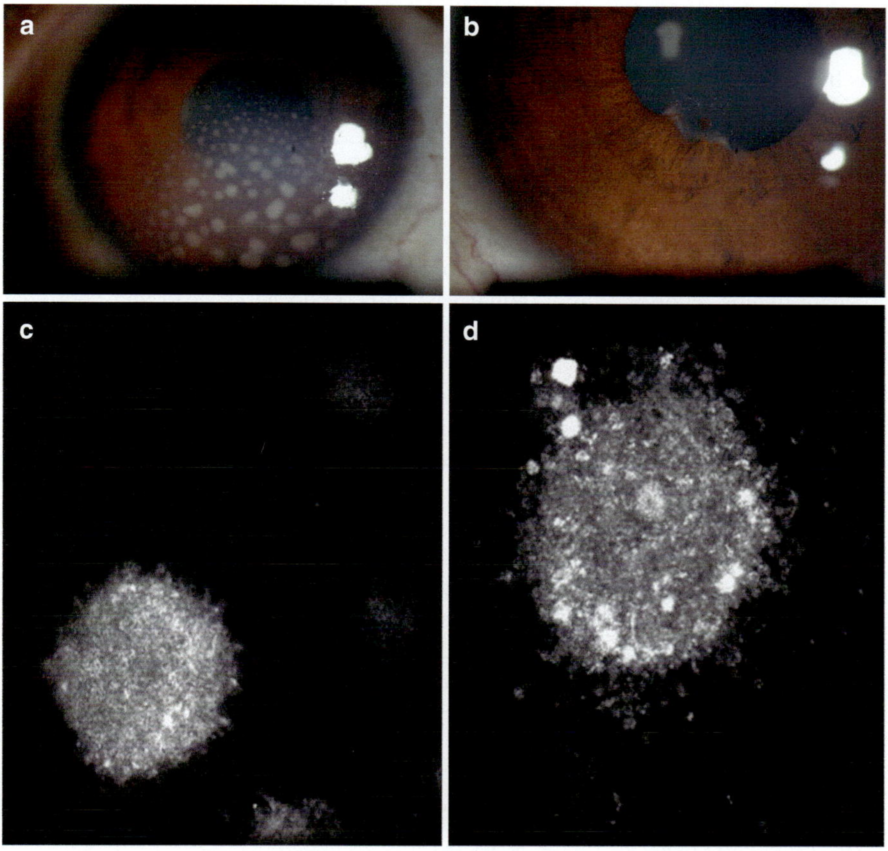

Fig. 5 A 25-year-old female as a case of bilateral granulomatous panuveitis due to sarcoidosis. Anterior segment photograph shows mutton-fat keratic precipitates in right eye (**a**) & broad based posterior synechiae (**b**). Confocal microscopy showed globular pattern of keratic precipitate in both eyes (**c**, **d**)

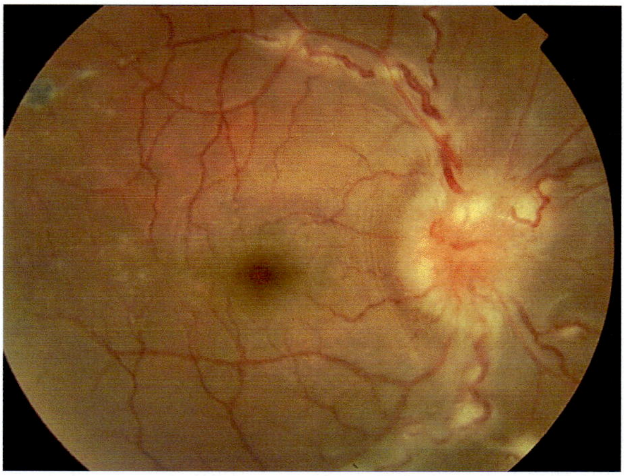

Fig. 6 Fundus photograph of the right eye showing optic disc granuloma with retinal vasculitis

consisting of epithelioid cells, Langerhans giant cells, lymphocytes, monocytes, and fibroblasts. CD4/CD8 ratio of lymphocytes were significantly higher in aqueous humour and vitreous humour of patients with ocular sarcoidosis [20, 21].

Differential Diagnosis

Sarcoidosis is generally amongst first few differential diagnosis in a case of granulomatous uveitis. Ocular manifestations of sarcoidosis like KPs, iris nodules, intermediate uveitis, chorioretinitis, retinal vasculitis, optic nerve head and choroidal granulomas and dacryoadenopathy, need to be differentiated from other causes.

I. *KPs*: Tuberculosis, VKH, Viral uveitis, Fuchs' uveitis and Hansen's disease.
II. *Iris nodules*: Tuberculosis, syphilis, leprosy, Fuchs' uveitis, primary iris neoplasms, metastatic carcinoma, seeding from retinoblastoma, and leukemic infiltrates.
III. *Intermediate uveitis*: Tuberculosis, Idiopathic intermediate uveitis, Lyme disease, and multiple sclerosis.
IV. *Chorioretinitis*: Tuberculosis, syphilis, toxoplasmosis, Vogt- Koyanagi-Harada disease, Bird Shot Choroidopathy and masquerade syndrome. Retinitis (rare): Epidemic retinitis and Behcet's disease.
V. *Vasculitis*: Tuberculosis, Toxolasmosis, Syphilis, Behcet's disease.
VI. *Optic disc granuloma*: Optic neuritis, papilledema.
VII. *Dacryoadenopathy and parotitis*: Tuberculosis, Hodgkin's disease, lymphoma, and brucellosis. Isolated lacrimal gland enlargement may mimic orbital pseudotumor or primary lacrimal gland tumor.
VIII. *Pulmonary disease*: Tuberculosis, berylliosis, pneumoconiosis, malignant lymphoma, hypersensitivity pneumonitis, metastatic lung tumor, and amyloidosis.
IX. *Cardiovascular disease*: Giant cell myocarditis.
X. *Skin diseases*: Cutaneous tuberculosis, granuloma annulare, annular elastolytic giant cell granuloma, necrobiosis lipoidica, Melkersson-Rosenthal syndrome, acne rosacea, and skin carcinoma.

Management

There are no preventive measures available for sarcoidosis. Family members of patients with sarcoidosis are at increased risk for developing sarcoidosis compared to general population. However, overall risk being extremely low, routine screening of family members is not advisable.

There is no definitive treatment for sarcoidosis. Up to one-third of patients resolve spontaneously without any treatment. Treatment is intended primarily to reduce the symptoms, lessen disability during periods of activity, and minimize the sequelae of inflammation. Treatment is warranted if (1) symptoms interfere with activities of daily living and cannot be controlled by simple measures and (2) organ function is threatened. Corticosteroids remain the mainstay of treatment for ocular sarcoidosis. Topical administration is effective for most patients with anterior uveitis, but periocular steroids may be required in severe cases. Posterior uveitis is managed with periocular and/or systemic corticosteroids. Choroidal infiltrates respond to systemic steroids. Pulsed intravenous methylprednisolone therapy is often required in cases with optic nerve involvement. Systemic immunomodulatory therapy or biologics are used to supplement steroid therapy for refractory disease or to allow a reduction in steroid dose or to achieve long term remission.

Oral corticosteroids remain the primary first-line therapy for systemic sarcoidosis [22–24].

Inhalational steroids are useful as maintenance therapy for pulmonary sarcoidosis [25]. Cytotoxic drugs, like methotrexate and azathioprine, are effective steroid-sparing agents and also useful in cases refractory to steroids [26]. Chloroquine and hydroxychloroquine are effective for pulmonary and cutaneous disease, hydroxychloroquine having higher ocular safety.

Prognosis

Prognosis is variable and depends on gender, race, age, organ involvement, signs and symptoms at presentation, etc. Majority of patients improve or stabilize within first 2 years of illness. Spontaneous remission occurs within 5 years in almost two-thirds of patients. There is less than 5% chance of disease recurrence. Progressive sarcoidosis leads to death in less than 5% of cases due to progressive respiratory insufficiency or cardiac or neurologic involvement [27]. Ocular inflammation is usually mild with favorable visual outcome. Cystoid macular edema, epiretinal membrane formation, and iris bombe due to the formation of posterior synechiae with secondary glaucoma may develop in cases with long-standing inflammation. Vitreous hemorrhage due to retinal neovascularization and choroidal neovascularization may also develop.

Ocular Imaging in Sarcoidosis

This chapter also highlights the role of anterior segment and fundus photography, confocal microscopy, ultrasound biomicroscopy, fundus autofluorescence, fundus fluorescein angiography including wide-field angiography, indocyanine green angiography, optical coherence tomography, and optical coherence tomography angiography in the diagnosis and management of eye manifestations of sarcoidosis.

Anterior Segment Imaging

Slit lamp photography is useful for documentation of anterior segment changes such as conjunctival congestion, scleral involvement, keratic precipitates, and iris nodules in the pupillary margin (Koeppe's nodules) and on the surface (Busacca nodules) in sarcoidosis [28]. Confocal microscopy can be used to study the keratic precipitates in uveitis. Sarcoidosis has characteristic globular pattern of keratic precipitates on confocal microscopy (Fig. 5) [29–31]. Anterior segment optical coherence tomography (ASOCT) can be used to document the changes in the iris and angle structures. High-frequency ultrasound biomicroscopy is required in patients with intermediate uveitis and complicated cataracts to rule out ciliary body membranes or atrophy of ciliary processes as the cause for hypotony. These findings would influence the surgical outcome [32].

Fundus Autofluorescence

Fundus autofluorescence (FAF) is a simple noninvasive imaging technique that uses the fluorescent properties of lipofuscin (LF) and similar metabolic end products of the outer photoreceptor segments that progressively accumulate in the retinal pigment epithelium (RPE) [33]. Abnormal accumulation of the LF in the RPE cells appears as hyperautofluorescence, and loss of the RPE cells appears as areas of hypoautofluorescence (Fig. 7) when the retina is excited by blue light. Used initially for monitoring retinal degenerative disorders [34], recent years have seen increasing use of FAF in posterior uveitis [35–37]. The exact source of the hyperautofluorescence is not well known in uveitis, and it is speculated that choroidal inflammation may induce accumulation of fluorophores in the retina [34]. Fundus autofluorescence in posterior segment manifestations of sarcoidosis has not been studied in detail. Gupta et al. have classified the evolution pattern of fundus autofluorescence in tuberculous serpiginous choroiditis [37]. FAF is a powerful noninvasive tool to monitor the disease course in posterior uveitis, and it scores over conventional FFA and ICG. It provides functional status of the RPE-photoreceptor complex. Active fundus lesions involving RPE

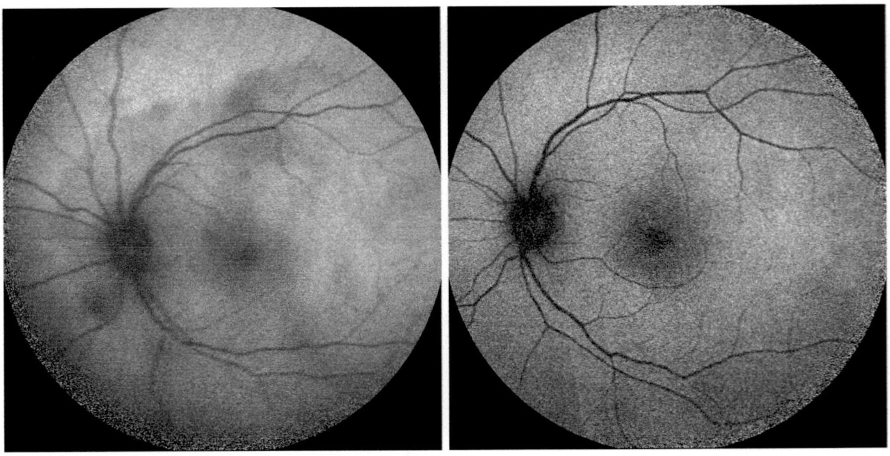

Fig. 7 Fundus autofluorescence in the left eye revealed multiple areas of hypoautofluorescence corresponding to the areas of vitreous opacities, and the posttreatment images showed decrease in the areas of hypoautofluorescence with normal pattern

present as hyperautofluorescent lesions, and healed lesions present as hypoautofluorescence due to death of the RPE and the overlying photoreceptors. Wide-field imaging techniques using optos help us to study the full extent of these lesions on FAF.

Fundus Fluorescein Angiography

Fundus fluorescein angiography (FFA) in sarcoidosis is used to demonstrate retinal vascular, macular, choroidal, and optic nerve head pathology. FFA also helps to pick up signs of subclinical inflammation; hence it is quite useful to monitor the response to therapy during follow-up and helps to decide on doses of immunomodulatory therapy.

Choroidal granulomas in active stage on FFA are seen as early hypofluorescence and late hyperfluorescence (Figs. 8 and 9). Larger choroidal granulomas are rarely associated with small subretinal fluid which can show pooling of dye along with hyperfluorescence of the granuloma in late phase on FFA [38]. In case of resolved granuloma, one can see an overlying window defect due to retinal pigment epithelium (RPE) atrophy. In completely atrophic choroidal granuloma, the whole area shows hypofluorescence on early frames which later becomes hyperfluorescent on late frames reflecting the bare sclera impregnated with fluorescein [39].

Inflamed retinal vessels are highly permeable to fluorescein which appears as leakage from the vessels on the FFA. This sign is well seen even in the absence of vascular sheathing on clinical examination, if the inflammation is not completely resolved. Multiple segmental leaks along the vessel are highly suggestive of sarcoid vasculitis. Occlusive vasculitis is uncommon in sarcoidosis. Hence capillary non-perfusion areas and neovascularization are not frequently observed on FFA.

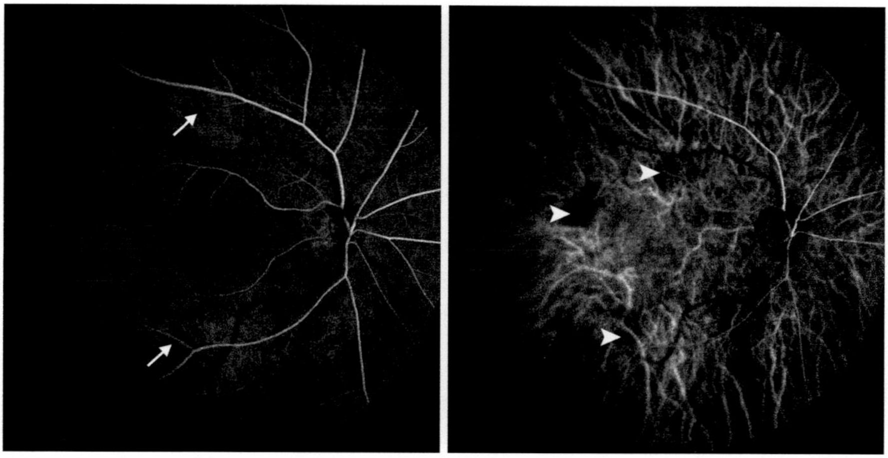

Fig. 8 Dual FFA and ICG of the right eye showing early hypofluorescence corresponding to choroidal granulomas in FFA and ICG showing areas of hypocyanescence corresponding to the areas of granulomas with staining and leakage of the choroidal vessels

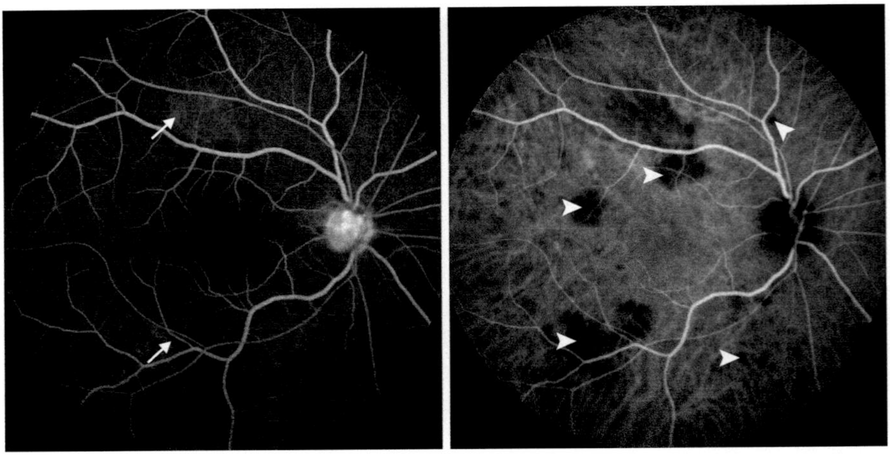

Fig. 9 Dual FFA and ICG of the late phase of the right eye angiograms showing disc hyperfluorescence with areas of hyperfluorescence (white arrows) and corresponding to the areas of choroidal granulomas and ICG showing hypocyanescence (white arrow heads) corresponding to the areas of granulomas

Apart from leakage from major retinal vessels, capillary leakage is also seen on FFA especially in case of intermediate uveitis when there is no clinically evident lesion in the retina or choroid. This also helps clinicians to differentiate old inactive vitritis from active vitreous inflammation. FFA can show capillary leakage if there is active inflammation in the vitreous.

FFA shows disc hyperfluorescence in inflammation of optic nerve or in case of disc granuloma. Sarcoid disc granulomas are visible clinically, but subclinical disc inflammation in intermediate uveitis and in vasculitis as well as cystoid macular edema can be well documented on FFA. But now with advent of noninvasive modality like OCT, clinicians now less rely on FFA to rule out macular edema.

Indocyanine Green Angiography

Indocyanine green angiography (ICG) has been used to study the choroidal vasculature. The ICG dye fluoresces at a near-infrared wavelength, making it easily detectable through the retinal pigment epithelium. Herbort et al. have studied ICG uses in posterior uveitis [40]. In contrast to fluorescein, ICG is almost completely protein bound (90%), so the ICG dye does not leak from the normal retinal capillaries, veins, or the arteries. It leaks slowly from the choriocapillaris and impregnates the choroidal stroma; however, it does not leak from the choroidal veins or the arteries. Thus, the slow wash-out effect of the ICG dye in the choroid is used to delineate the choroidal pathologies [40].

A typical ICG pattern comprised irregularly distributed, hypocyanescent, dark choroidal lesions (Figs. 8, 9 and 10) in the early and intermediate phases of angiography. The unique ICG signs of sarcoidosis uveitis were described and classified into four types [41].

First one consists of hypocyanescence in the intermediate phase and iso- or hypercyanescence in the late phase. The signs indicate the presence of "active" choroidal granulomas. Second pattern consists of hypocyanescence in the intermediate phase, which maintained in the late phase. Corticosteroids show no influence on these lesions; they represent "atrophic" changes. Third pattern consists of faint staining of choroidal granuloma in the intermediate phase and bright hypercyanescence in the late phase. Fourth pattern consists of clearly hypercyanescence in the intermediate phase, which is followed by diffuse zonal hypercyanescence in the late phase. Since these two types of staining may represent choroidal vasculitis, treatment with corticosteroids shows considerable effect on these lesions [41].

Optical Coherence Tomography (OCT)

It is now possible to study chorioretinal as well as vitreous involvement with great details using a noninvasive modality: SD – OCT. Various imaging modes on SD OCT can be used to study vitreoretinal interface, retina, and choroid layer by layer.

Enhanced vitreous imaging (EVI) helps in better visualization of posterior vitreous cavity [42, 43]. Normal mode OCT is useful for quantification of cystoid macular edema and to demonstrate subretinal fluid secondary to choroidal granuloma. It can also be used to differentiate preretinal nodules or exudates in sarcoidosis from intraretinal infiltrate seen in Behcet's disease. But Goldberg et al. have reported intraretinal hyper-reflective nodules even in sarcoidosis [44].

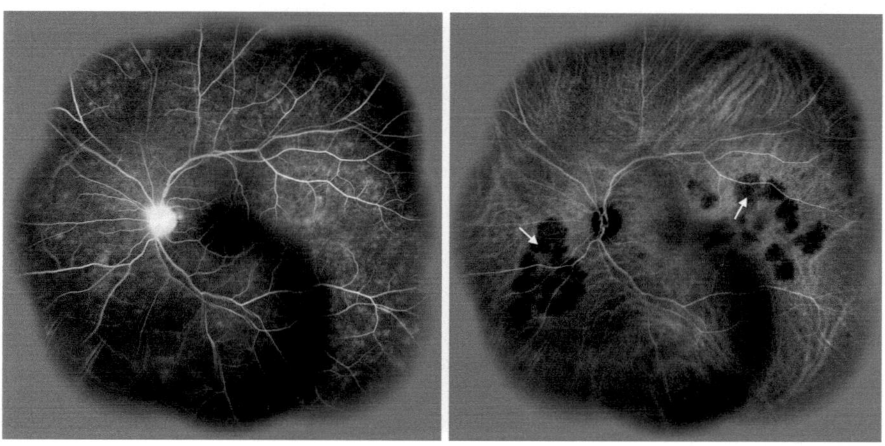

Fig. 10 Montage FFA of the left eye showing disc leak and diffuse perivascular leak, and ICG showing multiple areas of hypocyanescence corresponding to the areas of choroidal granulomas

Most useful is EDI mode, where choroidal granulomas are seen as homogeneous hyporeflective elevated lesions with choriocapillaries thinning (Fig. 11). The hypo-reflectivity is due to depigmentation and less scattering of light as reported in Birdshot retinopathy [45]. Sarcoid granulomas can be differentiated from tubercular

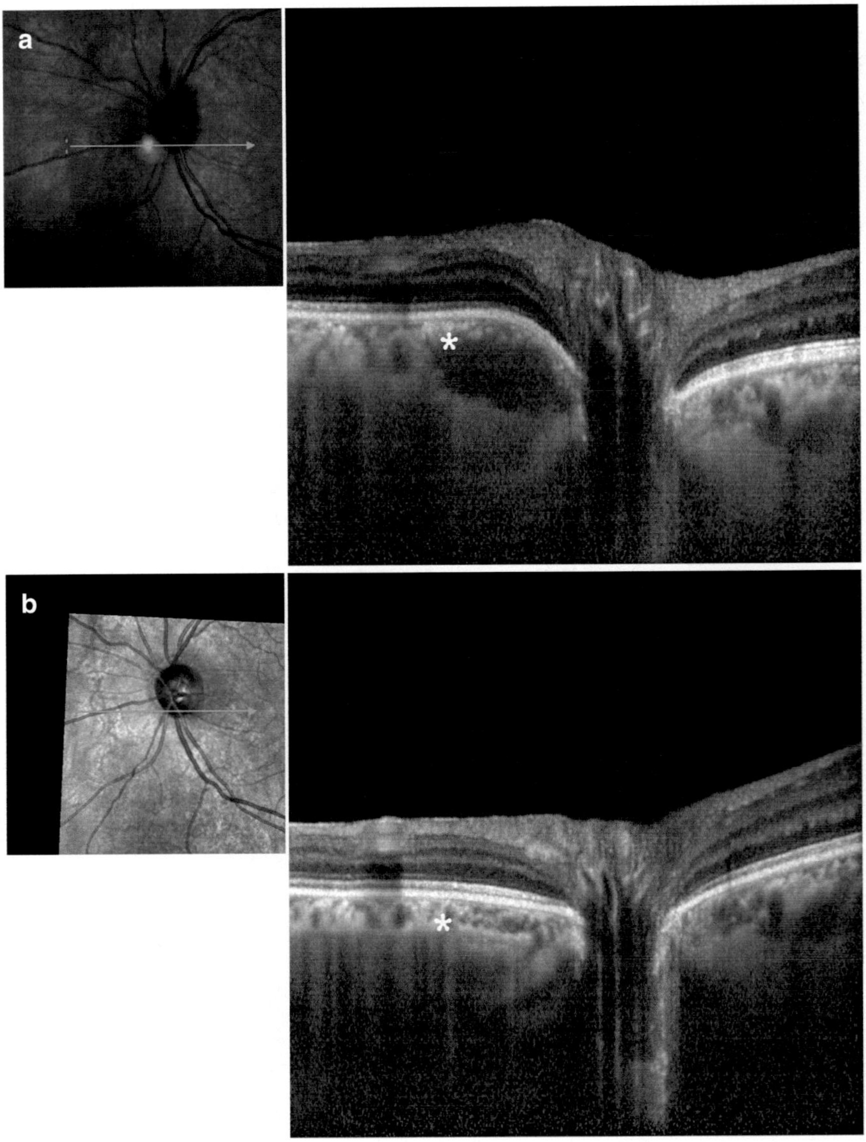

Fig. 11 EDI OCT of the left eye in a case of choroidal granulomas secondary to sarcoidosis showed well definied hyporelective granuloma (white asterix in figure **a**). Following treatment with systemic steroids and systemic methotrexate repeat OCT after 8 months showed healed complete granuloma. (white asterix in figure **b**)

by difference in homogenicity due to noncaseating nature of the granuloma [46]. Sattler's medium-sized vessel choroidal layer is disproportionately enlarged in sarcoidosis compared to tubercular uveitis [47]. In Vogt-Koyanagi-Harada (VKH) disease, there is diffuse choroidal thickening, whereas in sarcoidosis, choroid is thickened at the site of granuloma and appears healthy between granulomas on EDI-OCT [48]. Sarcoid granulomas have relatively well-defined margins and show more hyporeflectivity when compared with tubercular and VKH granulomas. The so-called increased transmission effects beneath the granuloma can be used to differentiate barely visible granulomas from normal large choroidal vessel lumens [46].

Posterior scleritis can rarely occur in sarcoidosis [49]. EDI OCT frequently shows diffuse choroidal thickening with RPE undulation and serous retinal detachment due to transmitted inflammation from inflamed posterior scleral tissue [50]. But recurrent posterior scleritis can cause choroidal atrophic changes and may show decreased thickness on EDI OCT [51].

Swept source OCT has added advantage over SD OCT in imaging peripheral choroidal granuloma of sarcoidosis completely and with greater depth [52].

Sarcoid granulomas immediately after treatment show decrease in size, but change in its homogenicity and hyporeflectivity takes a longer time, and after complete resolution, it may show subretinal fibrosis and outer retinal tubulations.

Thus, OCT is not only a noninvasive tool to monitor the inflammation but also useful to differentiate sarcoid granuloma from other similar entities.

OCT Angiography (OCTA)

Sarcoid granuloma is an infiltration of cells which displaces surrounding vasculature of choroid. On OCTA these granulomas are seen as dark spots or flow void areas in the choriocapillaries vasculature on OCTA (Fig. 12).

CNVM can be well documented on OCTA. A vascular network can be visualized arising from the choroid. It is also possible to locate exact level of involvement by changing segmentation margins on the OCTA machine. Regression of CNVM after anti-VEGF injections can be better monitored on OCTA rather than repeating invasive procedure of FFA.

In retinal vasculitis lower perifoveal vascular density has been described [53]. Current use of OCTA is limited due to small field of view, inability to show vascular leakage, and image artifact due to patient movement or blinking.

Summary and Conclusions of Ocular Imaging in Sarcoidosis

FFA is one of the most useful examinations to detect the retinal findings in patients with sarcoidosis. In sarcoidosis, FA can reveal optic disc leak, macular edema and focal or diffuse staining and leakage of dye from retinal vessels associated with the occlusion of retinal veins or arteries with retinal neovascularization in selected cases. ICG reveals useful information of choroidal changes in sarcoidosis. Choroidal

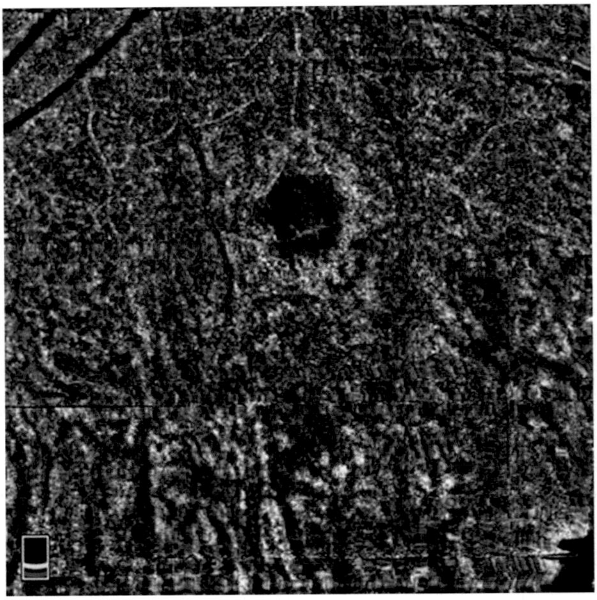

Fig. 12 OCT angiography shows hyporeflective ill defined lesion in the choroid due to sarcoid choroidal granuloma

involvements of sarcoidosis are characterized by hypocyanescence in the early to intermediate phase on ICG. The sign resolves in the late phase when the granulomas are fresh/active, however remain unchanged when they are atrophic. OCT helps to study the structural alterations of the choroidal granulomas in ocular sarcoidosis. OCTA is a new imaging technique with no contrast dye, and it provides en face imaging of all the layers of retina as well as choroid. All these imaging modalities complement each other to study the structural changes of the eyes in ocular sarcoidosis.

Compliance with Ethical Requirements Padmamalini Mahendradas, Anush Kawali, and Sujay Chauhan declare that they have no conflict of interest. All procedures followed were in accordance with the ethical standards of the responsible committee on human experimentation (institutional and national) and with the Helsinki Declaration of 1975, as revised in 2000. Informed consent was obtained from all patients for being included in the study. No animal studies were carried out by the authors for this chapter.

References

1. Rybicki BA, Major M, Popovich J Jr, et al. Racial differences in sarcoidosis incidence: a 5-year study in a health maintenance organization. Am J Epidemiol. 1997;145:234–41.
2. Newman LS, Rose CS, Bresnitz EA, et al. A case control etiological study of sarcoidosis: environmental and occupational risk factors. Am J Respir Crit Care Med. 2004;170:1324–30.
3. Smith G, Brownell I, Sanchez M, et al. Advances in the genetics of sarcoidosis. Clin Genet. 2008;73:401–12.
4. West SG. Sarcoidosis. In: Hochberg MC, Silman AJ, Smolen JS, Weinblatt ME, Weisman MH, editors. Rheumatology. 5th ed. Philadelphia: Elsevier Mosby; 2011. p. 1659–70.

5. Agostini C, Adami F, Semenzato G. New pathogenetic insights into the sarcoid granuloma. Curr Opin Rheumatol. 2000;12:71–6.
6. Iannuzzi MC, Rybicki BA, Teirstein AS. Sarcoidosis. N Engl J Med. 2007;357(21):2153–65.
7. Lynch JP, Kazerooni EA 3rd, Gay SE. Pulmonary sarcoidosis. Clin Chest Med. 1997;18:755–85.
8. Hunninghake GW, Costabel U, Ando M, Baughman R, Cordier JF, du Bois R, Eklund A, Kitaichi M, Lynch J, Rizzato G, Rose C, Selroos O, Semenzato G, Sharma OP. ATS/ERS/WASOG Statement on sarcoidosis. American Thoracic Society/European Respiratory Society/World Association of Sarcoidosis and other Granulomatous Disorders. Sarcoidosis Vasc Diffuse Lung Dis. 1999;16:149–73.
9. James DG. Life-threatening situations in sarcoidosis. Sarcoidosis Vasc Diffuse Lung Dis. 1998;15:134–9.
10. ATS, ERS, WASOG. Statement on sarcoidosis. Joint statement of the American Thoracic Society (ATS), the European Respiratory Society (ERS) and the World Association of Sarcoidosis and Other Granulomatous Disorders (WASOG) adopted by the ATS Board of Directors and by the ERS Executive Committee, February 1999. Am J Respir Crit Care Med. 1999;160:736–55.
11. Sharma OP. Diagnosis of cardiac sarcoidosis: an imperfect science, a hesitant art. Chest. 2003;123:18–9.
12. James DG, Sharma OP. Neurosarcoidosis. Proc R Soc Med. 1967;60:1169–70.
13. Stern BJ, Krumholz A, Johns C, et al. Sarcoidosis and its neurological manifestations. Arch Neurol. 1985;42:909–17.
14. McMahon JF, Adam MK, Dunn JP. Optical coherence tomography and management of a retinal granuloma in presumed ocular sarcoidosis. Ocul Immunol Inflamm. 2018;10:1–5.
15. Wachtel AS, Saunders M. Optic nerve sarcoidosis. Mayo Clin Proc. 1997;72:791.
16. Gelwan MJ, Kellen RI, Burde RM, et al. Sarcoidosis of the anterior visual pathway: successes and failures. J Neurol Neurosurg Psychiatry. 1988;51:1473–80.
17. Graham EM, Ellis CJ, Sanders MD, et al. Optic neuropathy in sarcoidosis. J Neurol Neurosurg Psychiatry. 1986;49:756–63.
18. JSSOG. Diagnostic guidelines and criteria for sarcoidosis-2006 (Japan Society for sarcoidosis and other granulomatous disorders and Japanese Ocular Inflammation Society). J Jpn Ophthalmol Soc. 2007;111:118–21.
19. Herbort CP, Rao NA, Mochizuki M, Members of Scientific Committee of First International Workshop on Ocular Sarcoidosis. International criteria for the diagnosis of ocular sarcoidosis: results of the first International Workshop on Ocular Sarcoidosis (IWOS). Ocul Immunol Inflamm. 2009;17(3):160–9.
20. Dave N, Chevour P, Mahendradas P, et al. Increased aqueous humor CD4+/CD8+ lymphocyte ratio in sarcoid uveitis. Ocul Immunol Inflamm. 2018;8:1–8.
21. Kojima K, Maruyama K, Inaba T, et al. The CD4/CD8 ratioin vitreous fluid is of high diagnostic value in sarcoidosis. Ophthalmology. 2012;119:2386–92.
22. Selroos O. Treatment of sarcoidosis. Sarcoidosis. 1994;11:80–3.
23. Newman LS, Rose CS, Maier LA. Sarcoidosis. N Engl J Med. 1997;336:1224–34.
24. Pietnalho A, Tukiainen P, Haahtela T, et al. Oral prednisone followed by inhaled budesonide in newly diagnosed pulmonary sarcoidosis: a double blind, placebo-controlled multicenter study. Finnish pulmonary sarcoidosis study group. Chest. 1999;116:424–31.
25. Baughman RP, Lower EE. Steroid-sparing alternative treatments for sarcoidosis. Clin Chest Med. 1997;18:853–64.
26. Gideon NM, Mannino DM. Sarcoidosis mortality in the United States 1979–1991: an analysis of multiple-cause mortality data. Am J Med. 1996;100:423–7.
27. Moschos MM, Guex-Crosier Y. Anterior segment granuloma and optic nerve involvement as the presenting signs of systemic sarcoidosis. Clin Ophthalmol. 2008;2(4):951–3.. PubMed PMID: 19668451; PubMed Central PMCID:PMC2699804).
28. Wertheim MS, Mathers WD, Planck SJ, et al. In vivo confocal microscopy of keratic precipitates. Arch Ophthalmol. 2004;122(12):1773–81.
29. Kanavi MR, Soheilian M, Naghshgar N. Confocal scan of keratic precipitates in uveitic eyes of various etiologies. Cornea. 2010;29(6):650–4.

30. Mahendradas P, Shetty R, Narayana KM, et al. In vivo confocal microscopyof keratic precipitates in infectious versus noninfectious uveitis. Ophthalmology. 2010;117(2):373–80.
31. Tran VT, LeHoang P, Herbort CP. Value of high-frequency ultrasound biomicroscopy in uveitis. Eye (Lond). 2001;15(Pt 1):23–30.
32. Yannuzzi LA, Ober MD, Slakter JS, et al. Ophthalmic fundus imaging: today and beyond. Am J Ophthalmol. Mar 2004;137(3):511–24.
33. Feeney L. Lipofuscin and melanin of human retinal pigment epithelium. Fluorescence, enzyme cytochemical, and ultrastructural studies. Invest Ophthalmol Vis Sci. 1978;17(7):583–600.
34. Yeh S, Forooghian F, Wong WT, et al. Fundus autofluorescence imaging of the white dot syndromes. Arch Ophthalmol (Chicago, Ill: 1960). 2010;128(1):46–56.
35. Haen SP, Spaide RF. Fundus autofluorescence in multifocal choroiditis and panuveitis. Am J Ophthalmol. 2008;145(5):847–53.
36. Gupta A, Bansal R, Gupta V, Sharma A. Fundus autofluorescence in serpiginouslike choroiditis. Retina (Philadelphia, Pa). 2012;32(4):814–25.
37. Rostaqui O, Querques G, Haymann P, et al. Visualization of sarcoid choroidal granuloma by enhanced depth imaging optical coherence tomography. Ocul Immunol Inflamm. 2014;22(3):239–41.
38. Herbort CP. Fluorescein and indocyanine green angiography for uveitis. Middle East Afr J Ophthalmol. 2009;16(4):168–87.
39. Herbort CP, LeHoang P, Guex-Crosier Y. Schematic interpretation of indocyanine green angiography in posterior uveitis using a standard angiographic protocol. Ophthalmology. 1998;105(3):432–40.
40. Wolfensberger TJ, Herbort CP. Indocyanine green angiographic features in ocular sarcoidosis. Ophthalmology. 1999;106(2):285–9.
41. Takahashi A, Nagaoka T, Yoshida A. Enhanced vitreous imaging optical coherence tomography in primary macular holes. Int Ophthalmol. 2016;36(3):355–63.
42. Pang CE, Freund K, Engelbert M. Enhanced vitreous imaging technique with spectral-domain optical coherence tomography for evaluation of posterior vitreous detachment. JAMA Ophthalmol. 2014;132(9):1148–50.
43. Goldberg NR, Jabs DA, Busingye J. Optical coherence tomography imaging of presumed sarcoid retinal and optic nerve nodules. Ocul Immunol Inflamm. 2015;24:1–4.
44. Baltmr A, Lightman S, Tomkins-Netzer O. Examining the choroid in ocular inflammation: a focus on enhanced depth imaging. J Ophthalmol. 2014;2014:459136.
45. Invernizzi A, Mapelli C, Viola F, et al. Choroidal granulomas visualized by enhanced depth imaging optical coherence tomography. Retina. 2015;35(3):525–31.
46. Mehta H, Sim DA, Keane PA, et al. Structural changes of the choroid in sarcoid and tuberculosis-related granulomatous uveitis. Eye (Lond). 2015;29(8):1060–8.
47. Modi YS, Epstein A, Bhaleeya S, et al. Multimodal imaging ofsarcoid choroidal granulomas. J Ophthalmic Inflamm Infect. 2013;3(1):58.
48. Pérez-Campagne E, Guex-Crosier Y, Schalenbourg A, et al. Giant nodular posterior scleritis compatible with ocular sarcoidosis simulating choroidal melanoma. Arch Soc Esp Oftalmol. 2007;82(9):563–6.
49. Hirukawa K, Keino H, Watanabe T, Okada AA. Enhanced depth imaging optical coherence tomography of the choroid in new-onset acute posterior scleritis. Graefes Arch Clin Exp Ophthalmol. 2013;251(9):2273–5.
50. Taki W, Keino H, Watanabe T, Okada AA. Enhanced depth imaging optical coherence tomography of the choroid in recurrent unilateral posterior scleritis. Graefes Arch Clin Exp Ophthalmol. 2013;251(3):1003–4.
51. Papavasileiou E, Miller JB, Sobrin L. Swept-source optical coherence tomography findings in convalescent phase of treated sarcoid choroidal granulomas. Retin Cases Brief Rep. 2016;10(1):32–6.
52. Sandhu R, Jia Y, Liang L, et al. Assessment of macular circulation in patients with retinal vasculitis using OCT angiography. Invest Ophthalmol Vis Sci. 2015;56:3359.
53. Sandhu R, Jia Y, Liu L, et al. Assessment of macular circulation in patients with retinal vasculitis using OCT angiography. Invest Ophthalmol Vis Sci. 2015;56:3359.

Vogt-Koyanagi-Harada Disease and Sympathetic Ophthalmia

Jeffrey J. Tan and Narsing A. Rao

Introduction

Vogt-Koyanagi-Harada disease (VKH) and sympathetic ophthalmia (SO) are clinically similar entities consisting of bilateral autoimmune granulomatous intraocular inflammation that can present with posterior or panuveitis associated with serous retinal detachments and optic disc edema. Later manifestations include Dalen-Fuchs nodules, sunset glow fundus, chorioretinal atrophy, subretinal fibrosis, and choroidal neovascularization. They also share similar theories of pathogenesis, which involve activated T-cells targeting uveal tissue [1, 2] and similar major histocompatibility antigen (MHC) haplotypes [3].

The most salient distinction between VKH and SO is the history of penetrating ocular trauma present in SO, with the uninjured eye acting is the sympathizing eye. Other important differences include greater systemic symptoms in VKH such as tinnitus, hearing loss, vertigo, meningismus, poliosis, and vitiligo. In terms of epidemiology, VKH is more prevalent in certain geographic regions (Asia, Latin America, and the Middle East) and in pigmented individuals with a mean age in the third decade [4, 5], while SO has no such predilections.

VKH can be divided into four different stages of disease: prodromal, uveitic, convalescent, and recurrent. The prodromal phase may present as a viral infection lasting anywhere from a few days to a few weeks and may demonstrate neurologic manifestations such as headache (82%), meningismus (55%), fever (18%), nausea (9%), and vertigo (9%), as well as auditory disturbances [6]. Cerebrospinal fluid

J. J. Tan
USC Roski Eye Institute, Department of Ophthalmology, Los Angeles, CA, USA

N. A. Rao (✉)
Ophthalmology, USC Roski Eye Institute Ophthalmology, Los Angeles, CA, USA
e-mail: narsing.rao@med.usc.edu

N. A. Rao et al. (eds.), *Posterior Uveitis*, Essentials in Ophthalmology,
https://doi.org/10.1007/978-3-030-03140-4_3

(CSF) may show pleocytosis in more than 80% of patients [7]. The uveitic phase occurs when patients develop acute ocular symptoms, and findings include bilateral granulomatous uveitis with pockets of subretinal fluid, choroidal thickening, optic nerve head hyperemia and swelling, vitritis, and anterior segment inflammation with mutton fat keratic precipitates, shallowing of the anterior chamber, and moderate intraocular pressure elevation [8, 9]. The convalescent phase occurs weeks to months thereafter with depigmentation of the choroid (eventually leading to sunset glow fundus over months), perilimbal depigmentation (Sugiura's sign), Dalen-Fuchs nodules, vitiligo, and poliosis [8]. Finally, some patients may develop chronic repeated bouts of inflammation in the recurrent phase. This may occur 6–9 months after initial presentation with complications such as retinal pigment epithelium (RPE) proliferation, subretinal fibrosis, choroidal neovascularization, posterior synechiae, cataract, band keratopathy, and glaucoma [8, 9].

SO shares many features in the acute and chronic phases of disease of VKH, but does not have as clear delineation between phases nor the extraocular findings. Moreover, SO can often start as an insidious mild non-granulomatous anterior chamber reaction [10]. SO can occur anywhere from days to years following trauma, and thus patients must be made aware of signs and symptoms that could arise after their injury.

The diagnosis for these diseases is made on clinical findings rather than serologic testing or histopathology. Multimodal imaging is instrumental in aiding in early and accurate diagnosis as the differential diagnosis is broad: infectious (tuberculosis, syphilis, bacterial, fungal, viral), malignant (intraocular lymphoma, diffuse uveal lymphoid hyperplasia, bilateral diffuse uveal melanocytic hyperplasia, monoclonal gammopathies), idiopathic (central serous chorioretinopathy, uveal effusion syndrome), and inflammatory (posterior scleritis, sarcoidosis, white dot syndromes, lupus choroidopathy).

In this chapter, we will review the most updated imaging modalities and their response to treatment in VKH and SO.

Vogt-Koyanagi-Harada Disease

Traditionally, fluorescein angiography (FA) was the primary ancillary test used in diagnosing VKH, and in certain countries (Europe, Japan), it was not uncommon to perform lumbar punctures to detect CSF pleocytosis. However, advances in optical coherence tomography (OCT) along with other imaging modalities such as fundus autofluorescence have allowed for non-invasive monitoring of changes to the retina, RPE, and choroid [11]. In the acute phase of the disease, OCT is most useful for evaluating the increased thickness of the choroid as well as the presence of subretinal fluid and exudative retinal detachments. Fluorescein angiography (FA) in the acute stage can demonstrate changes in choroidal perfusion and show pinpoint areas of hyperfluorescence and subsequent leakage into the subretinal space. Indocyanine green angiography (ICG) allows for evaluation of changes to choroidal perfusion as well. Fundus autofluorescence (FAF) is also useful in evaluating changes to the retinal pigment epithelium prior to changes evident on clinical exam. In the convalescent phase of disease, thinning of the choroid is apparent on OCT, as is blocked choroidal fluorescence on FA. OCT-enhanced depth imaging (OCT-EDI), ICG, and FAF are helpful in the chronic recurrent stage and during treatment, as they demonstrate subclinical disease in the choroid which can help tailor treatment with corticosteroids and immunomodulatory agents.

Although such imaging modalities have helped in diagnosis and monitoring response to treatment, it is not clear how often and which imaging modalities should be used in acute, convalescent, and chronic recurrent phases of VKH. It appears currently that most uveitis clinics use OCT and FAF during follow-up examinations, but further studies must be done to determine their clinical usefulness and appropriate timing for repeat imaging.

Optical Coherence Tomography (OCT)

Due to its ability to non-invasively identify changes to the retina, RPE, and choroid, OCT has become an essential tool in both acute and chronic VKH. Serous retinal detachments are a hallmark of acute VKH, such that when seen with bilateral intraocular inflammation, it carries a positive predictive value 100 and negative predictive value of 88.4 for diagnosis of VKH [8]. OCT technology enables identification of subclinical subretinal fluid that could otherwise be missed on fundus exam (Fig. 1). Furthermore, OCT allows objective measurements of subretinal fluid height and area which can be followed throughout the treatment course. Height of subretinal fluid on OCT correlates with visual acuity measured at the same visit, but does not correlate with resolution time or final visual acuity. Treatment with systemic corticosteroids in the acute phase can lead to reduction of the subretinal fluid height to 50% in a week and entire fluid resolution within 2–4 weeks (Fig. 2). Presence of choroidal folds and multifocal retinal detachment also correlates with

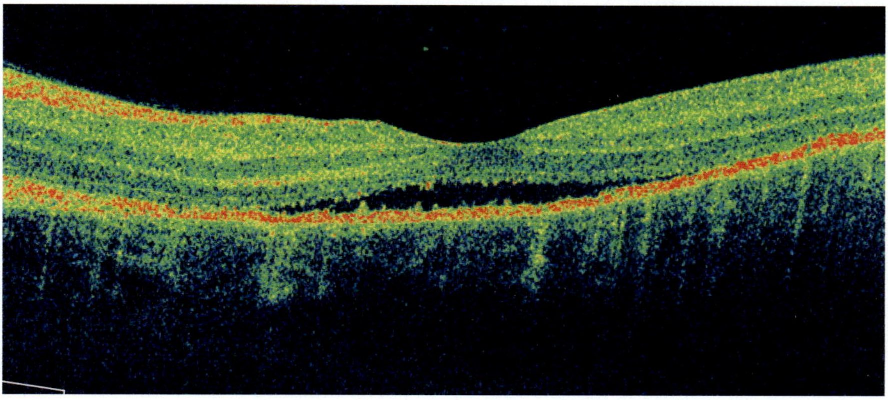

Fig. 1 Optical coherence tomography (OCT) of the macula showing subclinical subretinal fluid in the acute phase of VKH

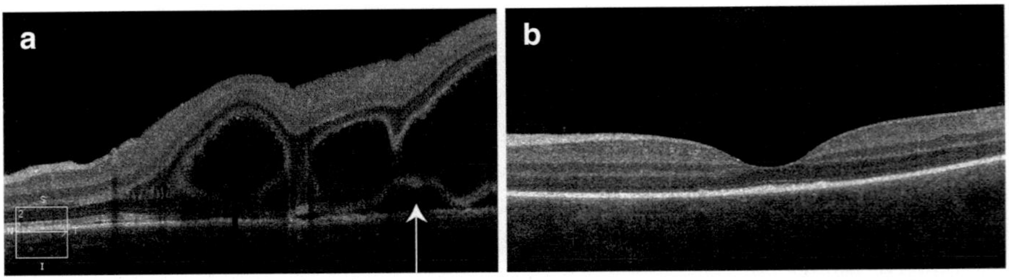

Fig. 2 OCT showing (**a**) subretinal (white arrow) and intraretinal (black arrow) fluid on presentation of acute VKH and (**b**) resolution of all fluid within 2 weeks of starting high-dose systemic corticosteroids

initial visual acuity but not with vision at the 3-month follow-up or time to resolution of subretinal fluid [12].

There can be macular edema in as high as 40% of patients in the acute stage of VKH [13]. This intraretinal fluid appears to be associated with severe dye leakage from the RPE on FA [13–15]. Additionally, patients in the acute phase may possess subretinal septae associated with exudative retinal detachments that can be seen on OCT [13, 16]. It is hypothesized that these subretinal septae are comprised of inflammatory products or are actually a separation of the inner and outer segments of the photoreceptors with the presence of fibrin among the outer segments [15, 17–19].

OCT technology has seen considerable advancement since its inception; however, there have been few direct comparisons among OCT technologies and machines. Newer enhanced spectral domain OCT (SD-OCT) imaging has the advantage of improved visualization of the ellipsoid zone and external limiting membrane (ELM) in acute VKH disease compared to prior modalities (Topcon OCT 2000 and Zeiss Stratus) [18]. Comparison between conventional OCT raster scans and enhanced depth imaging (EDI) raster scan protocol revealed high agreement between the two when measuring retinal thickness and volume [20]. When examining the choroid, SD-OCT instruments across similar generations (Zeiss Cirrus HD-OCT 1-line raster, Heidelberg Spectralis EDI, and Optovue RTVue retina cross) appear similar in their ability to produce accurate and reproducible measurements of choroidal thickness [21]. Based on the literature, SD-OCT technology currently provides a good view of the pertinent chorioretinal structures involved in the disease process.

Choroidal thickness is increased in the acute phase and decreased in the convalescent phase of VKH, and OCT can accurately reliably quantify these changes using various technologies to penetrate deeper into the choroid [22–24]. Mean choroidal thickness of patients with acute disease can be as high as 424–805 μm compared to controls of 287 μm [22, 23]. While in the convalescent phase, choroidal thickness is seen as low as 144–273 μm, especially in those eyes with sunset glow fundus and long-standing disease [22, 24–27]. The thinning of choroid as measured by OCT may reflect either choroidal melanocyte loss and or loss of choriocapillaris, which is evidenced by histopathological studies of eyes in the convalescent and

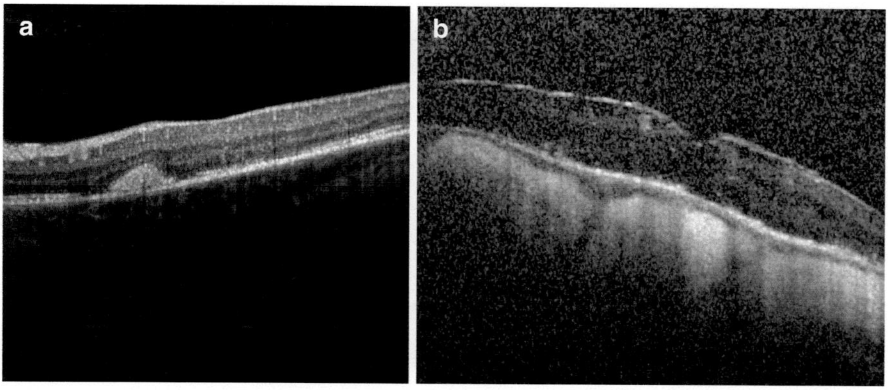

Fig. 3 OCT of chronic VKH: (**a**) subretinal fibrosis and photoreceptor disruption; (**b**) choroidal thinning with associated neurosensory retina, RPE loss, and epiretinal membrane

chronic recurrent phases [28, 29]. Other characteristics of chronic VKH include subretinal fibrosis, epiretinal membrane, RPE atrophy, and associated neurosensory retina atrophy (Fig. 3).

In response to treatment with systemic corticosteroids, choroidal thickness can also see dramatic decrease of greater than 50% by 2 weeks [23, 24]. OCT imaging of the choroid can also be used as an indicator of disease recurrence with findings of choroidal folds or an increase in choroidal thickness [24, 26]. More recent studies have shown that choroidal thickening can be seen even 1 month prior to anterior chamber inflammation, emphasizing the importance of repeat OCT imaging in VKH patients, especially those with history of recurrent inflammation [30]. Thus, OCT can be used to evaluate the stage of disease as well as monitor for tailored treatment.

Fluorescein Angiography (FA)

Fluorescein angiography (FA) is important for evaluating retinal and choroidal changes during the different stages of the disease, and it can help differentiate VKH from similar disease processes such as central serous chorioretinopathy (CSCR) or acute posterior multifocal placoid pigment epitheliopathy (APMPPE). The characteristic findings of acute VKH on FA are multiple deep hyperfluorescent spots and late leakage as the dye fills within serous detachments (Fig. 4). There may be optic disc hyperfluorescence as well if papillitis is present. However, as the disease process progresses to different phases, it may also reveal different findings on FA; thus, the phase of disease must be accounted for when interpreting these tests. The convalescent stage is marked by spotted hyper- and hypofluorescence and blockage of choroidal fluorescence due to retinal pigment epithelial migration. Additionally, there can be dot-like hyperfluorescence at the equator which clinically correlates with nummular white scars. In the chronic uveitic stage, the most common findings

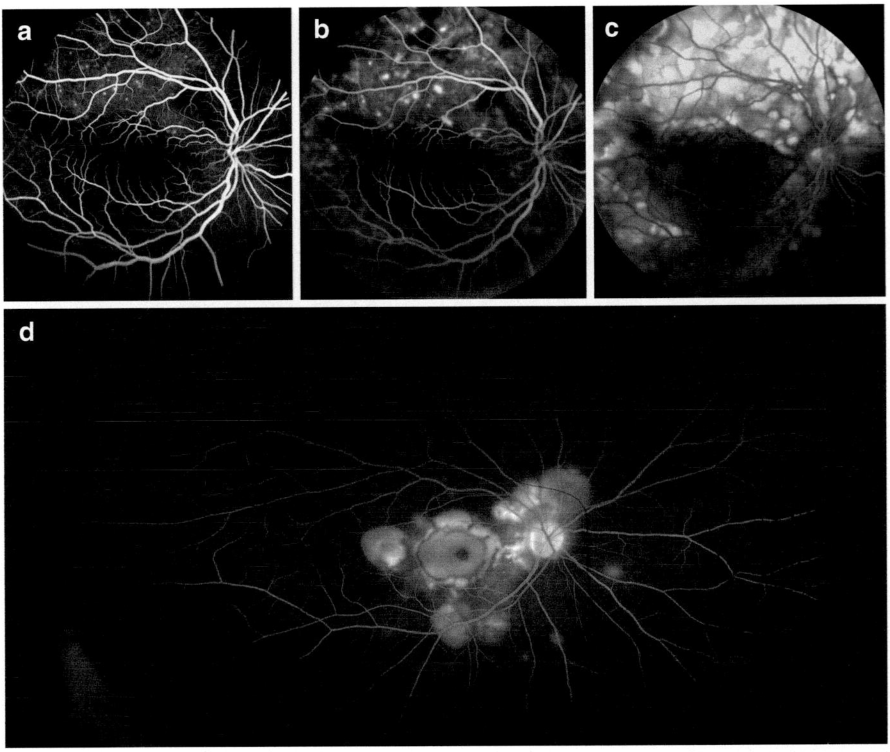

Fig. 4 Fluorescein angiogram (FA) demonstrating characteristic (**a**–**c**) early hyperfluorescent spots and late leakage in acute VKH. (**d**) Diffuse pooling on widefield fluorescein angiogram

are spotted hyper- and hypofluorescence and optic disc hyperfluorescence with almost one-fifth of patients showing retinal vascular hyperfluorescence [31]. One study noted early pinpoint peripapillary hyperfluorescence on FA only in patients in the hyperacute phase (those imaged less than 14 days after onset of symptoms), and these patients had significantly higher frequency of disease resolution. It is possible that this is a valuable prognostic sign whereby patients who lack this finding may indicate a later stage in their disease course and requirement of longer and more aggressive treatment [32].

Indocyanine Green Angiography (ICG)

As the choroid is affected early in VKH, indocyanine green angiography (ICG) can reveal diffuse delayed perfusion of the choroid as well as leakage, segmental hypercyanescence, and hypocyanescence areas which can be missed on FA (Fig. 5) [33, 34]. VKH, along with ocular sarcoidosis, tuberculosis, and birdshot chorioretinopathy, can show similar ICG findings of fuzzy indistinct choroidal

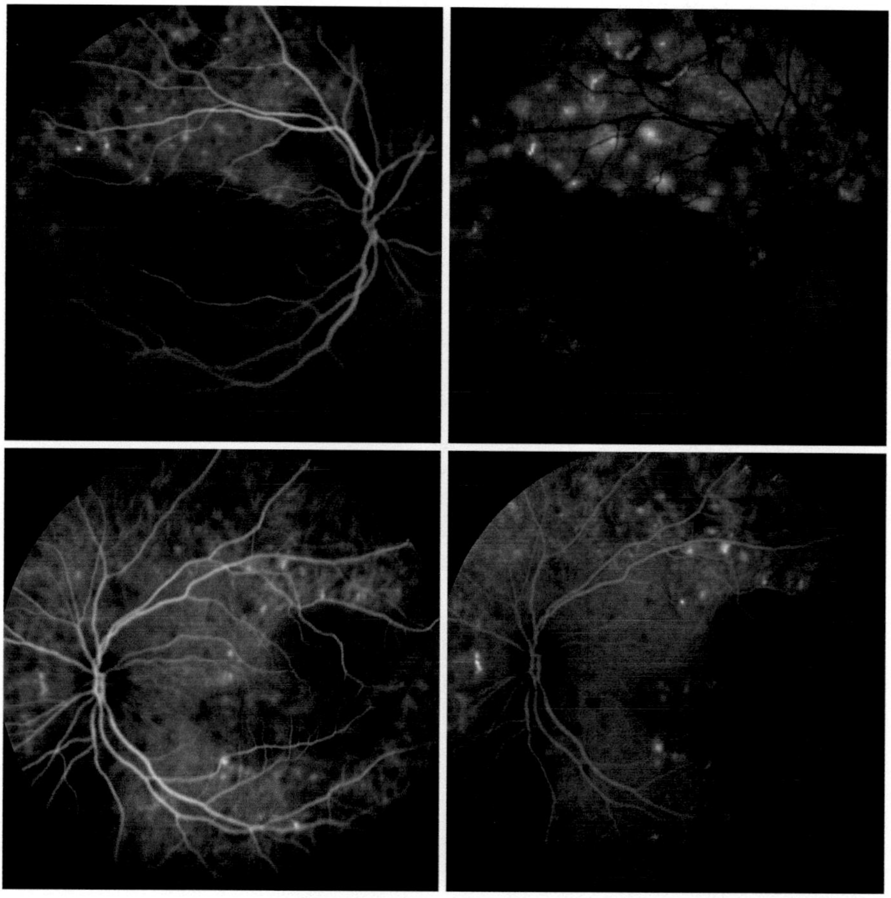

Fig. 5 Indocyanine green angiography (ICG) revealing fuzzy choroidal vessels and increased choroidal hypercyanescence in VKH

vessels and diffuse choroidal hypercyanescence, indicating stromal inflammatory vasculopathy [35].

ICG can be used to help titrate and taper immunosuppression effectively by showing subclinical disease during the treatment course. Lesions not seen on clinical exam or FA but seen on ICG can lead to earlier diagnosis and thus earlier treatment, decreasing the chance of development of chronic recurrent disease [36]. Hypocyanescence dark dots can be seen and used as a sign of early recurrence when only the anterior segment is involved, and these dots lessen in response to treatment [37]. The finding of persistent choroidal inflammation can make the duration of immunosuppression longer but results in lower incidence of long-term sequelae such as sunset glow fundus [35, 38]. In patients who have high propensity of frequent and severe recurrent inflammation, ICG can be a useful tool for periodic monitoring [37].

Fundus Autofluorescence (FAF)

Fundus autofluorescence (FAF) visualizes lipofuscin which accumulates in the retinal pigment epithelium (RPE) and can non-invasively detail areas of RPE dysfunction and loss. It can be useful in evaluating abnormalities in VKH that are not visible on clinical examination, and wide field scans can document the extent of disease.

In the acute phase, FAF shows diffuse increased hyperautofluorescence corresponding to the presence of exudative retinal detachments (Fig. 6a). These resolve in 6 months after treatment with high-dose intravenous steroids. However, in patients who present later in the acute phase, FAF shows a more diffuse and mottled hyperautofluorescence mixed with hypoautofluorescence, as well as lattice-like patterns [39–41].

In the chronic phase, FAF shows both decreased and increased autofluorescence patterns. The decreased autofluorescence pattern is related to the loss of RPE and involvement of the outer retina in the disease process. Peripapillary atrophy manifests as decreased autofluorescence as do nummular chorioretinal scars (Fig. 6b). An increased pattern is related to the development of cystoid macular edema, subretinal fibrosis, and areas of RPE proliferation (Fig. 6c). The appearance of a sunset

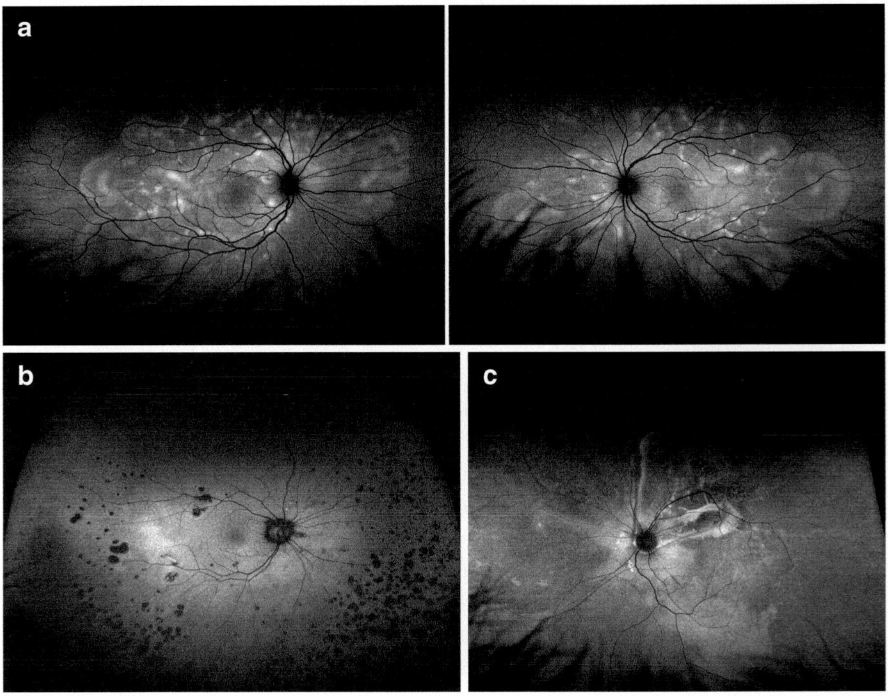

Fig. 6 Fundus autofluorescence (FAF) showing (**a**) increased signal corresponding to areas of exudative retinal detachment in acute VKH. Chronic VKH can show both (**b**) hypoautofluorescence in the form of peripapillary atrophy and nummular scars and (**c**) hyperautofluorescence in subretinal fibrosis and RPE proliferation

glow fundus does not correlate with abnormalities on FAF [11]. Since FAF can reflect the health of the RPE, recurrent bouts of inflammation and subclinical inflammation can be evaluated quickly and non-invasively.

Retinal Electrophysiologic Tests

Electroretinogram (ERG) can assess retinal function in acute and chronic VKH by showing diffusely diminished amplitudes and preserved implicit times [42]. Multifocal ERG (mfERG) can reveal recovery of macular function (i.e., improvement in latency and amplitude) before treatment and after treatment. However, mfERG recovery lags behind visual acuity improvements during testing and macular function is still significantly decreased compared to normal controls after treatment [43]. ERG may be useful in assessing retinal function in patients for which visual acuity cannot be obtained, but there have been no evidenced-based treatment regimens based on normalization of ERG.

Lumbar Puncture

The role of lumbar puncture in the diagnosis of VKH has been controversial. Cerebrospinal fluid pleocytosis, a diagnosis possible only by lumbar puncture, was included as an original major criterion required for the diagnosis of VKH [44]. The revised diagnostic criteria put forth in 2001 required a finding of CSF pleocytosis only in the absence of neurological or auditory findings [45]. However, multiple studies since have shown that 20–30% of patients diagnosed with VKH do not have CSF pleocytosis [46, 47]. The presence of clinical features consistent with VKH, especially if characteristic FA findings are present (disc edema, pinpoint hyperfluorescence, late leakage), suggests that CSF pleocytosis and lumbar puncture are not necessary for diagnosis but may be reserved for atypical presentations without the angiographic features. Finally, CSF pleocytosis cannot be used to differentiate among VKH, Lyme disease, neurosyphilis, multiple sclerosis, neurosarcoidosis, and Behcet's disease [47]. The presence of melanin-laden macrophages in CSF, however, is a feature of acute VKH and can be used to help narrow the diagnosis in these cases [48].

B-Scan Ultrasonography

When the view to the fundus is obscured by presence of dense vitritis, posterior synechiae, cataract, or corneal opacity, B-scan ultrasonography should be utilized to help make the diagnosis. The following features on ultrasound are noted to be consistent with the diagnosis of VKH: (1) diffuse, low to medium reflective thickening of the choroid posteriorly; (2) serous retinal detachment located inferiorly or in the posterior pole; (3) mild vitreous opacities with no posterior vitreous detachment;

and (4) thickening of the sclera and/or episclera posteriorly [49]. Furthermore, ultrasonography can also be used to follow response to treatment in the absence of a direct view as resolution of these findings occurs with appropriate steroid and immunomodulatory treatment.

Ultrasonography, however, must be used carefully to distinguish between several different entities such as posterior scleritis, benign reactive lymphoid hyperplasia of the uvea, and diffuse melanoma of the choroid. Ultrasonographic features of VKH and sympathetic ophthalmia are the same with the distinguishing feature being the absence of prior intraocular surgery or ocular trauma in the former.

VKH can also present with elevated intraocular pressure and shallow anterior chamber mimicking acute angle-closure glaucoma. However, ultrasound biomicroscopy in these cases can demonstrate detachment of the ciliary body and peripheral choroidals which resolve with immunosuppressive therapy, thereby differentiating the disease process from angle-closure glaucoma [50].

OCT-Angiography (OCT-A)

OCT-angiography (OCT-A) is a newer imaging modality that allows non-invasive viewing of retinochoroidal microvasculature through endoluminal flow changes. It is not yet widely available, and its clinical usefulness still being determined in various diseases. However, there is recent evidence suggesting that OCT-A flow voids in the choriocapillaris are representative of inflammatory foci, which can be used to diagnose and follow patients in acute VKH [51]. Furthermore, these true flow voids can be differentiated from shadowing effects from overlying subretinal fluid and pigment epithelial detachment such as in central serous chorioretinopathy [52].

Sympathetic Ophthalmia

As sympathetic ophthalmia (SO) is clinically nearly identical to VKH, they share many similar aspects in terms of multimodal imaging. Like VKH, SO reveals different findings during the acute and chronic phases of disease. However, due to SO's relative rarity, there are less studies and controlled trials examining imaging and response to treatment for this condition.

Optical Coherence Tomography (OCT)

OCT advancements have enabled non-invasive high-resolution imaging of posterior structures as deep as the choroid, making it particularly useful for SO. SO in the acute phase will reveal serous retinal detachments seen as empty spaces between the neurosensory retina and underlying RPE on OCT. Similar to VKH, these spaces may contain hyperreflective septa which are unique to these two disease entities. Due to the disconnection between photoreceptors and RPE, outer segment shedding can be interrupted resulting in photoreceptor outer segment elongation (Fig. 7a). Such alterations can regress and completely disappear if prompt therapy is started (Fig. 7b) [53]. Conversely, long-standing fluid can lead to cystoid macular edema formation and loss of photoreceptor function, similar to what is described in chronic central serous chorioretinopathy [53, 54].

OCT examination of the choroid also reveals changes resembling VKH: massive thickening, folds, and loss of the physiological architecture of the choroidal layers [55]. Dalen-Fuchs nodules can be captured and followed by OCT as they evolve, initially appearing as round hyperreflective areas located at the level of the outer retina and then regressing in response to therapy. Disruption of the RPE and outer retinal bands associated with the Dalen-Fuchs nodules may or may not recover with therapy [56]. During the chronic phase of SO, choroidal thinning and atrophy may be seen on OCT, but further studies are needed to confirm the reproducibility of these findings [57].

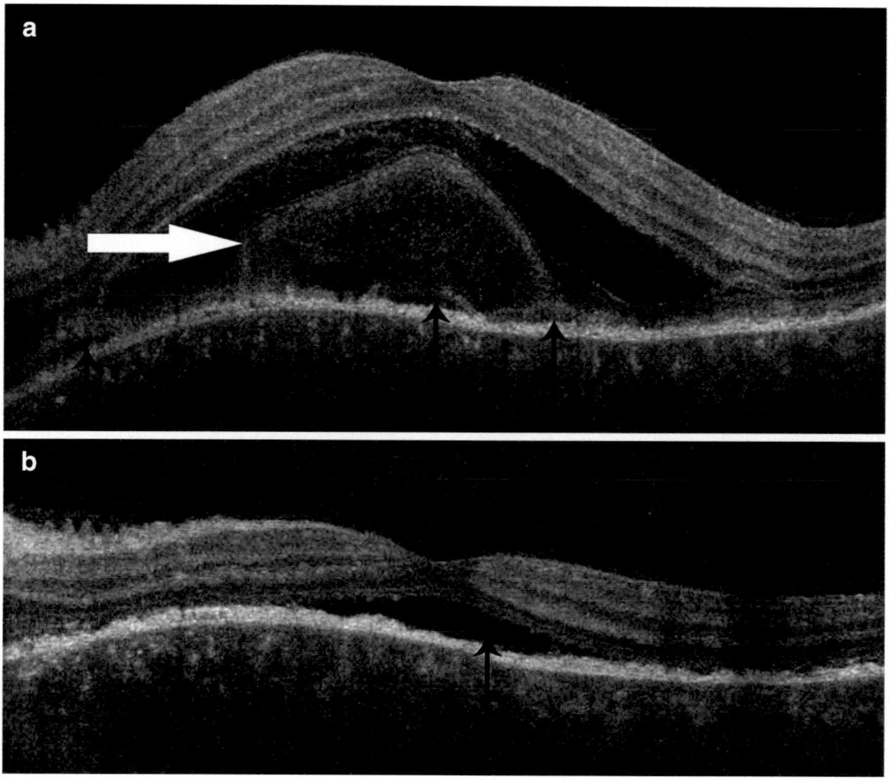

Fig. 7 OCT showing features of acute SO: (**a**) significant intraretinal fluid with elongation of photoreceptors (white arrow) and small pockets of subretinal fluid (black arrows). (**b**) Resolution of intraretinal fluid within 1 week of starting systemic corticosteroids but with residual subretinal fluid (black arrow)

Fluorescein Angiography (FA)

In the acute phase of SO, two distinct fluorescein angiography (FA) patterns are seen. The most frequent pattern is virtually identical to that of acute VKH with diffuse pinpoint hyperfluorescent spots at the level of the RPE with late leakage (Fig. 8a). The spots may coalesce as the dye fills under focal serous retinal detachments in severe cases, and there may be a hyperfluorescent disc even in the absence of clinically apparent papillitis [58]. In response to treatment, the hyperfluorescent spots are expected to see improvement. Additionally, disc leakage and petalloid leakage due to macular edema may also improve [59].

The second FA pattern is similar to what is seen in acute posterior multifocal placoid pigment epitheliopathy (APMPPE) with hypofluorescent foci during the early phase that become hyperfluorescent and stain late (Fig. 7b). However, unlike APMPPE, these lesions are slightly elevated, may have a mottled appearance, and likely represent Dalen-Fuchs nodules or inflammatory cells extending from the choroid [60, 61].

In the chronic phase of SO, FA findings are more variable depending on the presence of complications (Fig. 8b). Nummular scars and chorioretinal atrophy reveal window defects [61]. Subretinal fibrosis reflects proliferated metaplastic RPE which will hyperfluoresce and stain late [62]. Choroidal neovascularization is rare in chronic SO but would show dye leakage.

Indocyanine Green Angiography (ICG)

Indocyanine green angiography (ICG) is a useful adjunct to FA as it better images the choroid, which is a primary site of involvement in SO. Most commonly, ICG will reveal multiple hypocyanescence spots that correspond to hypercyanescence spots on FA. But as the ICG study progresses into later phases, the hypocyanescence spots may behave differently, giving clue to what type of lesions are involved. If the spots persist or become more prominent, they most likely represent areas of chorioretinal atrophy and cicatrization, which also correspond to yellow atrophic areas on fundus examination. On the other hand, if the hypofluorescent spots fade in the late phase, they are interpreted as areas of active choroiditis [63, 64]. Hypotheses of what these spots are include cellular infiltration, blockage from subretinal fluid, or Dalen-Fuchs spots, the last of which has been correlated by histopathology [65]. As such, these spots may attenuate or disappear after corticosteroid treatment [63, 64]. However, one study found that although the hypocyanescence spots disappear in the intermediate phase with corticosteroid treatment, they reappear in the late phase of ICG, possibly due to atrophy showing through underneath the resolving Dalen-Fuchs nodules [66].

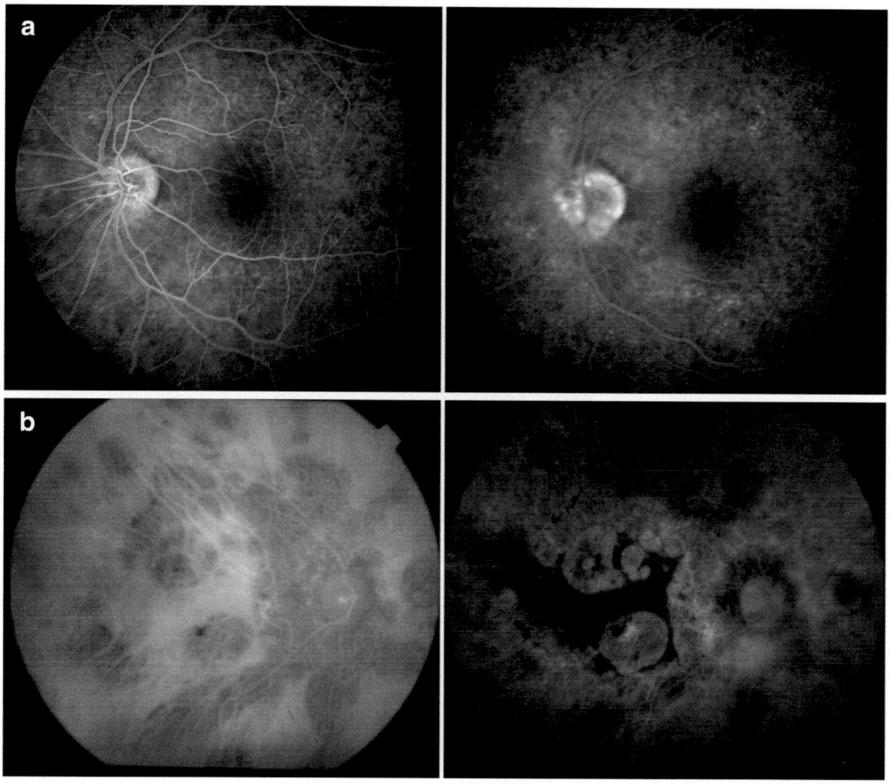

Fig. 8 Fluorescein angiogram (FA) patterns seen in acute SO include (**a**) multiple pinpoint hyperfluorescent dots and disc hyperfluorescence; and chronic SO may reveal (**b**) patchy areas of hypofluorescence corresponding to chorioretinal atrophy

Fundus Autofluorescence (FAF)

In acute disease, FAF may show hyperautofluorescence in areas of serous retinal detachment, suggesting increased metabolic activity and dysfunction of RPE (Fig. 9). These areas may evolve into speckled areas of hyper- and hypoautofluorescence described as "leopard spots" after subretinal fluid resorbs [67]. In chronic cases of SO, one would expect mixed findings of hypo- and hyperautofluorescence as described in the VKH FAF section due to their clinical and histopathological similarities; however, there are limited studies reporting application of FAF in SO to support this. Herein are images of chronic SO developing increasing areas of hypoautofluorescence as peripapillary atrophy and nummular scars progress over 5 years in the same eye (Fig. 10).

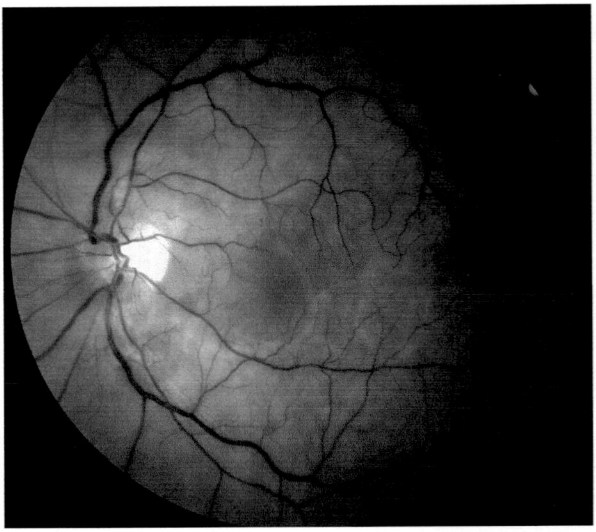

Fig. 9 Fundus autofluorescence (FAF) of acute SO revealing hyperautofluorescence corresponding to areas of exudate retinal detachment

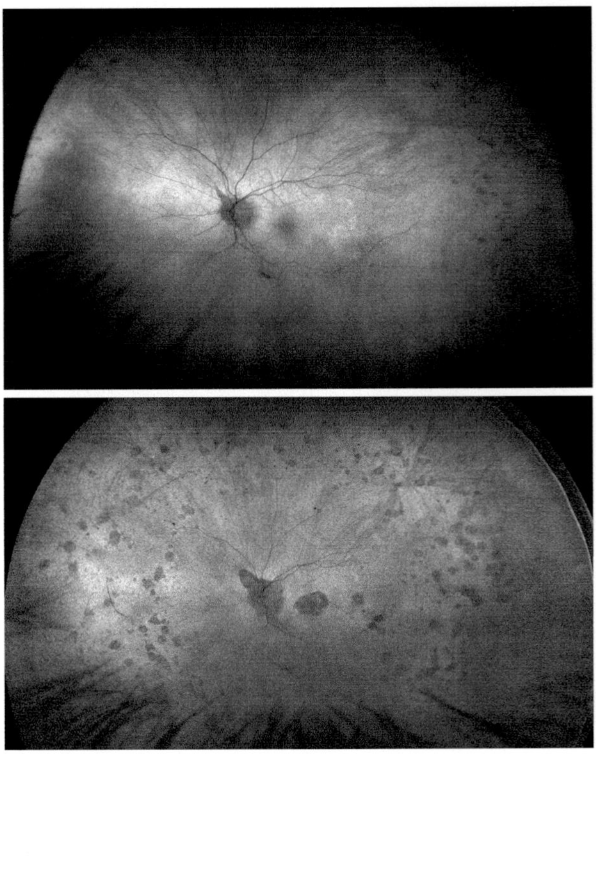

Fig. 10 Fundus autofluorescence (FAF) of chronic SO showing progression of hypoautofluorescent areas corresponding to peripapillary atrophy and nummular scars over 5 years in the same eye

B-Scan Ultrasonography

B-scan ultrasound can reveal diffuse choroidal thickening in the posterior pole due to choroidal inflammation and non-granulomatous infiltration [53]. It is particularly useful in cases where cataract, posterior synechiae, corneal opacities, and other pathologies preclude a view of the fundus.

Conflict of Interest Jeffrey J. Tan and Narsing A. Rao declare that they have no conflict of interest.

Informed Consent No human studies were carried out by the authors for this chapter.

Animal Studies No animal studies were carried out by the authors for this chapter.

References

1. Norose K, Yano A. Melanoma specific Th1 cytotoxic T lymphocyte lines in Vogt-Koyanagi-Harada disease. Br J Ophthalmol. 1996;80(11):1002–8.
2. Jakobiec FA, Marboe CC, Knowles DM, Iwamoto T, Harrison W, Chang S, et al. Human sympathetic ophthalmia: an analysis of the inflammatory infiltrate by hybridoma-monoclonal antibodies, immunochemistry, and correlative electron microscopy. Ophthalmology. 1983;90:76–95.
3. Davis JL, Mittal KK, Freidlin V, Mellow SR, Optican DC, Palestine AG, et al. HLA associations and ancestry in Vogt-Koyanagi-Harada disease and sympathetic ophthalmia. Ophthalmology. 1990;97:1137–42.
4. Beniz J, Forster DJ, Lean JS, Smith RE, Rao NA. Variations in clinical features of the Vogt-Koyanagi-Harada syndrome. Retina (Philadelphia, Pa). 1991;11(3):275–80.
5. Rubsamen PE, Gass JD. Vogt-Koyanagi-Harada syndrome. Clinical course, therapy, and long-term visual outcome. Arch Ophthalmol. 1991;109(5):682–7.
6. Rao NA, Sukavatcharin S, Tsai JH. Vogt-Koyanagi-Harada disease diagnostic criteria. Int Ophthalmol. 2007;27(2–3):195–9.
7. Damico FM, Kiss S, Young LH. Vogt-Koyanagi-Harada disease. Semin Ophthalmol. 2005;20(3):183–90.
8. Rao NA, Gupta A, Dustin L, Chee S-P, Okada AA, Khairallah M, et al. Frequency of distinguishing clinical features in Vogt-Koyanagi-Harada disease. Ophthalmology. 2010;117(3):591–9. 599.e1.
9. Forster DJ, Rao NA, Hill RA, Nguyen QH, Baerveldt G. Incidence and management of glaucoma in Vogt-Koyanagi-Harada syndrome. Ophtha. 1993;100(5):613–8.
10. Arevalo JF, Garcia RA, Al-Dhibi HA, Sanchez JG, Suarez-Tata L. Update on sympathetic ophthalmia. Middle East Afr J Ophthalmol. 2012;19(1):13–21.
11. Vasconcelos-Santos DV, Sohn EH, Sadda S, Rao NA. Retinal pigment epithelial changes in chronic Vogt-Koyanagi-Harada disease: fundus autofluorescence and spectral domain-optical coherence tomography findings. Retina (Philadelphia, Pa). 2010;30(1):33–41.
12. Nazari H, Rao NA. Resolution of subretinal fluid with systemic corticosteroid treatment in acute Vogt-Koyanagi-Harada disease. Br J Ophthalmol. 2012;96(11):1410–4.
13. Maruyama Y, Kishi S. Tomographic features of serous retinal detachment in Vogt-Koyanagi-Harada syndrome. Ophthalmic Surg Lasers Imaging. 2004;35(3):239–42.

14. Tsujikawa A, Yamashiro K, Yamamoto K, Nonaka A, Fujihara M, Kurimoto Y. Retinal cystoid spaces in acute Vogt-Koyanagi-Harada syndrome. Am J Ophthalmol. 2005;139(4):670–7.
15. Yamaguchi Y, Otani T, Kishi S. Tomographic features of serous retinal detachment with multilobular dye pooling in acute Vogt-Koyanagi-Harada disease. Am J Ophthalmol. 2007;144(2):260–5.
16. Parc C, Guenoun J-M, Dhote R, Brézin A. Optical coherence tomography in the acute and chronic phases of Vogt-Koyanagi-Harada disease. Ocul Immunol Inflamm. 2005;13(2–3):225–7.
17. Bordaberry MF. Vogt-Koyanagi-Harada disease: diagnosis and treatments update. Curr Opin Ophthalmol. 2010;21(6):430–5.
18. Ishihara K, Hangai M, Kita M, Yoshimura N. Acute Vogt-Koyanagi-Harada disease in enhanced spectral-domain optical coherence tomography. Ophthalmology. 2009;116(9):1799–807.
19. Lee JE, Park SW, Lee JK, Choi HY, Oum BS, Kim HW. Edema of the photoreceptor layer in Vogt-Koyanagi-Harada disease observed using high-resolution optical coherence tomography. Korean J Ophthalmol. 2009;23(2):74–9.
20. Park SY, Kim SM, Song Y-M, Sung J, Ham D-I. Retinal thickness and volume measured with enhanced depth imaging optical coherence tomography. Am J Ophthalmol. 2013;156(3):557–66. e2.
21. Branchini L, Regatieri CV, Flores-Moreno I, Baumann B, Fujimoto JG, Duker JS. Reproducibility of choroidal thickness measurements across three spectral domain optical coherence tomography systems. Ophthalmology. 2012;119(1):119–23.
22. Fong AHC, Li KKW, Wong D. Choroidal evaluation using enhanced depth imaging spectral-domain optical coherence tomography in Vogt-Koyanagi-Harada disease. Retina (Philadelphia, Pa). 2011;31(3):502–9.
23. Maruko I, Iida T, Sugano Y, Oyamada H, Sekiryu T, Fujiwara T, Spaide RF. Subfoveal choroidal thickness after treatment of Vogt-Koyanagi-Harada disease. Retina (Philadelphia, Pa). 2011;31(3):510–7.
24. Nakai K, Gomi F, Ikuno Y, Yasuno Y, Nouchi T, Ohguro N, Nishida K. Choroidal observations in Vogt-Koyanagi-Harada disease using high-penetration optical coherence tomography. Graefes Arch Clin Exp Ophthalmol. 2012;250(7):1089–95.
25. da Silva FT, Sakata VM, Nakashima A, Hirata CE, Olivalves E, Takahashi WY, et al. Enhanced depth imaging optical coherence tomography in long-standing Vogt-Koyanagi-Harada disease. Br J Ophthalmol. 2013;97(1):70–4.
26. Shinoda K, Imamura Y, Matsumoto CS, Mizota A, Ando Y. Wavy and elevated retinal pigment epithelial line in optical coherence tomographic images of eyes with atypical Vogt-Koyanagi-Harada disease. Graefes Arch Clin Exp Ophthalmol. 2012;250(9):1399–402.
27. Takahashi H, Takase H, Ishizuka A, Miyanaga M, Kawaguchi T, Ohno-Matsui K, Mochizuki M. Choroidal thickness in convalescent vogt-koyanagi-harada disease. Retina. 2014;34(4):775–80.
28. Inomata H, Rao NA. Depigmented atrophic lesions in sunset glow fundi of Vogt-Koyanagi-Harada disease. Am J Ophthalmol. 2001;131(5):607–14.
29. Nazari H, Hariri A, Hu Z, Ouyang Y, Sadda S, Rao NA. Choroidal atrophy and loss of choriocapillaris in convalescent stage of Vogt-Koyanagi-Harada disease: in vivo documentation. J Ophthalmic Inflamm Infect. 2014;4:9.
30. Tagawa Y, Namba K, Mizuuchi K, Takemoto Y, Iwata D, Uno T, Fukuhara T, Hirooka K, Kitaichi N, Ohno S, Ishida S. Choroidal thickening prior to anterior recurrence in patients with Vogt-Koyanagi-Harada disease. Br J Ophthalmol. 2016;100(4):473–7.
31. Arellanes-García L, Hernández-Barrios M, Fromow-Guerra J, Cervantes-Fanning P. Fluorescein fundus angiographic findings in Vogt-Koyanagi-Harada syndrome. Int Ophthalmol. 2007;27(2–3):155–61.
32. Chee S-P, Jap A, Cheung CMG. The prognostic value of angiography in Vogt-Koyanagi-Harada disease. Am J Ophthalmol. 2010;150(6):888–93.
33. Fardeau C, Tran THC, Gharbi B, Cassoux N, Bodaghi B, Lehoang P. Retinal fluorescein and indocyanine green angiography and optical coherence tomography in successive stages of Vogt-Koyanagi-Harada disease. Int Ophthalmol. 2007;27(2–3):163–72.

34. Harada T, Kanbara Y, Takeuchi T, Niwa T, Majima T. Exploration of Vogt-Koyanagi-Harada syndrome by infrared choroidal angiography with indocyanine green. Eur J Ophthalmol. 1997;7(2):163–70.
35. Bouchenaki N, Herbort CP. Indocyanine green angiography guided management of vogt-koyanagi-harada disease. J Ophthalmic Vis Res. 2011;6(4):241–8.
36. Bouchenaki N, Morisod L, Herbort CP. Vogt-Koyanagi-Harada syndrome: importance of rapid diagnosis and therapeutic intervention. Klin Monatsbl Augenheilkd. 2000;216(5):290–4.
37. Takemoto Y, Namba K, Mizuuchi K, Iwata D, Uno T, Ohno S, Hirooka K, Hashimoto Y, Saito W, Sugiyama K, Ishida S. Choroidal circulation impairment during the anterior recurrence of Vogt-Koyanagi-Harada disease confirmed with indocyanine green angiography and laser speckle flowgraphy. Acta Ophthalmol. 2016;94(7):e629–36.
38. Kawaguchi T, Horie S, Bouchenaki N, Ohno-Matsui K, Mochizuki M, Herbort CP. Suboptimal therapy controls clinically apparent disease but not subclinical progression of Vogt-Koyanagi-Harada disease. Int Ophthalmol. 2010;30(1):41–50.
39. Koizumi H, Maruyama K, Kinoshita S. Blue light and near-infrared fundus autofluorescence in acute Vogt-Koyanagi-Harada disease. Br J Ophthalmol. 2010;94(11):1499–505.
40. Ayata A, Dogru S, Senol MG, Unal M, Ersanli D, Bilge AH. Autofluorescence findings in Vogt-Koyanagi-Harada disease. Eur J Ophthalmol. 2009;19(6):1094–7.
41. Heussen FM, Vasconcelos-Santos DV, Pappuru RR, Walsh AC, Rao NA, Sadda SR. Ultra-wide-field green-light (532-nm) autofluorescence imaging in chronic Vogt-Koyanagi-Harada disease. Ophthalmic Surg Lasers Imaging. 2011;42(4):272–7.
42. da Silva FT, Hirata CE, Olivalves E, Oyamada MK, Yamamoto JH. Fundus-based and electro-retinographic strategies for stratification of late-stage Vogt-Koyanagi-Harada disease patients. Am J Ophthalmol. 2009;148(6):939–45. e3.
43. Yang P, Fang W, Wang L, Wen F, Wu W, Kijlstra A. Study of macular function by multifocal electroretinography in patients with Vogt-Koyanagi-Harada syndrome. Am J Ophthalmol. 2008;146(5):767–71.
44. Sugiura S. Vogt-Koyanagi-Harada disease. Jpn J Ophthalmol. 1978;22:9–35.
45. Read RW, Holland GN, Rao NA, Tabbara KF, Ohno S, Arellanes-Garcia L, et al. Revised diagnostic criteria for Vogt-Koyanagi-Harada disease: report of an international committee on nomenclature. Am J Ophthalmol. 2001;131:647–52.
46. Kitamura M, Takami K, Kitaichi N, Namba K, Kitamei H, Kotake S, Ohno S. Comparative study of two sets of criteria for the diagnosis of Vogt-Koyanagi-Harada's disease. Am J Ophthalmol. 2005;139(6):1080–5.
47. Tsai JH, Sukavatcharin S, Rao NA. Utility of lumbar puncture in diagnosis of Vogt-Koyanagi-Harada disease. Int Ophthalmol. 2007;27(2–3):189–94.
48. Kim LA, Khurana RN, Parikh JG, Rao NA. Melanin-laden macrophages in the CSF to diagnose Vogt-Koyanagi-Harada simulating ocular syphilis. Ocul Immunol Inflamm. 2008;16(1):59–61.
49. Forster DJ, Cano MR, Green RL, Rao NA. Echographic features of the Vogt-Koyanagi-Harada syndrome. Arch Ophthalmol. 1990;108(10):1421–6.
50. Yang P, Liu X, Zhou H, Guo W, Zhou C, Kijlstra A. Vogt-Koyanagi-Harada disease presenting as acute angle closure glaucoma at onset. Clin Exp Ophthalmol. 2011;39(7):639–47.
51. Aggarwal K, Agarwal A, Mahajan S, Invernizzi A, Mandadi SK, Singh R, Bansal R, Dogra MR, Gupta V, OCTA Study Group. The role of optical coherence tomography angiography in the diagnosis and management of acute Vogt-Koyanagi-Harada disease. Ocul Immunol Inflamm. 2016;20:1–12.
52. Aggarwal K, Agarwal A, Deokar A, Mahajan S, Singh R, Bansal R, Sharma A, Dogra MR, Gupta V, OCTA Study Group. Distinguishing features of acute Vogt-Koyanagi-Harada disease and acute central serous chorioretinopathy on optical coherence tomography angiography and en face optical coherence tomography imaging. J Ophthalmic Inflamm Infect. 2017;7(1):3.
53. Gupta V, Gupta A, Dogra MR, Singh I. Reversible retinal changes in the acute stage of sympathetic ophthalmia seen on spectral domain optical coherence tomography. Int Ophthalmol. 2011;31(2):105–10.

54. Iida T, Yannuzzi LA, Spaide RF, Borodoker N, Carvalho CA, Negrao S. Cystoid macular degeneration in chronic central serous chorioretinopathy. Retina. 2003;23(1):1–7. quiz 137-8.
55. Behdad B, Rahmani S, Montahaei T, Soheilian R, Soheilian M. Enhanced depth imaging OCT (EDI-OCT) findings in acute phase of sympathetic ophthalmia. Int Ophthalmol. 2015;35(3):433–9.
56. Muakkassa NW, Witkin AJ. Spectral-domain optical coherence tomography of sympathetic ophthalmia with Dalen-Fuchs nodules. Ophthalmic Surg Lasers Imaging Retina. 2014;45(6):610–2.
57. Tah V, Zarranz-Ventura J, Sim DA, Keane PA, Egan CA, Patel PJ, Lee RW, Tufail A, Pavesio CE, Westcott MC. Characterization of choroidal structure in sympathetic ophthalmia using optical coherence tomography. Invest Ophthalmol Vis Sci. 2012;53(14):1156.
58. Damico FM, Kiss S, Young LH. Sympathetic ophthalmia. Semin Ophthalmol. 2005;20(3):191–7.
59. Chan RV, Seiff BD, Lincoff HA, Coleman DJ. Rapid recovery of sympathetic ophthalmia with treatment augmented by intravitreal steroids. Retina. 2006;26(2):243–7.
60. Sharp DC, Bell RA, Patterson E, Pinkerton RM. Sympathetic ophthalmia. Histopathologic and fluorescein angiographic correlation. Arch Ophthalmol. 1984;102(2):232–5.
61. Gupta V, Gupta A, Dogra MR. Posterior sympathetic ophthalmia: a single centre long-term study of 40 patients from North India. Eye (Lond). 2008;22(12):1459–64.
62. Wang RC, Zamir E, Dugel PU, Sipperley JO, Thirkill CE, Shabatian B, Rao NA. Progressive subretinal fibrosis and blindness associated with multifocal granulomatous chorioretinitis: a variant of sympathetic ophthalmia. Ophthalmology. 2002;109(8):1527–31.
63. Bernasconi O, Auer C, Zografos L, Herbort CP. Indocyanine green angiographic findings in sympathetic ophthalmia. Graefes Arch Clin Exp Ophthalmol. 1998;236(8):635–8.
64. Saatci AO, Paşa E, Söylev MF, Koçak N, Durak I, Kaynak S. Sympathetic ophthalmia and indocyanine green angiography. Arch Ophthalmol. 2004;122(10):1568–9.
65. Casella AM, Farah ME, Martins MC, Hasegawa A, Oguido AP. Sympathetic ophthalmia – histopathological correlation with fluorescein and indocyanine green angiography: case report. Arq Bras Oftalmol. 2008;71(6):886–9.
66. Moshfeghi AA, Harrison SA, Ferrone PJ. Indocyanine green angiography findings in sympathetic ophthalmia. Ophthalmic Surg Lasers Imaging. 2005;36(2):163–6.
67. Fleischman D, Say EA, Wright JD, Landers MB. Multimodality diagnostic imaging in a case of sympathetic ophthalmia. Ocul Immunol Inflamm. 2012;20(4):300–2.

Multifocal Choroiditis/Serpiginous Choroiditis and Related Entities

Hossein Nazari Khanamiri and Narsing A. Rao

Introduction

Multifocal choroiditis (MFC), acute posterior multifocal placoid pigment epitheliopathy (APMPPE), Punctate Inner Choroidopathy (PIC), multiple evanescent white dot syndrome (MEWDS), serpiginous choroiditis (SC), multifocal serpiginoid choroiditis (MSC), birdshot retinochoroidopathy (BRC), and acute zonal occult outer retinopathy (AZOOR) are rare intraocular inflammatory disorders which are grouped under a clinical term of "white dot syndromes." These syndromes manifest variably with repeated bouts of multifocal retinal and choroidal inflammation and a primary pathologic process that occurs at or near the choroid, the retinal pigment epithelium (RPE), and the outer retina. Their etiology is generally not known, but it is suggested to be either a vasculitic occlusion of the choriocapillaris with secondary ischemia or infarction of the overlying RPE and photoreceptors or an immunologic response directed at the RPE with secondary damage to adjacent choriocapillaris and outer retina. The immunologic trigger for such immune activations is generally unknown.

The lack of knowledge about the pathogenesis is reflected in the descriptive names of these entities. Despite overlapping clinical features, the unique pattern of chorioretinitis initiation and propagation, association with systemic or local inflammations/infections, genetic predisposition, response to specific treatment modalities, and long-term course of the disease help to subclassify white dot syndromes to unique clinical entities as MFC, APMPPE, PIC, MEWDS, SC, MSC, BRC, and

H. Nazari Khanamiri
University of Texas Medical Branch, Department of Ophthalmology and Visual Sciences, Galveston, TX, USA

N. A. Rao (✉)
Ophthalmology, USC Roski Eye Institute Ophthalmology, Los Angeles, CA, USA
e-mail: narsing.rao@med.usc.edu

N. A. Rao et al. (eds.), *Posterior Uveitis*, Essentials in Ophthalmology,
https://doi.org/10.1007/978-3-030-03140-4_4

AZOOR. In this chapter, we will focus on more common clinical conditions with multifocal inflammatory lesions. Differentiation of these uveitis conditions is vital for preservation of vision as treatment approaches often vary drastically among them. A summary of clinical and imaging manifestations will be discussed (Tables 1 and 2).

Multifocal Choroiditis and Pan Uveitis

Clinical features and differential diagnosis. Multifocal choroiditis (MFC) is a bilateral, chronic, recurrent posterior uveitis characterized by discrete round chorioretinitis lesions at and around the macula in the absence of identifiable infectious (tuberculosis, syphilis, histoplasma capsulatum infection) or systemic inflammatory (sarcoidosis) condition. Patients are predominantly female and young who usually present with decreased vision and photopsia in one or both eyes. The clinical hallmark of MFC includes a variable number of 200–1000 μm, yellow-white chorioretinal inflammation spots distributed in the posterior pole and the equatorial area, sometimes in a linear arrangement (Fig. 1) [1]. They usually appear in different stages of development and, when detected in the active stage, are usually at the level of RPE and surrounded by swelling of overlying retina. Healed lesions are surrounded by variable pigmentation or subretinal fibrosis and appear atrophic or punched out. Anterior chamber and vitreous inflammation varies from mild to severe [2, 3]. Choroidal neovascularization arising from the lesions or optic nerve head occurs in about one third of the eyes and may be the presenting feature of the disease [4]. Permanent visual loss may develop if focal chorioretinitis lesions or secondary CNV involve the fovea (Fig. 2). Anecdotal reports indicated association with Epstein-Bar virus and sarcoidosis, but the underlying etiology remains elusive.

Episodes of active chorioretinitis lesions may resolve spontaneously or following the administration of immunosuppressive agents [4]. General rules for the use of systemic immunosuppressive regimen in uveitis applies for the use of such medications in MFC: inflammation activity, frequency and distribution of the new lesions, and development of complications such as CNV direct systemic immunosuppressive regimen.

Diagnosis. The diagnosis of MFC is based on the clinical presentation pattern and the distribution and the extent of the lesions. Imaging modalities define and document the extent of the disease and its complications such as foveal involvement and CNV. Laboratory tests to rule out infectious and systemic inflammatory causes of choroiditis should be requested. Clinical spectrum and respective prognosis may vary from patients with minimal vitreous inflammatory reaction and small punched out lesions (punctate inner choroidopathy – PIC) to patients with severe intraocular inflammation (multifocal choroiditis and panuveitis syndrome – MFCPU).

Imaging modalities. Color fundus photography is the traditional way to document the healed scars and active new lesions. Widefield imaging modalities are now more often utilized (Fig. 3). New active lesions appear as a grayish-yellow

Table 1 Imaging features of white dot syndromes in *acute phase*

	Fluorescein angiography	Indocyanine green angiography	Optical coherence tomography	Fundus autofluorescence	OCTA
MFC	Early hypofluorescence Late hyperfluorescence	Early hypocyanescence Late hypercyanescence	Ellipsoid zone disruption Subretinal infiltrate Sub-RPE deposits	Hyperautofluorescent lesions	Loss of homogeneity of the choriocapillaris network
SC	Early hypofluorescence Late speckled hyperfluorescence Lesions adjacent to old scars Disc hyperfluorescence	Hypocyanescence	Outer retina disruption Subretinal fluid and infiltrates Sub-RPE deposits	Hyperautofluorescent lesions at the margin of old scars	Choriocapillaris hypoperfusion patches
APMPPE	Early hypofluorescence with late staining	Early and late hypocyanescence	Outer retina hyperreflectivity and irregularities Ellipsoid zone disruptions	Iso- or hypoautofluorescent lesions	Choriocapillaris hypoperfusion corresponding to lesions
MEWDS	Early punctate hyperfluorescent lesions in a wreath-like pattern that stain in late phases Disc hyperfluorescence	Early and late hypocyanescence	Focal discontinuities of the ellipsoid zone and the deposition of refractile material between RPE and outer retina	Hyperautofluorescent dots	Patchy loss of the choriocapillary plexus
BRC	Disc hyperemia Early hypofluorescent lesions Subtle late staining Peripheral vasculitis Cystoid macular edema	Early and late hypocyanescence	Retina and choroid were thinner Increased choroidal reflectivity of acute lesions	Hyperautofluorescent spots	Decreased retinal vascular density and altered vascular architecture in superficial and deep retinal capillary layers

Table 2 Imaging features of white dot syndromes in *chronic/inactive phase*

	Fluorescein angiography	Indocyanine green angiography	Optical coherence tomography	Fundus autofluorescence	OCTA
MFC	Window defect and blockage corresponding to pigmentary changes Late staining of the margins of healed lesions	Hypocyanescent lesions	Decreased and nonhomogeneous reflectivity of outer retina Localized outer retinal atrophy Reconstruction of outer retina in well-treated lesions	Hypoautofluorescent lesions	Choriocapillaris network usually returns to normal with treatment OCTA may help with diagnosis of CNV
SC	Well-defined patch of hypofluorescence	Choroidal atrophy and hypocyanescence	Outer retinal disruption and atrophy in untreated lesions Pigment migration into retina Partial reconstruction of outer retina in well-treated lesions	Granular iso-/hypoautofluorescence	Choriocapillaris atrophy
APMPPE	Hyperfluorescence (window defect from RPE atrophy)	Hypocyanescence	Outer retina elevations flatten and hyperreflectivity gradually resolves Partial reconstitution of outer retina RPE often remains irregular	Slight hyper- and hypoautofluorescence corresponding to healed lesions	Reconstitution of choriocapillaris flow
BRC	Arterial narrowing	Early and late hypocyanescence	Outer retinal thinning and loss of normal architecture Outer retinal hyperreflective foci Focal hyperreflective foci, thinning or absence of Sattler's layer, and generalized thinning in the choroid	Macular and peripapillary confluent hypoautofluorescence	Possibly decrease choriocapillaris vascularity in old lesion areas

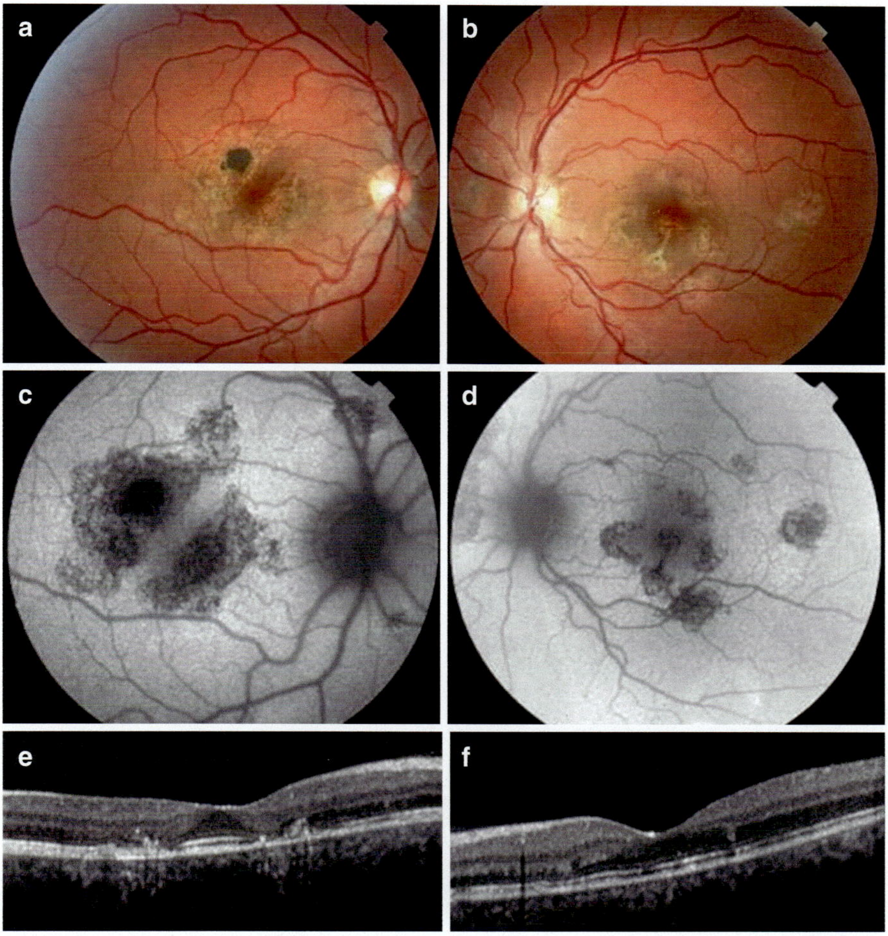

Fig. 1 Idiopathic multifocal choroiditis (MFC) in a middle-aged white woman. Right and left eye color photographs (**a** and **b**) and corresponding fundus autofluorescence images (**c** and **d**) demonstrate multiple, round, atrophic lesions associated with pigment alterations in the posterior pole. Unlike serpiginous choroiditis, lesions do not originate from peripapillary area. The size and distribution of the lesions further indicate MFC. Spectral domain-optical coherence tomography scans (**e** and **f**) show outer retinal destruction and pigment migration to the outer retina corresponding to healed chorioretinal lesions. (Part of the figure reproduced with permission from Nazari Khanamiri [6])

swollen retinal spot with or without surrounding edema and subretinal fluid. In fluorescein angiography (FA), active lesions are highlighted with their early hypofluorescence and late hyperfluorescence. The healed lesions, depending on the amount of atrophy or hyperpigmentation, is typically seen as window defects, blockage from pigment clumps, and late marginal staining. Examining FA images may be necessary for the diagnosis of CNV where leakage is noted.

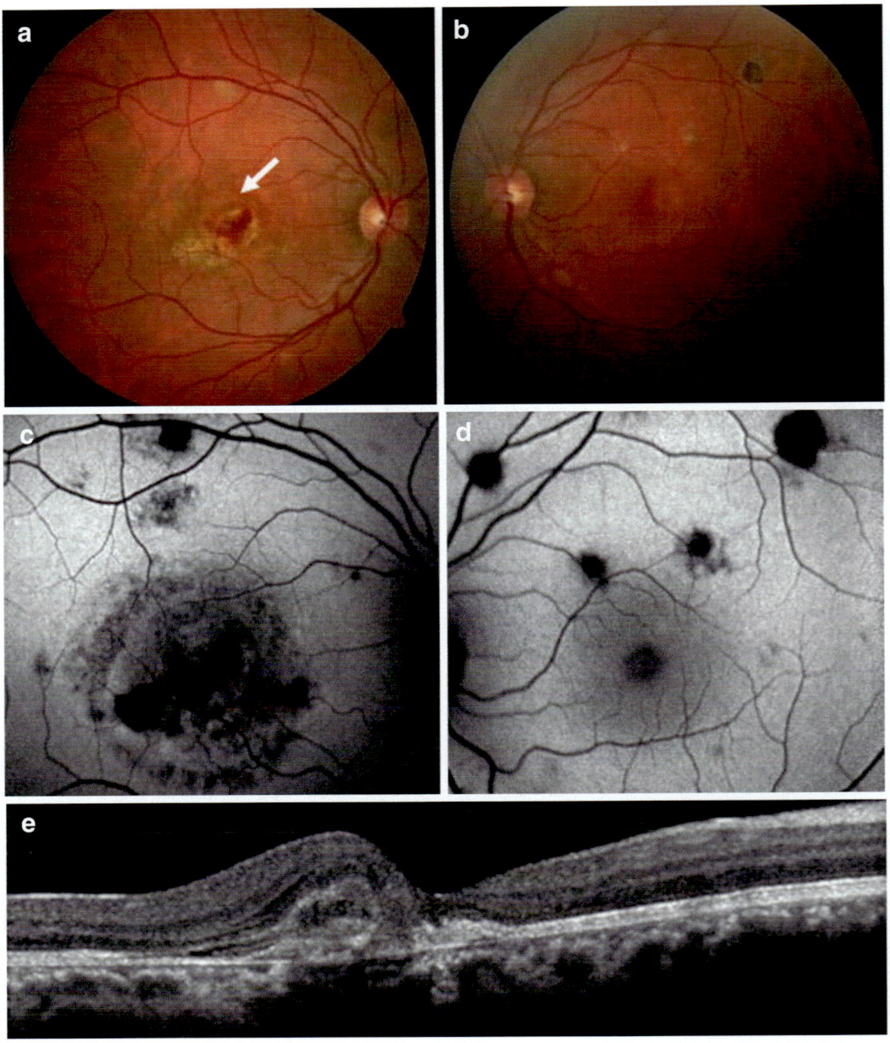

Fig. 2 A 41-year-old male with idiopathic multifocal choroiditis (MFC) presented with an acute decrease in vision due to the development of subfoveal choroidal neovascular membrane (CNV). The patient was previously treated for wet age-related macular degeneration. Multifocal nature of the lesions is more easily seen in fundus autofluorescence (FAF-**c** and **d**) compared to color fundus photography (**a** and **b**). Subretinal blood (white arrow) indicates the development of CNV, and optical coherence tomography scan (**e**) revealed subfoveal hyperreflective material along with a small amount of subretinal fluid

Similarly, indocyanine green angiography (ICGA) identifies active lesions with initial hypocyanescence and late hypercyanescence. In addition, ICGA may reveal hypocyanescent patches of subclinical lesions that are not visible by retinal fundus examination or FA.

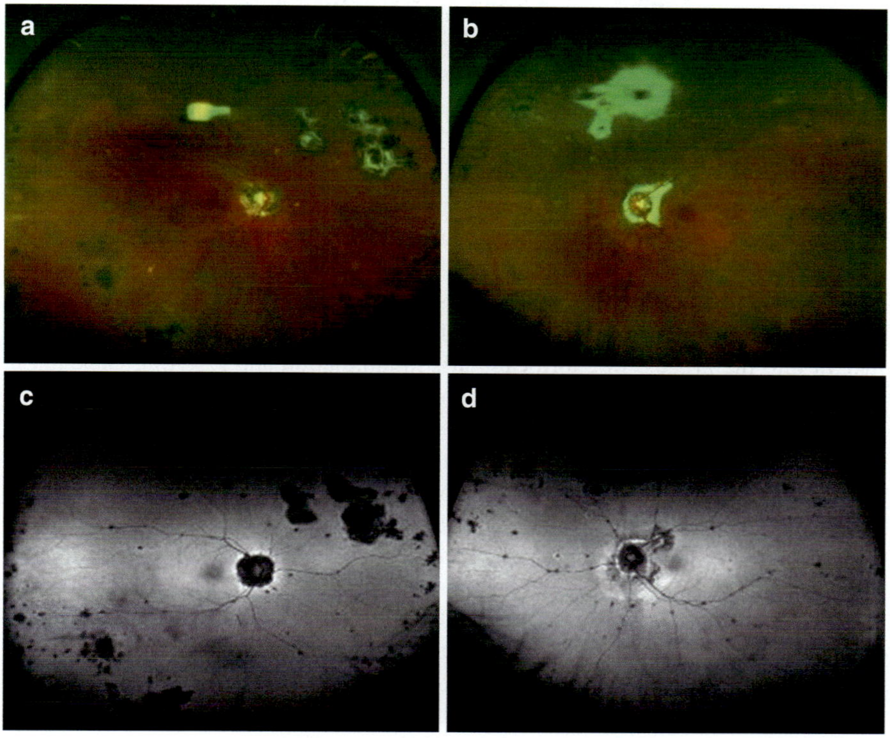

Fig. 3 Widefield pseudocolor fundus photography (**a** and **b**) and widefield fundus autofluorescence imaging (**c** and **d**) of idiopathic multifocal choroiditis (MFC). Fundus autofluorescence more readily identifies the extent of atrophic lesion compared to fundus photography

In optical coherence tomography (OCT), active lesions are identified as retinal ellipsoid zone disruption, subretinal infiltrations, sub-RPE elevations, dehiscence of the RPE, increased transmission of the OCT signal beyond the RPE band, and choriocapillaris hyporeflectivity (better seen in enhanced depth-OCT – see below) [5]. It is noted that retinal hyperreflectivity is full thickness in MFC and partial thickness in SC, but this is likely related to the severity and depth of inflammation in relation to outer retinal layers. More severe inflammation closer to the RPE may cause full-thickness retinal hyperreflectivity, and less severe inflammation may be only associated with outer retinal disturbances (Figs. 1 and 2) [6]. OCT is frequently used to monitor the evolution of active lesions as they heal and for the detection of complications such as CNV. As active lesions heal, the reflectivity of overlying retinal inflammation decreases and becomes less homogeneous. Depending on the severity of initial inflammation and the sufficiency of anti-inflammatory treatment, outer retinal hyperreflectivity of active lesions may turn to (1) localized outer retinal atrophy and loss of ellipsoid zone or (2) reconstitution of normal outer retina.

The development of CNV is often corroborated by studying OCT, FA, and fundus autofluorescence (FAF) (multimodal imaging). Typically, secondary CNV is identified with early hyperfluorescence and late leakage in FA along with intra- or subretinal fluid adjacent to the lesion in OCT scans. In OCT scans, sub-RPE or subretinal hyperreflectivity may represent CNV.

Enhanced depth-optical coherence tomography (EDI-OCT) allows detailed visualization of choroidal morphology. EDI-OCT may not only increase the clinician's insight into the process of uveitis involving the choroid, but it could also provide supportive information about the activity of the disease and guide the treatment and follow-up plan [7]. Choroidal vascular layer thickness and morphology including choriocapillaris structure and reflectivity, as seen in EDI-OCT, has been used as a proxy marker for blood flow and thus severity and/or activity of the choroidal inflammation. Correlation of EDI-OCT findings with ICGA has given a broader insight into the process of choriocapillaris inflammation and resulting ischemia in MFC and serpiginous choroiditis [7]. Choriocapillaris hypoperfusion seen in ICGA manifests as a thickened and hyporeflective choriocapillaris layer in EDI-OCT [7]. This may be accompanied by hyperreflectivity of the overlying retina depending on the severity of the hypoperfusion. Invernizzi et al. presented cases where lesions with overlying outer retina reflectivity resulted in outer retina atrophy but those without signs of inflammation of overlying retina recovered with no retina sequela in OCT [7]. The healing of active lesions with leaving an atrophic scar results on reconstitution of isoreflective choriocapillaris in EDI-OCT, but ICGA hypocyanescence remains. However, in the lesions that heal with no scar (restitutio ad integrum), choriocapillaris flow (as seen in ICGA) returns to normal [7].

Fundus autofluorescence is a noninvasive imaging system that is mainly used to show the integrity and function of the RPE layer. FAF signals originate mostly from lipofuscin molecules in RPE. Active lesions of MFC show hyperautofluorescence about 2–5 days after the clinical appearance of the lesions. The autofluorescence of the lesions decreases gradually as they progress to atrophic scars and become less active (Figs. 3 and 4). While FAF is helpful in delineating the lesions, the diagnostic and prognostic utility of this information is not clear [8]. Patients with MFC may demonstrate an enlarged blind spot in visual field testing. Electroretinography (ERG) and electrooculography (EOG) signals are usually normal indicating the localized nature of multifocal choroiditis lesions. Quantification of retinal sensitivity and fixation pattern by microperimetry may offer new data about the impact of the disease on visual function [9].

Optical coherence tomography angiography (OCTA) is an evolving noninvasive imaging tool that allows visualization of the retinal and choroidal microvasculature. OCTA delineates vascular blood flow without any dye injection based on split-spectrum amplitude-decorrelation angiography and/or "en face" OCT-derived techniques. Multiple recent publications have shown OCTA findings of chorioretinal inflammatory disease in correlation with other imaging modalities in the diagnosis and monitoring of active inflammatory lesions and their complications such as CNV. Being a noninvasive and dyeless rapid image acquisition method is the major advantage of OCTA compared to conventional angiography methods. In addition, stratification of retinal and choroidal vascular network that allows better localization of the plane of the lesion is possible with OCTA. Active

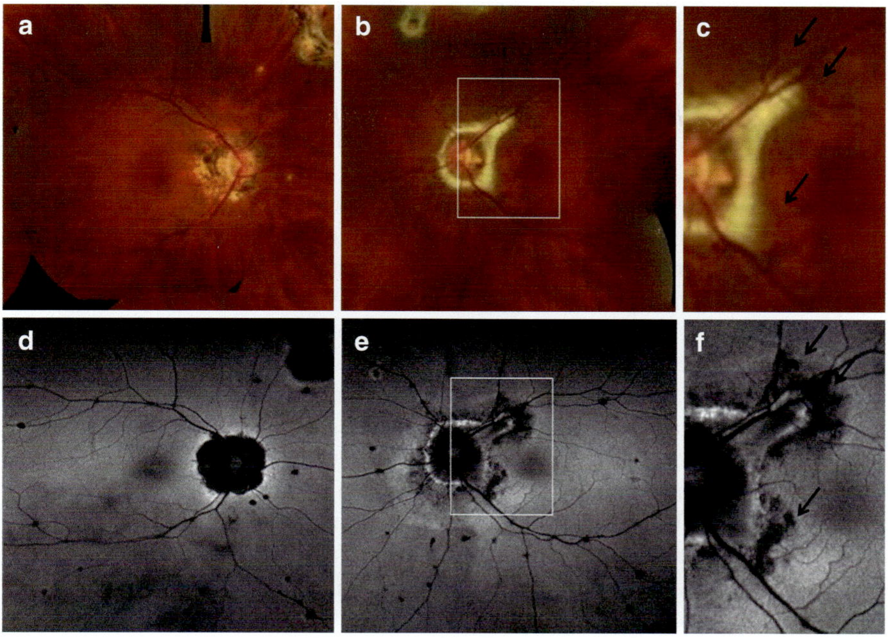

Fig. 4 Montage color fundus photography (**a** and **b**) and widefield fundus autofluorescence imaging (**d** and **e**) of the same patient with idiopathic multifocal choroiditis (MFC) shown in Fig. 3. **c** and **f** denotes magnified view of the area marked in **b** and **d** showing areas of RPE damage (black arrow)

MFC lesions show loss of homogeneity of the choriocapillaris network in OCTA. The loss of the choriocapillaris network returns to normal with appropriate treatment in about 4 weeks. Zahid et al. showed that 83% of the lesions in MFC contain CNV [5]. CNV was observed with higher frequency in subretinal lesions compared to sub-RPE lesions [5]. A limitation of current OCTA imaging systems is their inability to show the leakage. Thus, it is generally difficult to identify active leaking CNV lesions solely based on OCTA. Other limitations of the available OCTA devices include projection artifacts, poor signal strength, motion artifacts, segmentation errors, and flow masked by overlying material reducing signal penetration.

Serpiginous Choroiditis

Clinical features and differential diagnosis. Serpiginous choroiditis (SC) is a posterior uveitis characterized by a geographic pattern of choroiditis extending from the peripapillary area and spreading intermittently to the periphery [6]. SC usually involves both eyes of otherwise healthy, middle-aged individuals. There is no familial or ethnic predilection, though women are involved slightly more frequently. The disease may cause severe and permanent visual loss if inflammatory lesions involve the fovea [6].

Pathogenesis of SC is unclear, but based on limited histopathologic studies showing inflammatory infiltrate in the choroid, favorable response to immunosuppressive treatment, and the absence of association with systemic or local infectious or noninfectious diseases, an autoimmune inflammation directed at the RPE or choroidal vessels or both is the likely primary event. The underlying specific trigger for this inflammatory process is unknown [6]. On the other hand, patients with a history of exposure to tuberculosis may present with fundus lesions simulating SC. The condition often referred as tuberculosis-associated multifocal serpiginoid choroiditis (TB-MSC) shows evidence of previous exposure to tuberculosis and/or the presence of mycobacterial DNA in the aqueous humor. Other infectious agents such as HSV, VZV, and syphilis may cause similar multifocal serpiginoid choroiditis (MSC) lesions. Chorioretinal lesions of MSC are more likely to be multifocal and originate or extend to the retinal periphery [6]. The distinction between SC and MSC is crucial as the treatment for the latter should include specific antimicrobial agents in addition to immunosuppressive treatment. As clinical features are often inconclusive and tissue diagnosis is not practical, identification of the pattern of retinal and choroidal involvement as seen by multimodal imaging studies along with specific laboratory tests to rule out infectious etiologies play a crucial role in the differentiation of SC and MSC. In addition, diagnostic and imaging modalities often help with early detection of the reactivation of inflammation and the development of complications such as CNV.

Diagnosis. Laboratory tests are often requested to differentiate SC from mimicking MSC lesions in patients with a possibility of exposure to mycobacterium tuberculosis, HSV, VZV, and syphilis. Clinical and multimodal imaging patterns of chorioretinal lesions are indispensable for the differentiation and follow-up. SC may manifest with irregular serpentine or helicoid choroiditis, typically starting at the juxtapapillary area, grayish yellow discoloration of the retina, minimal vitreous inflammatory cells, and recurrences of the lesions at the margins of the healed scars (Fig. 5). Retina and RPE outside the areas of active or healed lesions appear normal, and examination of the other eye may show similar atrophic lesions. The intermittently advancing choroiditis can usually be stopped with aggressive anti-inflammatory treatment with corticosteroids and immunomodulatory agents.

FA delineates early hypofluorescence and late speckled hyperfluorescence of the active lesions that often develop at the borders of previously scarred areas. These atrophic inactive lesions show a well-defined patch of hypofluorescence caused by a combination of loss of retinal and choroidal vasculature and blockage from hyperpigmentation. Choroidal nonperfusion seen in ICGA indicates active or subclinical lesions that may be more extensive than clinically visible retinal lesions. As the choriocapillaris layer is the presumed site of inflammation, ICGA or OCTA may be the preferred imaging modality for following and monitoring the patients with SC [10, 11]. In ICGA and OCTA, choroidal nonperfusion of active lesions, seen as dark patches bordering atrophic areas, is usually larger than the corresponding retinal lesions [11]. In addition, subclinical lesions of inflammatory choriocapillaropathies maybe detectable with ICGA or OCTA even when signs of active inflammation are absent [11, 12]. In a study of six eyes with SC, OCTA showed choroidal hypoperfusion in all eyes and helped to identify a CNV lesion that was not detected on FA

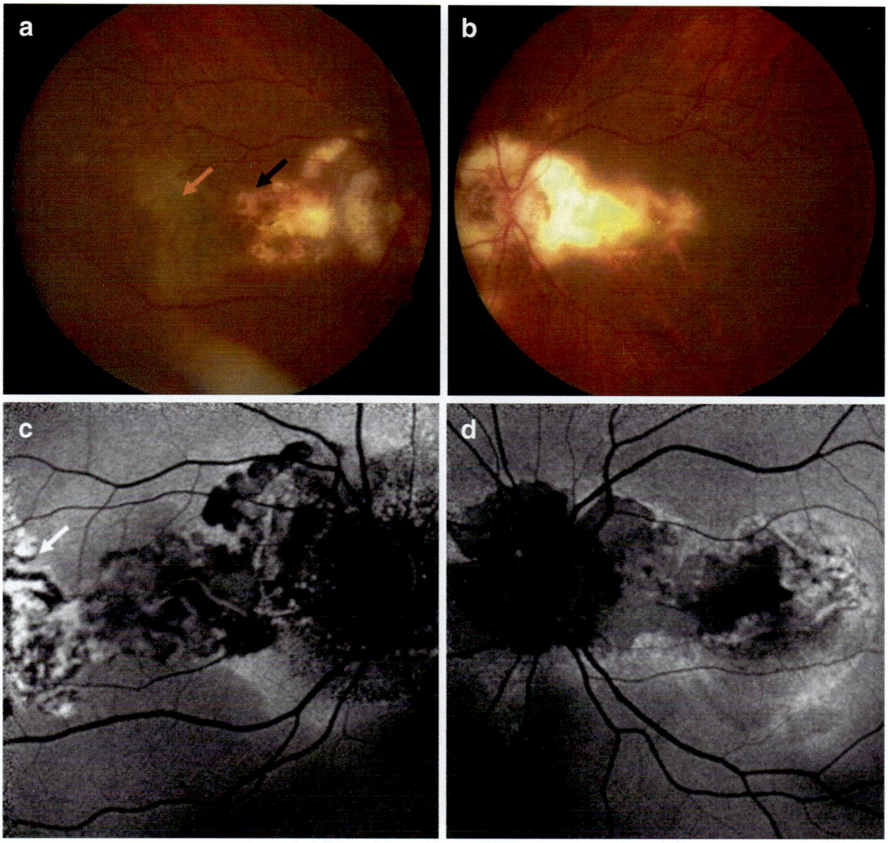

Fig. 5 Serpiginous choroiditis (SC). Note that the lesions originate from the peripapillary area and extend in a serpentine manner to macula and periphery (**a** and **b**). New activation (red arrow) starts at the margins of old scars (black arrow). Fundus autofluorescence (**c** and **d**) indicates the hyperautofluorescence of active lesions (white arrow) in contrast to hypoautofluorescence of the old scars

[13]. In another study of 18 eyes with TB-MSC, Mandadi et al. detected patches of choriocapillaris flow void suggestive of focal hypoperfusion, especially in the chronic phase [14]. The choriocapillaris hypoperfusion areas corresponded well with the hypocyanescent patches seen in ICGA. The authors suggested that the areas of choriocapillaris atrophy appeared better defined on OCTA compared with ICGA. Choriocapillaris atrophy as seen by OCTA correlated well with EDI-OCT (Fig. 6) [14].

FAF is an excellent tool for evaluation of disease burden and extent of lesion. Widefield FAF is particularly valuable for showing the peripheral lesions. Active lesions may demonstrate hyperautofluorescence which usually appear few days after the earliest ICGA indications of a new lesion. These hyperautofluorescent areas usually appear at the edge of old scars. Healed lesions usually have a granular iso-/hypoautofluorescence appearance (Fig. 5) [6].

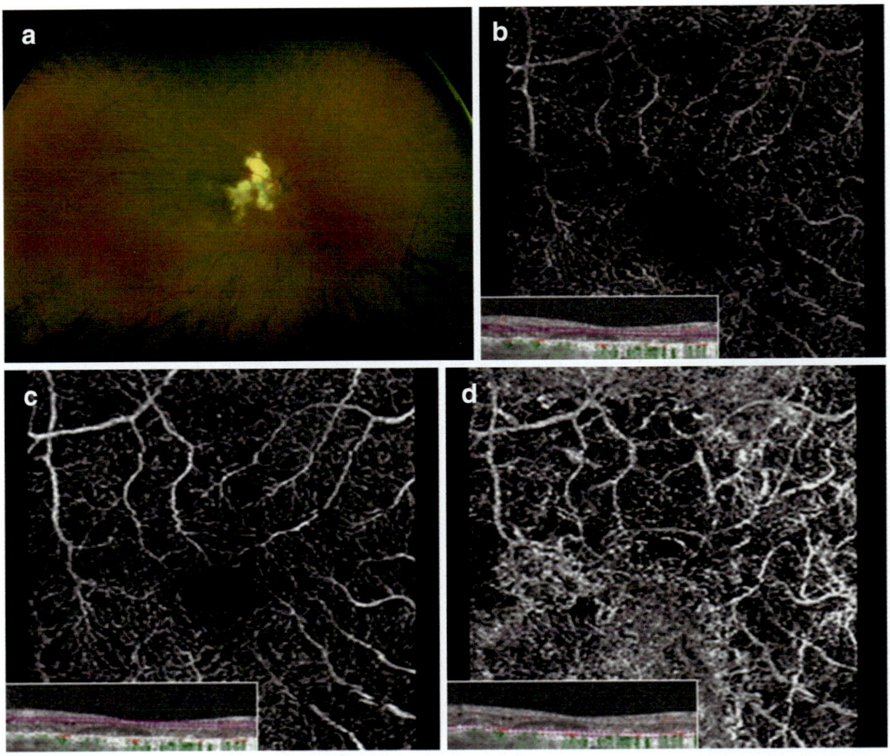

Fig. 6 Fundus photography (**a**) and optical coherence tomography angiography (OCTA-**b** to **d**) of a patient with tuberculosis-related multifocal serpiginoid choroiditis (TB-MSC). While superficial (**b**) and middle (**c**) retinal vascular plexus are mostly undisturbed, choriocapillaris slab (**d**) shows patchy areas of choriocapillaris hypoperfusion. (Images courtesy of Dr. Debarshi Mustafi)

Birdshot Retinochoroidopathy

Birdshot retinochoroidopathy is a chronic bilateral posterior uveitis with characteristic retinal hypopigmented lesions, ¼–½ disc diameter in size and clustered around the optic nerve, radiating toward the periphery. The lesions almost always involve inferior and nasal peripapillary area (Fig. 7). The disease has a strong association with HLA-A29 and is thought to be due to autoimmunity to retinal S antigen. Most patients experience a gradual decline in visual acuity due to cystoid macular edema and retinal atrophy. Treatment includes immunomodulatory therapy for chronic disease and oral or intravitreal corticosteroids for acute flare-ups.

Fluorescein angiography features of active disease include disc hyperemia and an initially hypofluorescent lesions with subtle late staining (Fig. 7). In addition, cystoid macular edema and vasculitis may indicate active disease. ICGA may reveal more fundus lesions with early and late hypocyanescence (Fig. 7). Electrophysiology studies (30 Hz flicker implicit time in particular) are valuable for evaluating the adequacy of immunomodulatory treatment.

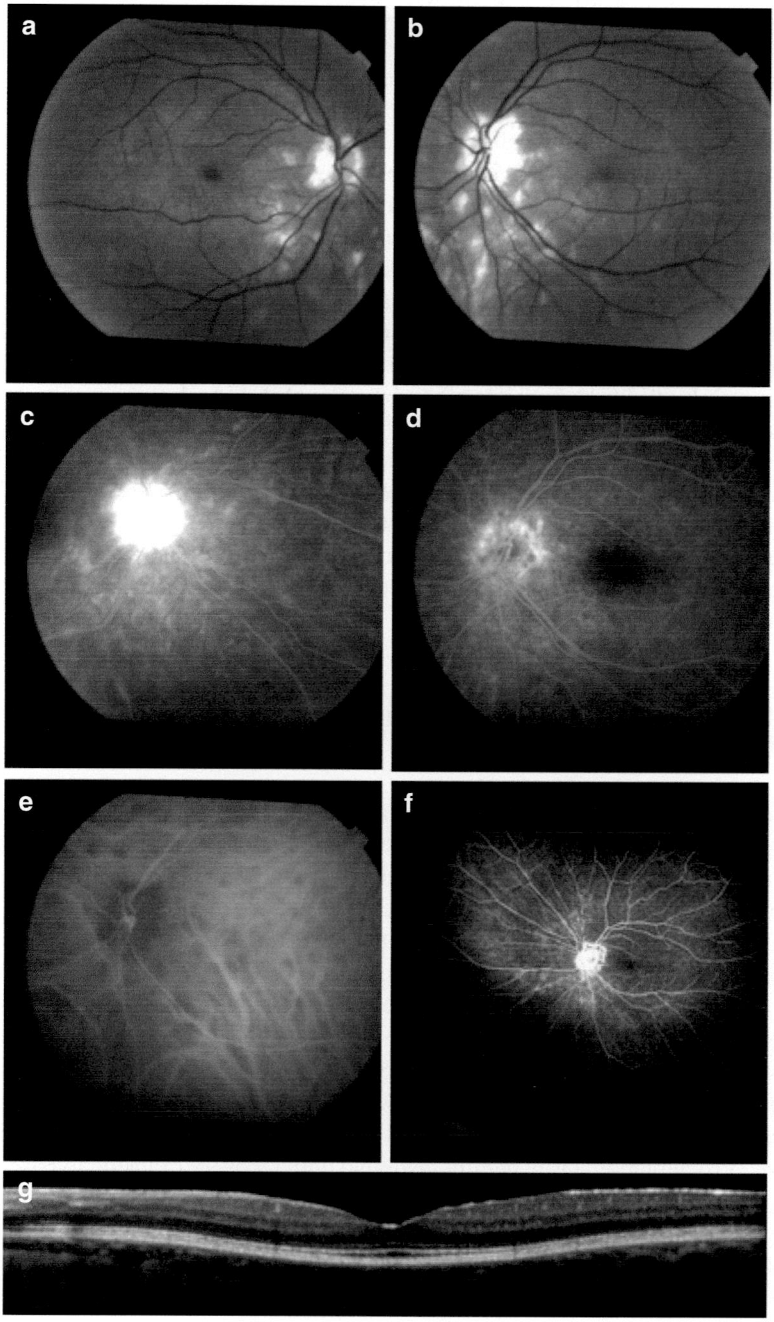

Fig. 7 Birdshot retinochoroidopathy (BRC) is characterized by multiple round oval lesions commonly seen at least in inferior and inferonasal retina (**a** and **b**). FA (**c** and **d**) may show disc hyperfluorescence and peripheral vasculitis. ICGA (**e**) may show hypocyanescent spots as an indicator of subclinical lesions not detected by clinical examination and other diagnostic modalities. Widefield imaging (**f**) is indispensable for evaluating peripheral vasculitis. OCT scan (**g**) did not show cystoid macular edema (that may indicate disease activity) in this patient

OCT may show retinal and choroidal thinning in individuals with active and inactive diseases. Active lesions in OCT present with thinning and loss of normal architecture of outer retina along with the presence of outer retinal hyperreflective foci [15]. Decreased choroidal reflectivity as seen in EDI-OCT may indicate disease activity in contrast to inactive disease that may show increased choroidal reflectivity [15]. In addition, focal hyperreflective foci, thinning or absence of Sattler's layer, and generalized thinning may be seen in the choroid.

FAF abnormalities are present in about 80% and macular FAF lesions are present in about 50% of the eyes with BRC suggesting FAF as a valuable tool for long-term structure/function correlation in patients with BRC [16]. In addition, the presence of macular confluent hypoautofluorescence is shown to be associated with lower vision [16]. However, the utility of FAF signal changes in identifying active inflammation, disease progression, or monitoring of patient responses to therapy has not been clearly shown [16, 17].

In an OCTA analysis of 64 eyes from 32 patients with BRC, capillary loops (58%), telangiectatic vessels (44%), increased intercapillary spaces (52%), altered vascular architecture (53%), and rarefication of C-scans (63%) were detected in retinal layers. It was also shown that decreased retinal vascular density and altered vascular architecture in superficial and deep capillary layers significantly correlated with disease activity [18].

Acute Posterior Multifocal Placoid Pigment Epitheliopathy (APMPPE)

Clinical features and differential diagnosis. Acute posterior multifocal placoid pigment epitheliopathy (APMPPE) is another rare inflammatory choriocapillaropathy with unknown etiology that manifests with photopsia, decreased vision, paracentral scotoma, or metamorphopsia in an otherwise healthy middle-aged person [19]. Frequently, a flu-like prodrome precedes the ocular presentation. No gender or ethnic predilection is reported. Typically, anterior segment inflammation is minimal, and retinal examination reveals multiple creamy or yellow-white subretinal plaque-like lesions with indistinct borders and ½–1 disc diameter in size [20]. The disease is usually self-limited, and visual recovery occurs in 4–8 weeks. Individual chorioretinal lesions fade in 1–2 weeks, and new lesions appear in a course of 3–4 weeks. Choroidal atrophy and RPE mottling and atrophy may be left in the wake of active lesions. Visual outcome is generally favorable with recovery of vision to baseline in most patients. In a small fraction of patients with foveal involvement or in the presence of complications such as CNV, visual loss may be permanent. Recurrences may be seen in almost half of the patients over time.

The retinochoroidal lesions of APMPPE are believed to be either (1) a focal inflammation at the level of the RPE associated with secondary inflammatory damage to overlying outer retina and occlusion of underlying choriocapillaris or (2) a vasculitis process primarily involving terminal choriocapillaris lobules causing interruption of choroidal perfusion that results in an ischemic-inflammatory damage to the overlying RPE and photoreceptors. The inciting source of these inflammatory processes is not known. Association with HLA-B7 and HLA-DR2 haplotypes in a fraction of patients supports an immune driven mechanism. In addition, infrequent associations with systemic vasculitis have been also reported [21, 22].

Clinical resolution can be observed in most cases without therapeutic intervention. However, in cases with severe ocular inflammation/subretinal exudation or in the presence of neurologic manifestations (such as headache or focal neurologic deficits), systemic corticosteroids with gradual taper are shown to be beneficial.

Diagnosis. Diagnosis of APMPPE is suggested with typical clinical presentation and is supported with imaging studies. The disease is frequently bilateral, and lesions are typically seen in various stages of evolution. Active inflammatory lesions resolve in weeks leaving circumscribed areas of RPE alterations. Early-phase hypofluorescence and late-phase staining lesions are typically seen in FA imaging of the acute lesions. Inactive lesions typically show hyperfluorescence resulting from window defect from RPE atrophy [23]. Active and healed lesions show hypocyanescence in ICGA likely from disturbed perfusion in an inflamed capillary bed [24].

OCT demonstrates outer retinal inflammation with dome-shaped disruptions of the ellipsoid zone and hyperreflectance of the overlying retinal layers [25, 26]. As the lesions heal, outer retina dome-shaped lesions flatten, and hyperreflectivity gradually resolves leaving outer retina thinning [25]. In a few months, outer retina partially reconstitutes the ellipsoid band, but RPE often remains irregular.

FAF imaging shows isoautofluorescence or hypoautofluorescence corresponding to acute lesions. Hypoautofluorescent areas may be due to the blocking effect of overlying retinal edema or direct RPE damage with decreased lipofuscin production. After resolution, lesions show irregular increased autofluorescence likely due to lipofuscin accumulation in the RPE and photoreceptor outer segments.

OCTA is a dyeless imaging tool to help to understand the pathophysiology of the disease and monitor retinochoroidal inflammation and response to treatment. Observing the evolution of lesions from acute to subacute and to healed stages with OCTA shows choriocapillaris and deep choroidal hypoperfusion in acute lesions [13, 27] and choroidal reperfusion in subacute and healed stages of the lesions [13, 27–29]. Heiferman et al. showed that the choroidal perfusion in healed lesions shows distinct small vascular channels with intervening no-flow zones, which appeared differently compared with surrounding unaffected zones of the choriocapillaris [27]. The preservation of medium-sized choroidal vessels in the choriocapillaris layer may explain recovery of vision in APMPPE [27]. In addition, choroidal hypoperfusion patches outside the clinically apparent chorioretinitis lesions are reported in APMPPE and BCR [27, 30]. This is unlike more limited choroidal hypoperfusion patterns seen only at the clinically evident lesions in MEWDS and POHS [30] and may indicate a more widespread inflammation in APMPPE and BCR. Superficial and deep retinal capillary networks are less defined with OCTA, but retinal vascular density and diameter are shown to decrease in uveitic eyes compared to normal control retinas [31].

Adaptive optics scanning laser ophthalmoscopy (AOSLO) imaging systems correct for higher-order aberrations of the cornea and lens and improve the image resolution of the retina up to 2–3 μm enabling visualization of individual cone photoreceptors [32]. Roberts et al. studied the photoreceptor layer with AOSLO and SD-OCT in patients with APMPPE. AOSLO showed hyporeflectivities and loss of photoreceptor in subacute lesions. These hyporeflectivities corresponded to outer retinal irregularities seen in SD-OCT. Follow-up exams showed partial recovery of these hyporeflectivities along with the recovery of outer retinal layers in SD-OCT. In inactive lesions, diffuse hyper- and hyporeflective areas seen on AOSLO corresponded to hyper- and hypopigmented areas observed clinically. In areas of pigmented scarring, AOSLO showed loss of visible photoreceptors [32].

Multiple Evanescent White Dot Syndrome (MEWDS)

Clinical features and differential diagnosis. MEWDS is a white dot syndrome that often involves one eye in healthy female aged 15–50. Patients usually present with a prodrome of photopsia, dyschromatopsia, and temporal or paracentral scotoma before an acute painless drop in vision. The disease is typically self-limited, and complete visual recovery with no recurrence is a rule. Anterior segment inflammation is mild if present, and fundus examination shows 25–50 flat, gray-white lesions (100–200 micrometers - smaller than the lesions of APMPPE) at the level of outer retina and RPE in the posterior pole. The fovea typically appears granular, but the chorioretinal lesions do not usually involve the foveal center. Optic disc edema, mild posterior vitreous cells, retinal venous sheathing, and superficial retinal hemorrhages may be seen in some patients. Some patients may have a relative afferent pupillary defect and an enlarged blind spot. The pathogenesis of MEWDS is unknown. Infectious activation of the immune system may be the mechanism given that about one third of the patients report a viral prodrome. Hormonal status may contribute to the disease given female predominance.

MEWDS lesions resolve in 3–10 months, and patients recover their baseline visual acuity. Therefore, no treatment is recommended for patients with MEWDS. Retinal lesions usually resolve without visible scar. Scotoma and enlarged blind spot may persist longer and may not resolve in some patients. Recurrences rarely occur. A small proportion of patients may develop choroidal neovascularization that needs treatment with intravitreal anti-vascular endothelial growth factor agents.

Diagnosis. Typical clinical presentation and imaging features of the retinal lesions support the diagnosis (Fig. 8). FA reveals early punctate hyperfluorescent lesions in a wreath-like pattern that stain in late phases. This is in differentiation to slightly larger lesions of APMPPE where early hypofluorescence is followed by late hyperfluorescence. Optic nerve head and retinal vascular staining maybe seen in some patients with MEWDS. Early and late hypocyanescence characterize acute lesions in ICGA [33]. These hypocyanescent spots may outnumber the clinical lesions.

Fundus autofluorescence (FAF) shows hyperautofluorescent dots corresponding to the lesions seen in fundus exam [33]. FAF may be the most practical ancillary test to follow the patients with MEWDS.

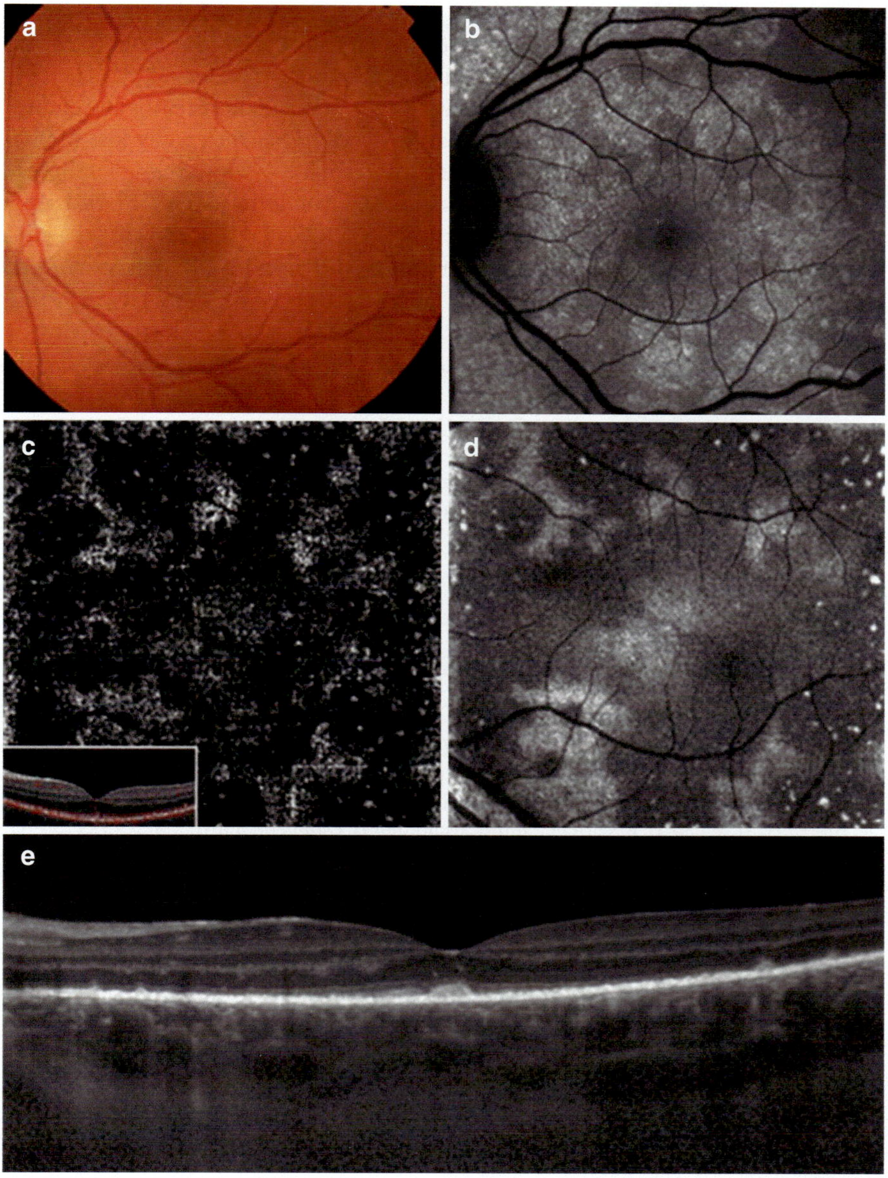

Fig. 8 Multiple evanescent white dot syndrome (MEWDS) . (**a**) Color photography of the left eye showing temporal disc edema and multifocal white lesions in the temporal midperiphery. (**b**) Fundus autofluorescence showing multiple hyperautofluorescent areas. (**c**) Optical coherence tomography angiography showing areas of photoreceptor slab blackout corresponding to areas of ellipsoid zone disruption and, in the bottom left corner, the OCT B-scan showing OCTA segmentation lines. (**d**) En face OCT showing hyporeflective areas at the level of ellipsoid zone with hyperreflective dots in the outer nuclear layer. (**e**) SD-OCT demonstrating disruption of the ellipsoid zone and a subfoveal accumulation of a hyperreflective material. (Reproduced with permission from Veronese et al. [33])

OCT reveals focal discontinuities of the ellipsoid zone and the deposition of refractile material between RPE and outer retina (Fig. 8). Recurrent episodes are rare and may show outer nuclear layer thinning.

OCTA shows patchy loss of the capillary plexus at the photoreceptor and choriocapillaris slabs (Fig. 8) [33]. In an observation by Veronese, the patchy loss of photoreceptor and choriocapillaris vasculature corresponded with areas of ellipsoid zone disruption in OCT and choriocapillaris blackout areas in ICGA [33]. In a separate observation, choriocapillaris hypoperfusion in OCTA correlated well with clinically observed pathology in MEWDS, but in APMPPE and BCR, they were more widespread [30].

Acknowledgment We would like to thank Austin Nakatsuka, MD for critically reviewing the manuscript.

Compliance with Ethical Requirements Hossein Nazari Khanamiri, MD and Narsing Rao, MD declare that they have no conflict of interest.

No human studies were carried out by the authors for this article.

No animal studies were carried out by the authors for this article.

References

1. Spaide RF, Yannuzzi LA, Freund KB. Linear streaks in multifocal choroiditis and panuveitis. Retina. 1991;11(2):229–31.
2. Dreyer RF, Gass DJ. Multifocal choroiditis and panuveitis. A syndrome that mimics ocular histoplasmosis. Arch Ophthalmol. 1984;102(12):1776–84.
3. Thorne JE, et al. Multifocal choroiditis with panuveitis incidence of ocular complications and of loss of visual acuity. Ophthalmology. 2006;113(12):2310–6.
4. Morgan CM, Schatz H. Recurrent multifocal choroiditis. Ophthalmology. 1986;93(9):1138–47.
5. Zahid S, et al. Optical coherence tomography angiography of chorioretinal lesions due to idiopathic multifocal choroiditis. Retina. 2017;37(8):1451–63.
6. Nazari Khanamiri H, Rao NA. Serpiginous choroiditis and infectious multifocal serpiginoid choroiditis. Surv Ophthalmol. 2013;58(3):203–32.
7. Invernizzi A, et al. Enhanced depth imaging optical coherence tomography features in areas of choriocapillaris hypoperfusion. Retina. 2016;36(10):2013–21.
8. Cardillo Piccolino F, Grosso A, Savini E. Fundus autofluorescence in serpiginous choroiditis. Graefes Arch Clin Exp Ophthalmol. 2009;247(2):179–85.
9. Pilotto E, et al. Retinal function in patients with serpiginous choroiditis: a microperimetry study. Graefes Arch Clin Exp Ophthalmol. 2010;248(9):1331–7.
10. De Luigi G, et al. Tuberculosis-related choriocapillaritis (multifocal-serpiginous choroiditis): follow-up and precise monitoring of therapy by indocyanine green angiography. Int Ophthalmol. 2012;32(1):55–60.
11. El Ameen A, Herbort CP. Serpiginous choroiditis imaged by optical coherence tomography angiography. Retin Cases Brief Rep. 2016;12(4):279–85.
12. Cimino L, Auer C, Herbort CP. Sensitivity of indocyanine green angiography for the follow-up of active inflammatory choriocapillaropathies. Ocul Immunol Inflamm. 2000;8(4):275–83.
13. Mangeon M, et al. Multimodal evaluation of patients with acute posterior multifocal placoid pigment epitheliopathy and serpiginous choroiditis. Ocul Immunol Inflamm. 2018;26(8):1212–8.
14. Mandadi SKR, et al. Novel findings on optical coherence tomography angiography in patients with tubercular serpiginous-like choroiditis. Retina. 2017;37(9):1647–59.

15. Dastiridou AI, et al. Choroidal imaging with swept-source optical coherence tomography in patients with birdshot chorioretinopathy: choroidal reflectivity and thickness. Ophthalmology. 2017;124(8):1186–95.
16. Böni C, et al. Fundus autofluorescence findings in eyes with birdshot chorioretinitis. Invest Ophthalmol Vis Sci. 2017;58(10):4015–25.
17. Yeh S, et al. Fundus autofluorescence imaging of the white dot syndromes. Arch Ophthalmol. 2010;128(1):46–56.
18. Pohlmann D, et al. Multimodal imaging in birdshot retinochoroiditis. Ocul Immunol Inflamm. 2017;25(5):621–32.
19. Gass JD. Acute posterior multifocal placoid pigment epitheliopathy. Arch Ophthalmol. 1968;80(2):177–85.
20. Fiore T, et al. Acute posterior multifocal placoid pigment epitheliopathy: outcome and visual prognosis. Retina. 2009;29(7):994–1001.
21. Hsu CT, et al. Acute posterior multifocal placoid pigment epitheliopathy associated with a systemic necrotizing vasculitis. Retina. 2003;23(1):64–8.
22. Chiquet C, et al. Acute posterior multifocal placoid pigment epitheliopathy associated with Wegener's granulomatosis. Retina. 1999;19(4):309–13.
23. Jones NP. Acute posterior multifocal placoid pigment epitheliopathy. Br J Ophthalmol. 1995;79(4):384–9.
24. Howe LJ, et al. Choroidal hypoperfusion in acute posterior multifocal placoid pigment epitheliopathy. An indocyanine green angiography study. Ophthalmology. 1995;102(5):790–8.
25. Goldenberg D, et al. Spectral domain optical coherence tomography classification of acute posterior multifocal placoid pigment epitheliopathy. Retina. 2012;32(7):1403–10.
26. Branisteanu D, Bilha A. Acute posterior multifocal placoid pigment epitheliopathy following influenza vaccination. Rom J Ophthalmol. 2015;59(1):52–8.
27. Heiferman MJ, et al. Acute posterior multifocal placoid pigment epitheliopathy on optical coherence tomography angiography. Retina. 2017;37(11):2084–94.
28. Werner JU, et al. Multi-modal imaging including optical coherence tomography angiography in patients with posterior multifocal placoid pigment epitheliopathy. Ophthalmic Surg Lasers Imaging Retina. 2017;48(9):727–33.
29. Burke TR, et al. Application of OCT-angiography to characterise the evolution of chorioretinal lesions in acute posterior multifocal placoid pigment epitheliopathy. Eye (Lond). 2017;31(10):1399–408.
30. Wang JC, et al. Distinguishing white dot syndromes with patterns of choroidal hypoperfusion on optical coherence tomography angiography. Ophthalmic Surg Lasers Imaging Retina. 2017;48(8):638–46.
31. Kim AY, et al. Quantifying retinal microvascular changes in uveitis using spectral-domain optical coherence tomography angiography. Am J Ophthalmol. 2016;171:101–12.
32. Roberts PK, et al. Characterizing photoreceptor changes in acute posterior multifocal placoid pigment epitheliopathy using adaptive optics. Retina. 2018;38(1):39–48.
33. Veronese C, et al. Bilateral multiple evanescent white dot syndrome. Int Ophthalmol. 2017;38(5):2153–8.

Part III

Infectious Posterior or Panuveitis

Ocular Toxoplasmosis

Daniel Vitor Vasconcelos-Santos

Introduction

Toxoplasmosis is an ubiquitous zoonosis that affects nearly one third of the human population [1]. Ocular involvement may be present in congenital or postnatally acquired disease but is more frequent and severe in the former [2]. Despite its self-limited course in immunocompetent individuals, toxoplasmic retinochoroiditis may complicate with irreversible visual loss, particularly when the macula or optic nerve head is involved. Ocular disease is typically recurrent, and reactivation of intraretinal *Toxoplasma gondii* cysts, with subsequent bouts of intraocular inflammation, may occur anytime in life [3–5].

Etiology

T. gondii is an intracellular apicomplexan parasite, capable of establishing lifelong chronic infection of virtually any warm-blooded animal [6]. The parasite has three main evolving forms:

- Tachyzoites: are the infective/proliferative form, involved in the active phase of the disease.
- Bradyzoites: are the latent form, involved in the chronic phase of the disease. They constitute cysts that may be viable in muscular and neural tissue (retina and rest of the central nervous system) of intermediate hosts for decades.
- Sporozoites: are formed by sexual reproduction in the intestine of felines (definite hosts), being eliminated in their feces and potentially contaminating soil, water, fruits, and vegetables. These sporozoites may be infective for up to 1 year in water or soil.

D. V. Vasconcelos-Santos (✉)
Universidade Federal de Minas Gerais, Faculdade de Medicina, Belo Horizonte, Brazil
e-mail: dvitor@ufmg.br

N. A. Rao et al. (eds.), *Posterior Uveitis*, Essentials in Ophthalmology,
https://doi.org/10.1007/978-3-030-03140-4_5

Felines are infected by ingesting meat containing bradyzoites/tachyzoites of intermediate hosts or by ingestion of sporulated oocysts present in contaminated soil. Humans are mainly infected orally, through ingestion of contaminated water or fruits/vegetables contaminated by oocysts and of raw/undercooked meat containing tissue cysts [3, 6].

After crossing enterocytes, the parasite disseminates as tachyzoites through the bloodstream until an adaptive immune response is mounted to contain parasite replication/dissemination. Remaining parasites eventually encyst in tissues, establishing chronic lifelong infection mainly in skeletal muscle and CNS, including the retina. These *T. gondii* cysts are resistant to antiparasitic therapy and may later rupture, releasing bradyzoites that convert to tachyzoites, locally reactivating the disease [3, 6].

Other modes of human infection include transplacental transmission, organ transplantation, blood transfusion, and laboratory accidents [1, 3, 6].

Epidemiology

T. gondii is present in all continents but is more prevalent in tropical areas. In South America, including Brazil, prevalence rates may be as high as 80% [4, 5, 7].

Seroprevalence increases with age [3–5], with more frequent and early seroconversion being identified in populations with poor sanitation or ingesting raw/undercooked meat, unwashed fruits/vegetables, and/or unfiltered water [4–6, 8].

Rates of ocular involvement in congenital toxoplasmosis may be as high as 80% [9]. Transplacental transmission typically occurs in the setting of recently acquired infection of pregnant women, being more frequent but less severe at the end of gestation [1, 10, 11]. Even though postnatally acquired disease less frequently leads to ocular manifestations, recent studies have been reinforcing its importance worldwide, especially in highly endemic areas [12, 13].

Pathogenesis of Ocular Disease

Toxoplasmic retinochoroiditis results from a delicate balance between parasite and host factors [2, 14, 15]. In immunocompetent patients, an exuberant reactive granulomatous response is frequently present, eventually controlling parasite replication but also potentially leading to local damage to the retina and adjacent structures [14].

Recent evidence suggests that different strains of *T. gondii* may lead to more severe systemic and even ocular disease [16–19]. Parasite genotype may also be determinant, at least in part, of response to antiparasitic drugs [2, 20]. The host immunoimmaturity in the neonatal period, or even immunosuppression in individuals with AIDS or under immunomodulatory therapy, may be associated with more frequent and severe systemic and ocular disease [1, 21].

Clinical Presentation

Congenital Toxoplasmosis

Women with primary toxoplasmic infection during pregnancy can transmit the parasite to the fetus, more frequently when seroconversion occurs later in pregnancy. Severity of fetal involvement, however, is greater in the first trimester and may include neurologic sequelae (microcephaly, hydrocephalus, and intracranial calcifications), anemia, thrombocytopenia, cutaneous rash, hepatitis, pneumonitis, myocarditis, encephalitis, and even abortion [1, 10, 11].

In the third trimester, subclinical forms are common, but ocular disease is frequently present. Retinochoroiditis is the major clinical manifestation of congenital toxoplasmosis, being disclosed in up to 80% of infected newborns, either as retinochoroidal scars, with macular tropism (Figs. 1 and 2), or even as active lesions (Fig. 3), mainly in offspring of previously untreated mothers. Bilateral lesions are also very frequent in this context [4, 5, 9, 10, 22].

New active foci of retinochoroiditis may develop anytime in life, accompanied by variable degree of vitritis, retinal and/or optic disc edema, periphlebitis, and

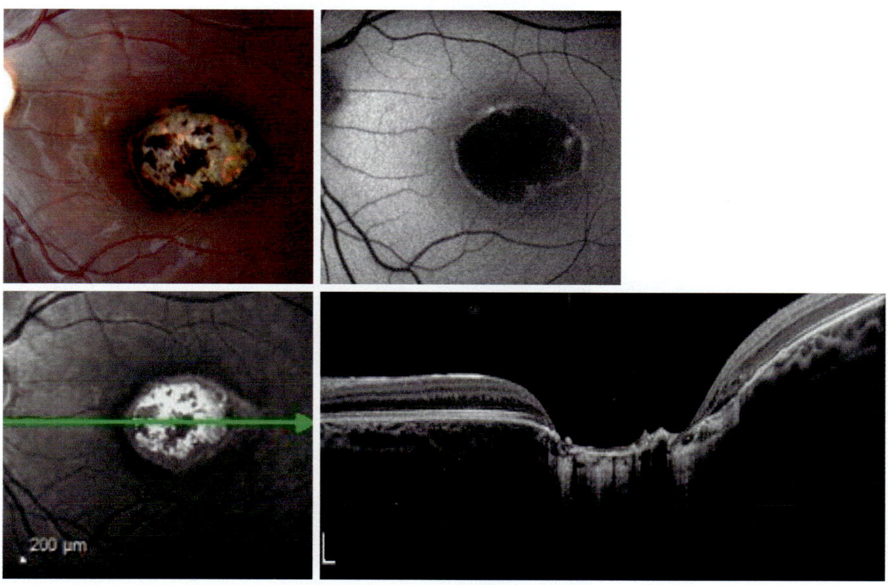

Fig. 1 Typical "wagon-wheel scar" in the left macula of a child with congenital toxoplasmosis (top left). The lesion displays sharply demarcated decreased autofluorescence signal (top right) with correspondent colobomatous change involving the retina/choroid on spectral-domain optical coherence tomography (bottom)

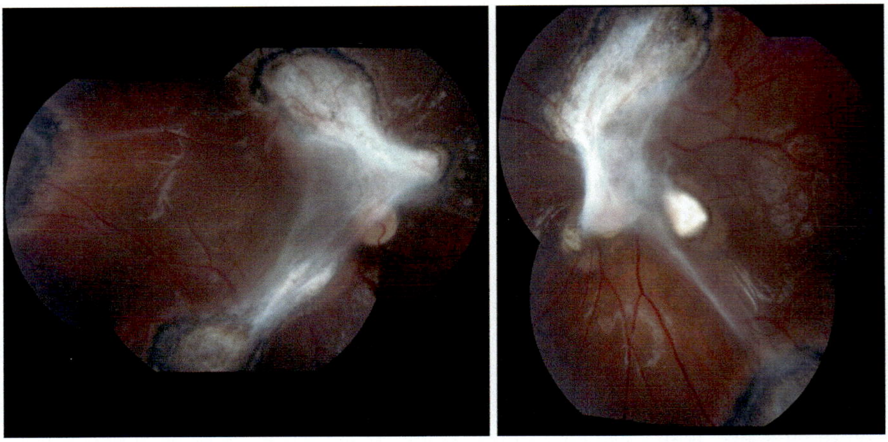

Fig. 2 Multiple bilateral retinochoroidal scars connected by epiretinal fibrotic bands in a child with congenital toxoplasmosis

Fig. 3 Active retinochoroiditis in the right macula of a newborn with congenital toxoplasmosis

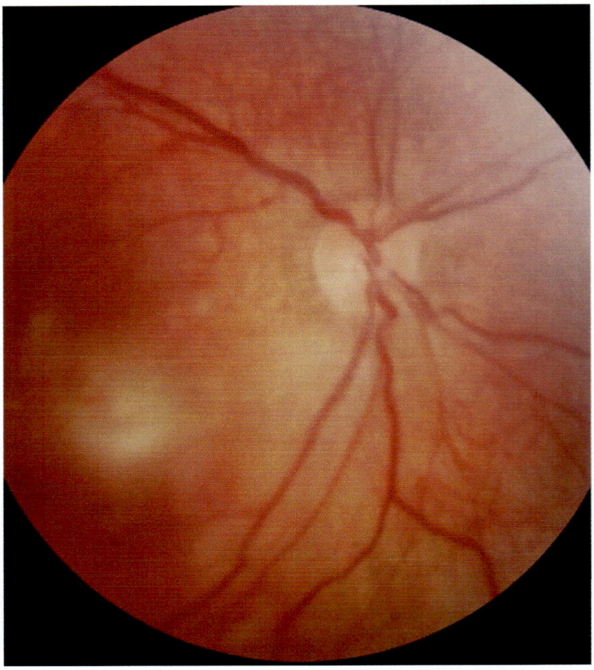

hemorrhages. This focus of reactivation may arise in the margins of a preexistent scar (so-called "satellite" lesion) (Fig. 4), or as an isolated focal lesion, distant to or even in the absence of other retinochoroidal scars (Fig. 5) [4, 5].

Ocular complications including cataract, vitreous bands, tractional/rhegmatogenous retinal detachment, strabismus, nystagmus, and microphthalmia can also develop [4, 5, 9].

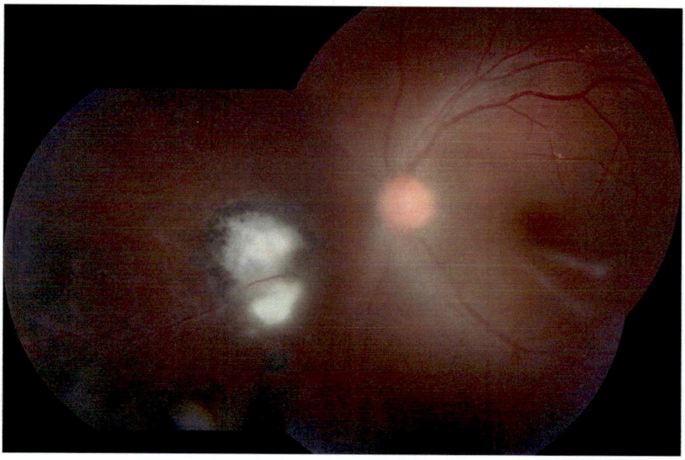

Fig. 4 Active focus of retinochoroiditis adjacent to preexistent scars. Vitreous haze and perivenular sheathing can also be seen

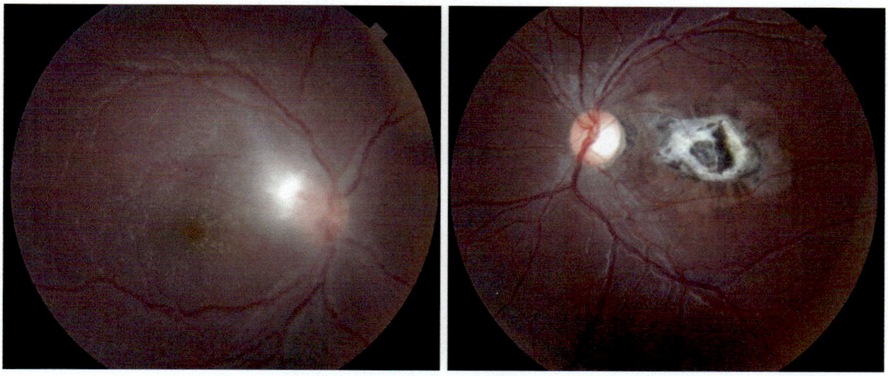

Fig. 5 Juxtadiscal focus of retinochoroiditis leading to neuroretinitis, with formation of an incomplete macular star in the right macula. An old pigmented scar is seen in the left eye

Postnatally Acquired Toxoplasmosis

Immunocompetent individuals with postnatal toxoplasmosis are usually asymptomatic. When present, symptoms are frequently non-specific, including fever, myalgia, cutaneous rash, and lymphadenopathy [1, 21]. More severe systemic involvement, characterized by hepatitis, pneumonitis, myocarditis, and even encephalitis, is rare in the absence of immunosuppression but may be associated with more virulent *T. gondii* strains [23]. Toxoplasmosis in immunosuppressed individuals is also more severe and may be progressive. In patients with AIDS, toxoplasmic encephalitis may precede, coincide with, or even follow ocular toxoplasmosis [24].

Ocular involvement in postnatally acquired toxoplasmosis may take days to years to primarily infection. Retinochoroiditis early after seroconversion is present in only 2–20%, but up to 60% may develop rupture of intraretinal cysts later in life, leading to local reactivation of the disease (Fig. 6) [2, 4, 5, 13, 21, 25].

Individuals with active toxoplasmic retinochoroiditis often complain of decreased vision and/or floaters. Conjunctival hyperemia, photophobia, and ocular pain may be present in the setting of involvement of the anterior segment of the eye. In these cases, keratic precipitates (Fig. 7), anterior chamber cells/flare and even ocular hypo-/hypertension may be disclosed [4, 5, 21].

Active toxoplasmic retinochoroiditis is characterized by a focal white-yellowish exudate of variable size in the retina, typically with ill-defined borders (Fig. 8). It may initially affect the inner retina, often progressing to involve its full thickness. Reactive choroidal thickening is also frequently noted, as well as inflammatory

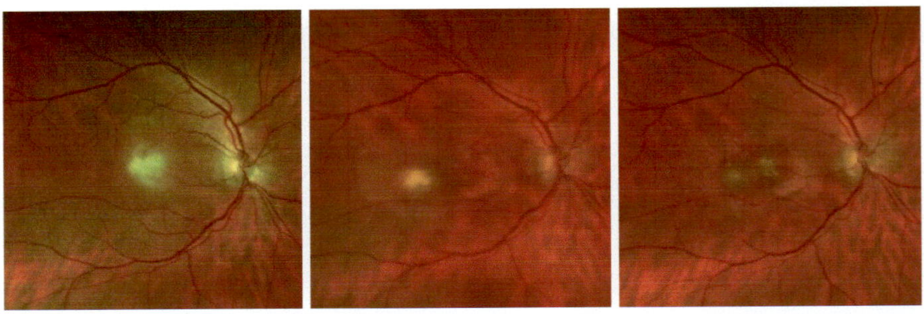

Fig. 6 Recurrent toxoplasmic retinochoroiditis. First episode occurred soon after seroconversion, with involvement of the foveal center (left). Eleven months later, a new active lesion was detected temporal do the fovea (middle), eventually resolving after antiparasitic therapy, 5 weeks later (right)

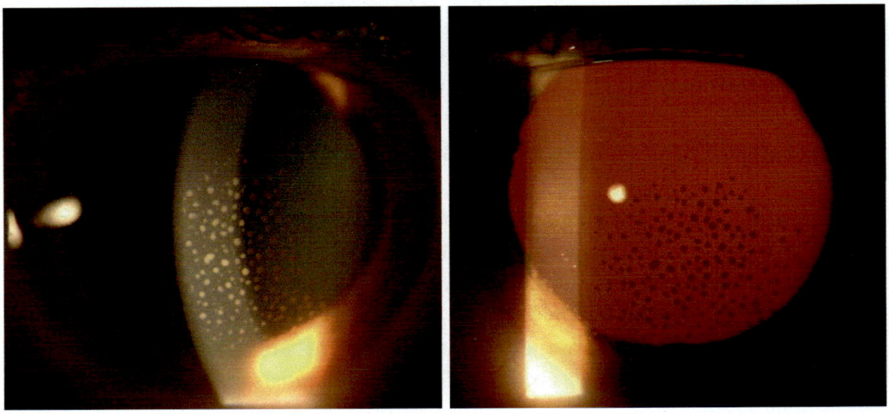

Fig. 7 Direct and indirect slit-lamp illumination of keratic precipitates in active toxoplasmic retinochoroiditis

exudation to the vitreous and macular and/or optic disc edema, depending on the location of the inflammatory focus. In the setting of more severe vitritis, the active lesion may assume a "headlight-in-the-fog" appearance (Fig. 9).

Inflammatory precipitates in the surface of the posterior hyaloid, as well as along retinal blood vessels, can also be noted [4, 5, 21, 26]. Perivenular sheathing, as well as Kyrieleis plaques (exudates overlying arteriolar wall), can also be appreciated. More rarely, vascular occlusion may also develop [4, 5, 21].

As intraocular inflammation resolves, a retinochoroidal scar is formed, often with some degree of pigmentation, associated with hyperplasia/hypertrophy of the retinal pigment epithelium (RPE). Atrophic/depigmented scars can also be formed.

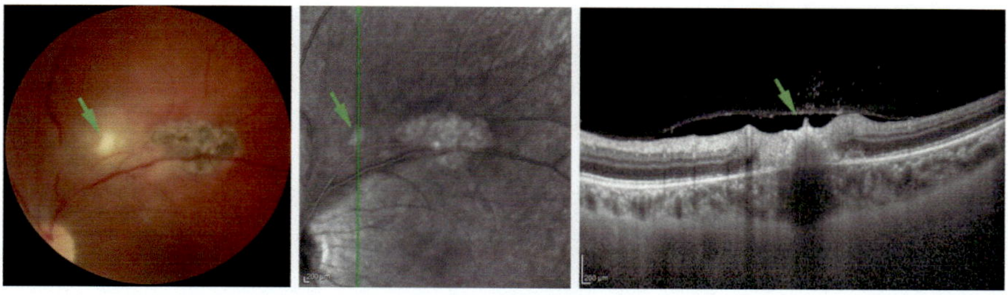

Fig. 8 Clinical and tomographic aspect of active recurrent ocular toxoplasmosis. The active focus is indicated by green arrows. Posterior hyaloid is thickened and partially detached. Vitreous cells, as well as reactive inflammatory fusiform thickening of the underlying choroid, can also be appreciated

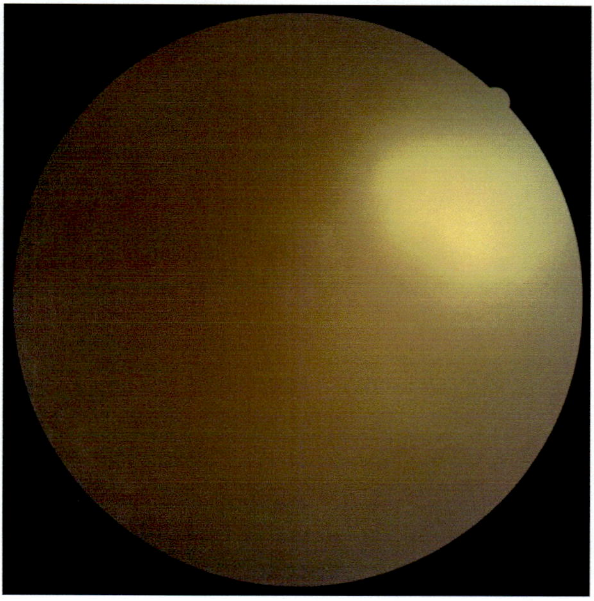

Fig. 9 Active toxoplasmic lesion displaying appearance of "headlight in the fog," because of significant vitritis

In the setting of reactivation of retinochoroiditis, the new active lesion frequently arises in the margins of a preexistent scar, and this "satellite lesion" is regarded as an important finding for the diagnosis of ocular toxoplasmosis [4, 5] (Figs. 4 and 8). A focal active lesion, in the absence of previous scarring, can also be observed (Figs. 6 and 9).

Atypical forms of ocular toxoplasmosis include [4, 5, 26, 27]:

- Neuroretinitis, often when the active focus arises in the juxtadiscal retina, leading to edema of the optic disc and macular, culminating with formation of macular star (Fig. 10).
- Punctate outer retinal toxoplasmosis, when the active lesion presumably affects the outer retina, leading to subretinal exudation and minimal vitritis (Fig. 11).
- Extensive necrotizing lesions, single or multiple, which may resemble herpetic retinitis, predominantly occurring in immunosuppressed individuals, those of older age, as well as in the setting of recently postnatally acquired toxoplasmosis (Figs. 12 and 13). Prior inadvertent use of systemic and/or local corticosteroids without proper antibiotic coverage may also be another culprit.

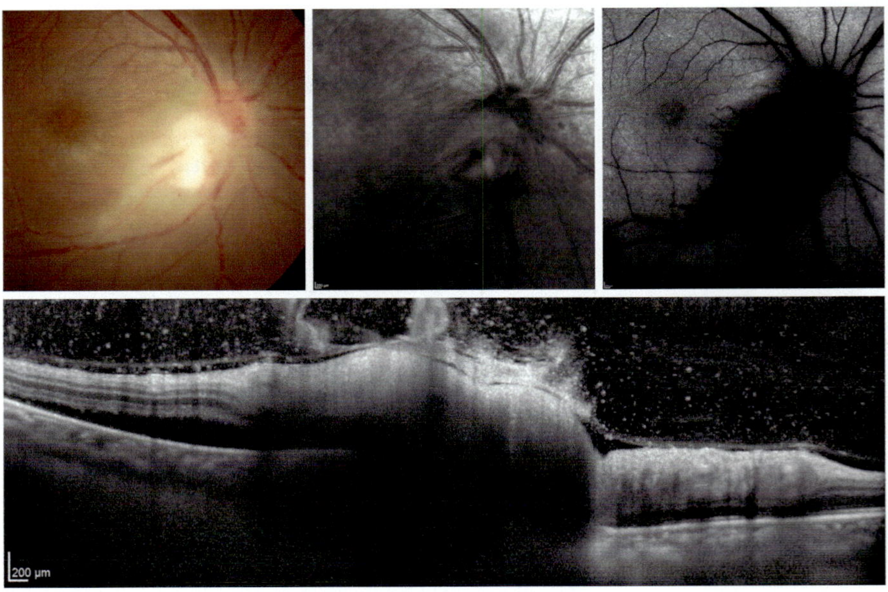

Fig. 10 Aspect of active toxoplasmic lesion close to the optic disc leading to significant disc edema, macular exudates, and subretinal fluid (neuroretinitis). Fundus autofluorescence is not remarkable, except for the area of decreased signal surrounding the lesion (top right). Near-infrared guided (top middle)-optical coherence tomography shows dense vitreous inflammatory exudation, local hyper-reflectivity of the retina at the level of the active lesion (with deep shadowing), as well as fusiform thickening of the underlying choroid (bottom)

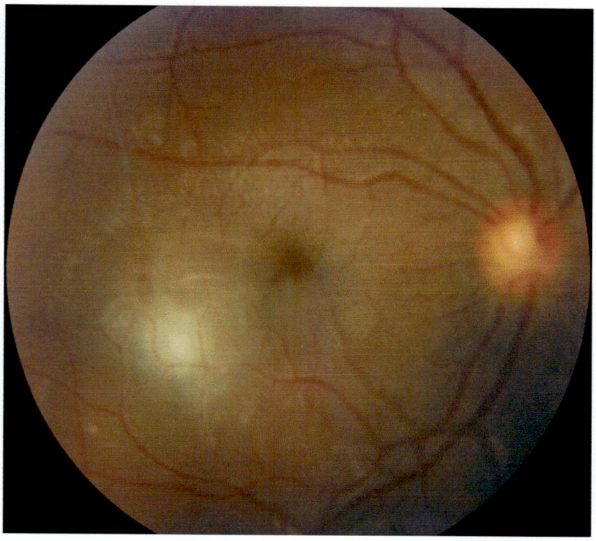

Fig. 11 Aspect of punctate outer retinal toxoplasmosis, in which inflammatory exudation led to focal serous retinal detachment. Vitritis is also minimal

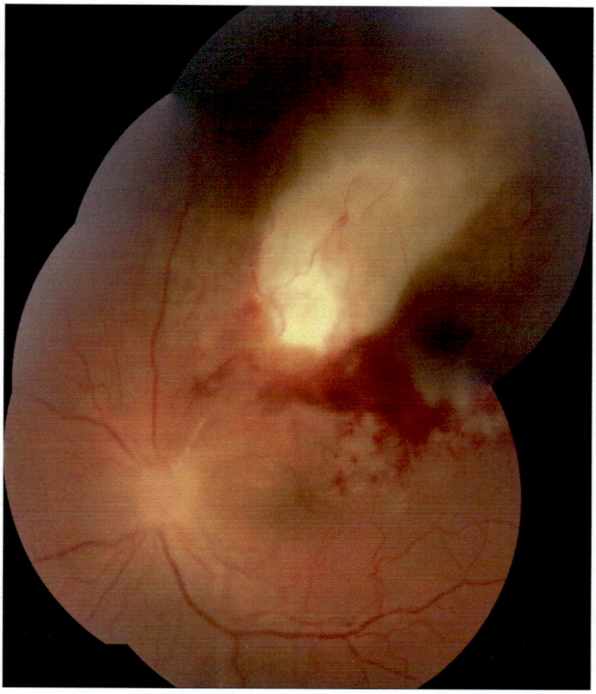

Fig. 12 Large exudative toxoplasmic lesion in the superotemporal arcade, simulating herpetic retinitis. Hemorrhages associated with venular occlusions, as well as Kyrieleis arteriolitis, are also seen

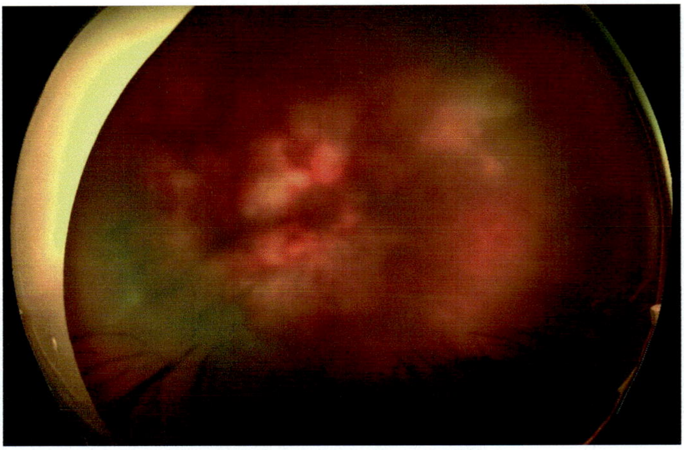

Fig. 13 Extensive hemorrhagic retinitis initially suspicious of herpetic etiology. PCR of aqueous humor was positive for *T. gondii* and negative for herpesviruses. HIV testing eventually came with positive results

– Ocular toxoplasmosis in the absence of retinochoroiditis has also been reported, mostly in the context of recent seroconversion. Isolated iridocyclitis, papillitis, retinal vasculitis, and even vitritis have been rarely reported [4, 5, 27, 28].

Diagnosis

Diagnosis of ocular toxoplasmosis is essentially clinical, based on the observation of focal necrotizing retinochoroiditis, typically in the presence of adjacent/distant retinochoroidal scarring [4, 5] (Figs. 6 and 8).

Serology may be supportive, but also help to exclude ocular toxoplasmosis, when specific antibodies (IgG and IgM) are absent [29, 30]. High titers of anti-*T. gondii* IgM and/or IgA, as well as IgG with low avidity, are suggestive of recently acquired toxoplasmosis. Residual IgM levels should be interpreted with caution, as they may persist months to years after seroconversion. Congenital toxoplasmosis is diagnosed by detection of specific IgM and/or IgA (that do not cross the placenta) in the neonatal period and/or persistently high levels of *anti-T gondii* IgG beyond 12 months of life [9, 10].

In most cases of recurrent toxoplasmic retinochoroiditis, however, patients do only display anti-*T. gondii* IgG, denoting chronic infection. In these individuals, titers of IgG do not correlate to disease activity.

Other laboratory investigations may be important to exclude other infectious etiologies, particularly syphilis and tuberculosis among others. HIV coinfection should also be investigated in the setting of more severe and even refractory toxoplasmic retinochoroiditis.

In atypical cases, invasive investigations such as intraocular fluid polymerase chain reaction (PCR) DNA analysis may be employed, not only to confirm toxoplasmosis but also to entertain other etiologies considered in the differential diagnosis [29, 31]. Detection of *T. gondii* DNA through PCR does confirm toxoplasmosis (Fig. 13), but a negative PCR result of aqueous humor is not able to exclude it. In this context, positivity of vitreous is usually greater than of aqueous samples [29, 31].

Intraocular antibody synthesis can be assessed by the Goldmann-Witmer coefficient, based on the correlation of specific antibody and total globulin titers in aqueous humor versus serum. A positive result (>3) indicates intraocular synthesis of anti-*T. gondii* antibodies, supporting the diagnosis of ocular toxoplasmosis [29].

Imaging

Imaging modalities, including spectral-domain optical coherence tomography (SD-OCT), fluorescein angiography, fundus autofluorescence and reflectance, indocyanine green angiography, and even B-scan, may be highly helpful to delineate vitreous, retinal, and choroidal changes, both at baseline and during follow-up. They may also be very relevant to the assessment of local complications, including macular edema, epiretinal membranes, vitreoretinal traction, vascular occlusions, and choroidal neovascularization, among others. The combination of these techniques in the *multimodal imaging* approach clearly defines patterns of active, regressive, and cicatricial lesions [2, 4, 5].

SD-OCT recapitulates histopathological changes in toxoplasmic retinochoroiditis. The active focus is typically characterized by focal hyper-reflectivity/edema of the neurosensory retina, with posterior shadowing and focal elevation/detachment of the RPE. SD-OCT also shows inflammatory exudation to the vitreous, local detachment of the posterior hyaloid and fusiform thickening of the underlying choroid. Other local changes, such as retinal edema and even subretinal fluid, can also be promptly delineated by SD-OCT (Figs. 8, 10, and 14). After resolution, the retinochoroidal lesion progressive flattens, leaving an area of focal disorganization or retinal layers and variable hyper-reflectivity associated with subretinal fibrosis (Fig. 14) [4, 5].

In fluorescein angiography, the retinochoroiditis focus is initially hypofluorescent, with progressive staining/leakage in the latter phases (Fig. 15). Fluorescein angiography is also valuable to assess vascular occlusions and choroidal neovascularization. Cicatricial lesions may display hypofluorescence (blockage by RPE hypertrophy/hyperplasia) or hyperfluorescence (RPE atrophy leading to window defect of staining of subretinal fibrotic change) (Fig. 16).

Fundus autofluorescence is typically unremarkable in acute lesions but may indicate their regression, signaled as increased autofluorescence. After complete scarring, autofluorescence signal then decreases, eventually delineating the area of the scar (Figs. 16 and 17).

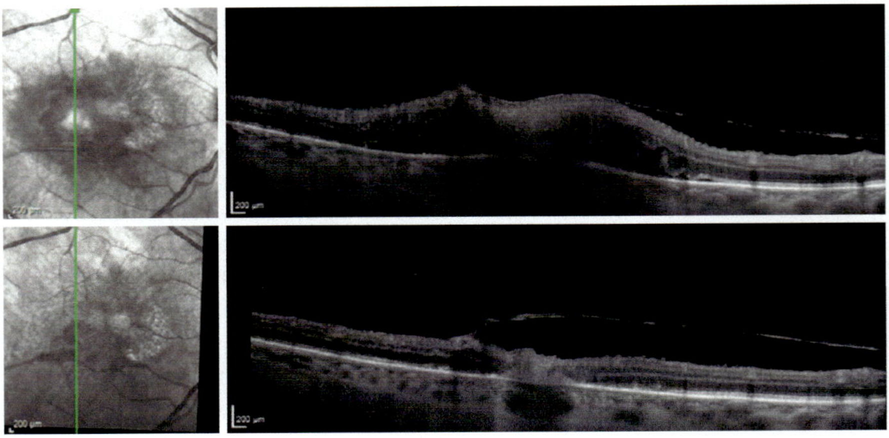

Fig. 14 Tomographic evidence of improvement before (top) and 5 weeks after triple therapy (bottom) for the second recurrence of patient shown in Fig. 6. The infiltrated area progressively flattens, and edema is completely resorbed; choroid also returns to normal thickness. A central scar is left, with disorganization of retinal layers. Partially detached and thickened hyaloid is also seen

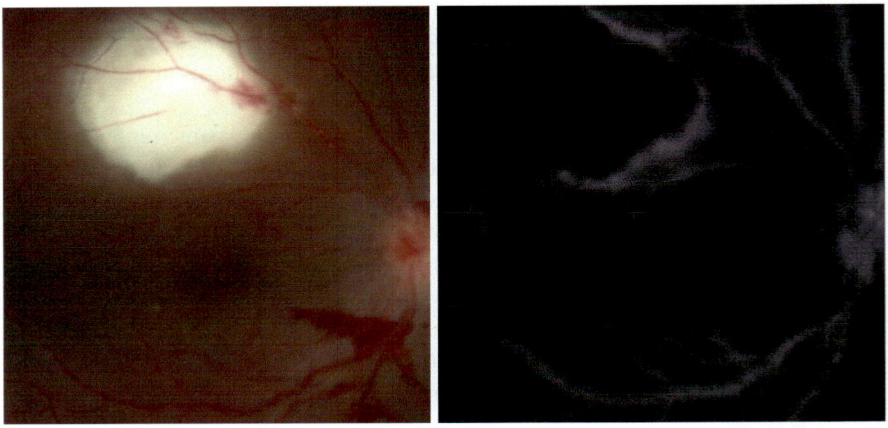

Fig. 15 Angiographic aspect of active toxoplasmic retinochoroiditis. Fluorescein angiography discloses hypofluorescence of the active lesion, with leakage at the margins. Diffuse venular and disc leakage can also be seen, as well as arteriolar occlusion temporal to the active lesion

In indocyanine green angiography, local or distant hypocyanesence is frequently seen, associated with inflammatory infiltration of the underlying choroid (Fig. 17). Multiple dark dots may indicate more diffuse choroidal involvement.

B-scan may reveal vitreous changes, notably inflammatory echoes, vitreous schisis, vitreous detachment, and even vitreoretinal traction. At the level of the active lesion, focal retinochoroidal thickening can typically be appreciated on B-scan (Fig. 18). It is also particularly useful in the setting of severe vitritis, precluding fundus examination, as well as in the suspicion of retinal detachment.

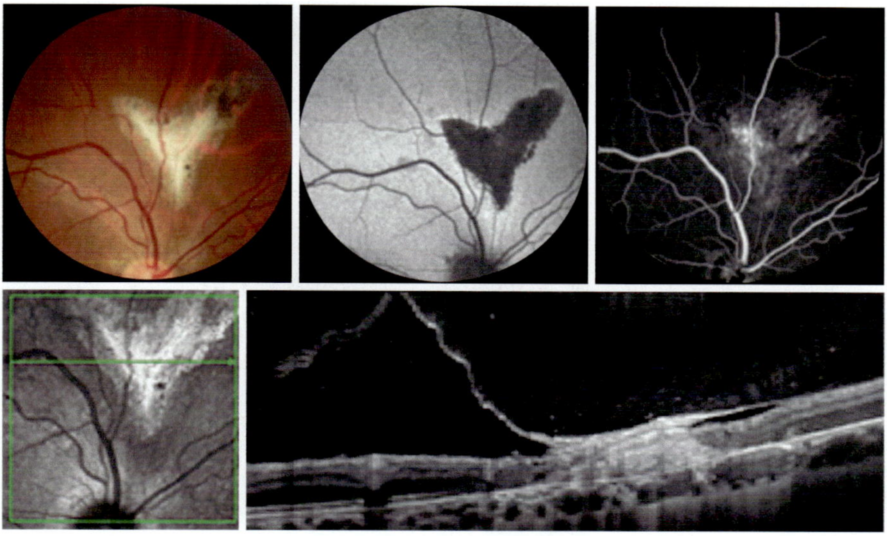

Fig. 16 Aspect of regressed toxoplasmic lesion. Decreased autofluorescence signal sharply demarcates the retinochoroidal scar (top middle). Mixed hypo-/hyperfluorescence is seen at the level of the scar (top right). Spectral-domain optical coherence tomography displays thickened posterior hyaloid partially attached to the scar, indicated by focal reflectivity with thinning/disorganization of retinal layers (bottom)

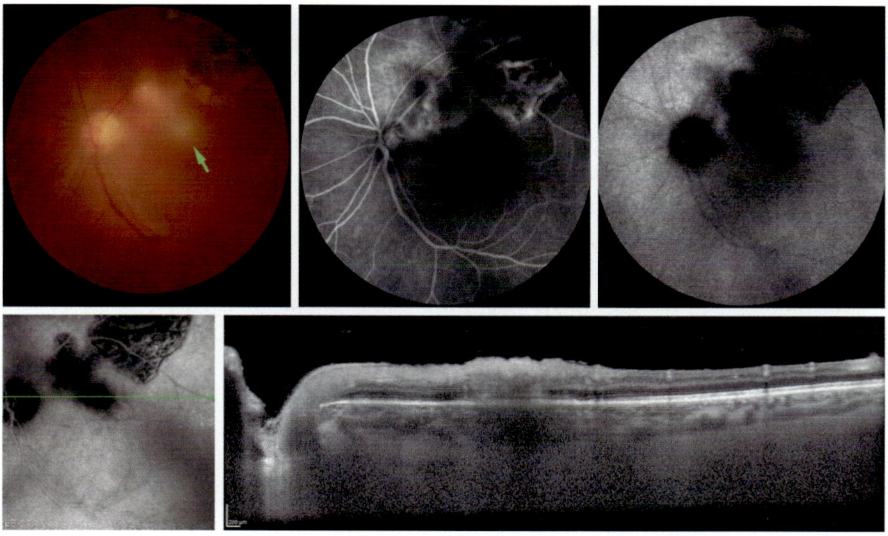

Fig. 17 Aspect of recurrent focus of toxoplasmic retinochoroiditis (top left, green arrow). On fluorescein angiography (top middle), the hypofluorescence of this active focus is contiguous with the foveal avascular zone; preexistent scars show mixed hypo-/hyperfluorescence. On indocyanine green angiography (ICG, top right), focal hypocyanescence is clearly seen at the level of the active lesion. ICG-guided spectral-domain optical coherence tomography delineates the correspondence between the hypocyanescent focus and the fusiform thickening of the choroid underlying the active retinal lesion

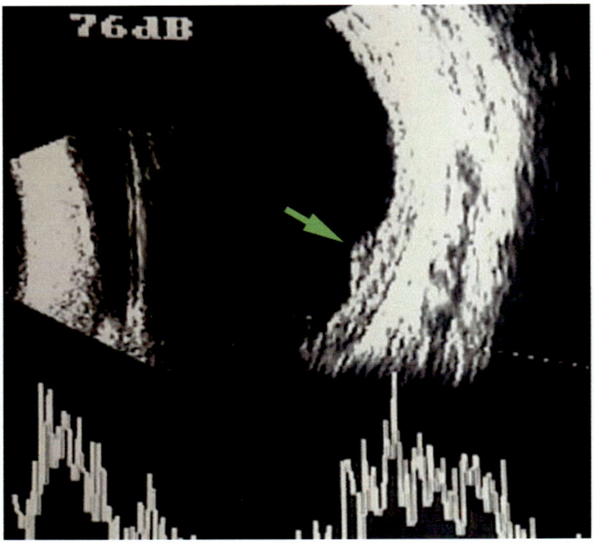

Fig. 18 Ultrasonographic aspect of a large active toxoplasmic lesion, with focal thickening of the retinochoroidal complex (arrow)

Differential Diagnosis

In newborns suspected of congenital toxoplasmosis, other infections of the *TORCHS* acronym (toxoplasmosis, rubella, cytomegalovirus, herpes, syphilis) are to be considered [10]. More recently, congenital Zika virus infection has been associated with lesions in the retina and optic nerve, some of which may resemble toxoplasmic scars [32]. Retinocytoma, retinoblastoma, retinochoroidal coloboma, and persistent hyperplastic primary vitreous are also part of the differential diagnosis of ocular toxoplasmosis in the neonatal period [33].

In older children and in adults, toxoplasmic retinochoroiditis should be differentiated from other infectious (bacteria, viruses, fungi, and protozoa), noninfectious, and even neoplastic conditions [33].

In immunosuppressed individuals, differential diagnosis includes acute retinal necrosis (ARN), progressive outer retinal necrosis (PORN), CMV retinitis, fungal infection, and even primary vitreoretinal lymphoma [4, 5, 21].

Treatment

Because of its possibly self-limited course in immunocompetent patients, toxoplasmic retinochoroiditis may not initially demand treatment for all cases. Treatment however is frequently recommended to accelerate resolution of intraocular inflammation, reducing extent of damage to the retina and the optic disc and minimizing structural complications [2, 4, 5, 34]. It is important to note that currently available antiparasitic drugs are not able to eliminate *T. gondii* tissue cysts, thus not preventing further reactivations of toxoplasmic retinochoroiditis, unless continuous chemoprophylaxis is employed (see below).

Treatment decision should be individualized, based on several factors, including:

- Patient immune status
- Clinical course and visual acuity
- Location / size of the active lesion
- Degree of vitritis
- Macula and/or optic disc edema
- Vascular occlusion
- Special circumstances (newborns, pregnant women, drug allergy)

Side effects of the medications should also be considered and monitored for each case [2, 4, 5, 34, 35].

Treatment is based on a combination of antiparasitic drugs, as well as systemic corticosteroids, for a period of 5–8 weeks. Topical corticosteroids, mydriatic, and hypotensive agents are also employed as needed.

Different antiparasitic drugs and therapeutic regimens are available (Table 1) [4, 5, 32]. Even though few controlled studies support the possible equivalence of some of these regimens, the combination of sulfadiazine and pyrimethamine (with folinic acid supplementation) is still regarded as the standard "classic therapy" (also called *triple therapy)*, employed in critical situations, such as immunosuppressed patients and newborns with congenital toxoplasmosis. This is also supported by the superiority of this regimen over alternative ones, not only in vitro but also in experimental models of toxoplasmosis [1, 2].

Table 1 Main therapeutic regimens for ocular toxoplasmosis

Regimen	Observations
Sulfadiazine + pyrimethamine + folinic acid	Known as classic/triple therapy Well-reputed among specialists, it is the regimen of first choice in severe cases, in immunosuppressed individuals and for congenital toxoplasmosis
Sulfadiazine + pyrimethamine + clindamycin + folinic acid	Known as quadruple therapy. The possible advantage of adding clindamycin apparently does not outweigh higher frequency of adverse effects
Azithromycin + pyrimethamine + folinic acid	Better tolerated than triple therapy. Good option for individuals allergic to sulfa
Clindamycin + pyrimethamine + folinic acid	Another alternative for individuals allergic to sulfa
Sulfamethoxazole/ trimethoprim	Better tolerated than triple therapy but possibly less efficacious for severe cases. Regimen of choice for primary/ secondary prophylaxis
Azithromycin	Alternative for primary/secondary prophylaxis in individuals allergic to sulfa
Clindamycin	Option for primary/secondary prophylaxis in individuals allergic to sulfa Drug of choice for intravitreal therapy, in combination with dexamethasone

Immunosuppressed patients with active lesions should invariably be treated, usually for 6 to up to 12 weeks, because of progressive nature of retinochoroiditis in these individuals, with high risk of complications and even loss of the eye. Newborns with congenital toxoplasmosis should also be always treated during their first year of life, regardless of the presence of retinochoroiditis. Pregnant women recently seroconverting for toxoplasmosis also need therapy with spiramycin (regardless of retinochoroiditis) to minimize risk of transplacental transmission. As spiramycin does not cross the placenta, when fetal infection is confirmed by PCR of amniotic fluid or suspected by ultrasound, other antiparasitic drugs are indicated to reach the fetus (avoiding pyrimethamine in the first trimester and sulfadiazine in the last 8 weeks of pregnancy) [1, 10, 36]. Because of the low risk of fetal infection, reactivation of retinochoroiditis in a chronically infected immunocompetent woman during pregnancy may be initially followed, as long as the posterior pole is not threatened.

Oral corticosteroids (prednisone 0.5–1 mg/kg/day or equivalent) in a tapering regimen are frequently added to the antiparasitic regiment, to better control intraocular inflammation and to possibly minimize risk of permanent visual-threatening damage to ocular structures [34, 35]. These systemic corticosteroids should however be deferred until proper differential diagnosis has been made with other infectious etiologies (viral, bacterial [including syphilis], and even fungal). In uncertain cases, deferring the steroid until initial response to antiparasitic therapy is recommended [4, 5].

Intravitreal injections of clindamycin and dexamethasone may also be used in selected cases, particularly in the setting of intolerance, contraindication, or even resistance to systemic therapy [35, 37]. Depot corticosteroids or even corticosteroid implants are contraindicated in ocular toxoplasmosis.

Laser photocoagulation may occasionally be attempted for active extramacular lesions with chronic exudation partially resistant to systemic therapy.

Pars plana vitrectomy may be needed for removal of persistent vitreous opacities, vitreoretinal traction, and/or epiretinal membranes. Rhegmatogenous retinal detachment is also another indication for PPV. Pre- and even postoperative antiparasitic treatment should be individualized, being usually not needed in the setting of inactive lesions [38].

It is very important to monitor treatment toxicity but also response. Resolution of retinochoroiditis is typically centripetal, with progressive flattening of the margins, absorption of retinal edema, and reduction of vitreal inflammatory infiltration [26, 39] (Figs. 14 and 19). Lesion pigmentation is variable and may develop only late.

Prophylaxis

Primary prophylaxis is recommended for immunosuppressed individuals and pregnant women (or those on pregnancy planning) not previously infected with *T. gondii*, as follows:

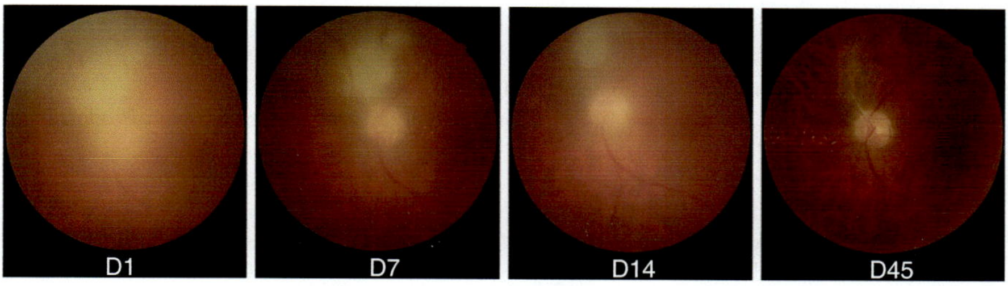

Fig. 19 Progressive resolution of a large active toxoplasmic lesion superior to the optic disc, over the course of triple therapy. Systemic corticosteroid was deferred until signs of initial response. PCR of aqueous humor for herpesviruses had negative results

- Avoiding ingestion of undercooked/raw meat (freezing at −20 °C/−4 °F overnight also destroys tissue cysts)
- Drinking only well-filtered/boiled water
- Carefully washing vegetables/fruits prior to consumption
- Using gloves and washing hands/kitchen utensils after manipulating meat/soil
- Avoiding contact with felines and their feces (even in soil/litter boxes)

Regular monthly serologic screening of susceptible pregnant women is also highly recommended, to allow prenatal treatment in case of seroconversion [1, 2, 10]:

Secondary prophylaxis with double-strength sulfamethoxazole/trimethoprim (800/160 mg 3x/week or every other day) has been shown to prevent recurrences of toxoplasmic retinochoroiditis in immunocompetent adults [40, 41]. This may be particularly helpful for individuals with multiple recurrences threatening the macula and is also employed in immunosuppressed patients. Ideal duration of such treatment has however not been established.

Prognosis

Despite being self-limited in immunocompetent patients, ocular toxoplasmosis is typically a recurrent disease, with new episodes being possible anytime in life. Risk of reactivation is especially greater in the first 12 months that follow the last episode of retinochoroiditis. Prognosis depends upon immune status of the individual, size, and location of active lesion. Presence of ocular complications is also critical to the visual prognosis, including persistent vitreous opacities, macular edema, epiretinal membranes, extensive retinochoroidal scarring, choroidal neovascularization, optic atrophy, and even retinal detachment [4, 5, 21, 42].

Conflict of Interest The author declares that he does not have any conflict of interest.

No human studies were carried out by the author for this article.

References

1. Montoya JG, Liesenfeld O. Toxoplasmosis. Lancet. 2004;363(9425):1965–76.
2. Vasconcelos-Santos DV. Ocular manifestations of systemic disease: toxoplasmosis. Curr Opin Ophthalmol. 2012;23(6):543–50.
3. Holland GN. Ocular toxoplasmosis: a global reassessment. Part I: epidemiology and course of disease. Am J Ophthalmol. 2003;136(6):973–88.
4. Oréfice F, Vasconcelos-Santos DV, Cordeiro CA, Oréfice JL, Costa RA. Toxoplasmosis. In: Foster CS, Vitale AT, editors. Diagnosis and treatment of uveitis. New Delhi: Jaypee-Highlights; 2013. p. 544–68.
5. Orefice JL, Costa RA, Scott IU, Calucci D, Orefice F, Grupo Mineiro de Pesquisa em Doencas Oculares I. Spectral optical coherence tomography findings in patients with ocular toxoplasmosis and active satellite lesions (MINAS report 1). Acta Ophthalmol. 2013;91(1):e41–7.
6. Dubey JP. The history and life cycle of Toxoplasma gondii. In: Weiss LM, Kim K, editors. Toxoplasma gondii – the model apicomplexan: perspectives and methods, vol. 2007. 1st ed. Amsterdam: Elsevier Academic Press; 2007. p. 1–17.
7. Dubey JP, Lago EG, Gennari SM, Su C, Jones JL. Toxoplasmosis in humans and animals in Brazil: high prevalence, high burden of disease, and epidemiology. Parasitology. 2012;139(11):1375–424.
8. Bahia-Oliveira LM, Jones JL, Azevedo-Silva J, Alves CC, Orefice F, Addiss DG. Highly endemic, waterborne toxoplasmosis in North Rio de Janeiro state, Brazil. Emerg Infect Dis. 2003;9(1):55–62.
9. Vasconcelos-Santos DV, Azevedo DOM, Campos WR, Oréfice F, Queiroz-Andrade GM, Carellos EVM. Congenital toxoplasmosis in southeastern Brazil: results of early ophthalmologic examination of a large cohort of neonates. Ophthalmology. 2009;116(11):2199–205.e1.
10. Peyron F, Wallon M, Kieffer F, Garweg JG. Toxoplasmosis. In: Wilson CB, Nizet V, Maldonado YA, Remington JS, Klein JO, editors. Remington and Klein's infectious diseases of the fetus and newborn infant. 8th ed. Philadelphia: Saunders; 2016. p. 949–1042.
11. Dunn D, Wallon M, Peyron F, Petersen E, Peckham C, Gilbert R. Mother-to-child transmission of toxoplasmosis: risk estimates for clinical counselling. Lancet. 1999;353(9167):1829–33.
12. Silveira C, Belfort R Jr, Muccioli C, Abreu MT, Martins MC, Victora C, Nussenblatt RB, Holland GN. A follow-up study of Toxoplasma gondii infection in southern Brazil. Am J Ophthalmol. 2001;131(3):351–4.
13. Arantes TE, Silveira C, Holland GN, Muccioli C, Yu F, Jones JL, Goldhardt R, Lewis KG, Belfort R Jr. Ocular involvement following postnatally acquired Toxoplasma gondii infection in Southern Brazil: a 28-year experience. Am J Ophthalmol. 2015;159(6):1002–1012.e1002.
14. Pavesio CE, Lightman S. Toxoplasma gondii and ocular toxoplasmosis: pathogenesis. Br J Ophthalmol. 1996;80(12):1099–107.
15. Bhopale GM. Pathogenesis of toxoplasmosis. Comp Immunol Microbiol Infect Dis. 2003;26(4):213–22.
16. Saeij JP, Boyle JP, Boothroyd JC. Differences among the three major strains of Toxoplasma gondii and their specific interactions with the infected host. Trends Parasitol. 2005;21(10):476–81.
17. Pena HF, Gennari SM, Dubey JP, Su C. Population structure and mouse-virulence of Toxoplasma gondii in Brazil. Int J Parasitol. 2008;38(5):561–9.
18. Bottos J, Miller RH, Belfort RN, Macedo AC, Belfort R Jr, Grigg ME. Bilateral retinochoroiditis caused by an atypical strain of Toxoplasma gondii. Br J Ophthalmol. 2009;93(11):1546–50.
19. Carneiro AC, Andrade GM, Costa JG, Pinheiro BV, Vasconcelos-Santos DV, Ferreira AM, Su C, Januario JN, Vitor RW. Genetic characterization of Toxoplasma gondii revealed highly diverse genotypes for isolates from newborns with congenital toxoplasmosis in southeastern Brazil. J Clin Microbiol. 2013;51(3):901–7.
20. Silva LA, Reis-Cunha JL, Bartholomeu DC, Vitor RW. Genetic polymorphisms and phenotypic profiles of sulfadiazine-resistant and sensitive Toxoplasma gondii isolates obtained from newborns with congenital toxoplasmosis in Minas Gerais, Brazil. PLoS One. 2017;12(1):e0170689.

21. Holland GN. Ocular toxoplasmosis: a global reassessment. Part II: disease manifestations and management. Am J Ophthalmol. 2004;137(1):1–17.
22. Mets MB, Holfels E, Boyer KM, Swisher CN, Roizen N, Stein L, Stein M, Hopkins J, Withers S, Mack D, Luciano R, Patel D, Remington JS, Meier P, McLeod R. Eye manifestations of congenital toxoplasmosis. Am J Ophthalmol. 1997;123(1):1–16.
23. Demar M, Hommel D, Djossou F, Peneau C, Boukhari R, Louvel D, Bourbigot AM, Nasser V, Ajzenberg D, Darde ML, Carme B. Acute toxoplasmoses in immunocompetent patients hospitalized in an intensive care unit in French Guiana. Clin Microbiol Infect. 2012;18(7):E221–31.
24. Bowen LN, Smith B, Reich D, Quezado M, Nath A. HIV-associated opportunistic CNS infections: pathophysiology, diagnosis and treatment. Nat Rev Neurol. 2016;12(11):662–74.
25. Balasundaram MB, Andavar R, Palaniswamy M, Venkatapathy N. Outbreak of acquired ocular toxoplasmosis involving 248 patients. Arch Ophthalmol. 2010;128(1):28–32.
26. Oréfice F, Bahia-Oliveira LM. Toxoplasmose. In: Oréfice F, editor. Uveíte clínica e cirúrgica. Rio de Janeiro: Cultura Médica; 2005. p. 699–804.
27. Smith JR, Cunningham ET Jr. Atypical presentations of ocular toxoplasmosis. Curr Opin Ophthalmol. 2002;13(6):387–92.
28. Holland GN, Muccioli C, Silveira C, Weisz JM, Belfort R Jr, O'Connor GR. Intraocular inflammatory reactions without focal necrotizing retinochoroiditis in patients with acquired systemic toxoplasmosis. Am J Ophthalmol. 1999;128(4):413–20.
29. Garweg JG, de Groot-Mijnes JD, Montoya JG. Diagnostic approach to ocular toxoplasmosis. Ocul Immunol Inflamm. 2011;19(4):255–61.
30. Montoya JG. Laboratory diagnosis of Toxoplasma gondii infection and toxoplasmosis. J Infect Dis. 2002;185(Suppl 1):S73–82.
31. Montoya JG, Parmley S, Liesenfeld O, Jaffe GJ, Remington JS. Use of the polymerase chain reaction for diagnosis of ocular toxoplasmosis. Ophthalmology. 1999;106(8):1554–63.
32. Vasconcelos-Santos DV, Andrade GM, Caiaffa WT. Zika virus, microcephaly, and ocular findings. JAMA Ophthalmol. 2016;134(8):946.
33. Vasconcelos-Santos DV, Dodds EM, Orefice F. Review for disease of the year: differential diagnosis of ocular toxoplasmosis. Ocul Immunol Inflamm. 2011;19(3):171–9.
34. Morais FB, Arantes TE, Muccioli C. Current practices in ocular toxoplasmosis: a survey of Brazilian uveitis specialists. Ocul Immunol Inflamm. 2018;26(2):317–23.
35. Kim SJ, Scott IU, Brown GC, Brown MM, Ho AC, Ip MS, Recchia FM. Interventions for toxoplasma retinochoroiditis: a report by the American Academy of ophthalmology. Ophthalmology. 2013;120(2):371–8. https://doi.org/10.1016/j.ophtha.2012.07.061.
36. Petersen E. Toxoplasmosis. Semin Fetal Neonatal Med. 2007;12(3):214–23.
37. Soheilian M, Ramezani A, Azimzadeh A, Sadoughi MM, Dehghan MH, Shahghadami R, Yaseri M, Peyman GA. Randomized trial of intravitreal clindamycin and dexamethasone versus pyrimethamine, sulfadiazine, and prednisolone in treatment of ocular toxoplasmosis. Ophthalmology. 2011;118(1):134–41.
38. Heringer GC, Oueghlani E, Dell'Omo R, Curi AL, Orefice F, Pavesio CE. Risk of reactivation of toxoplasmic retinitis following intraocular procedures without the use of prophylactic therapy. Br J Ophthalmol. 2014;98(9):1218–20.
39. Orefice JL, Costa RA, Orefice F, Campos W, da Costa-Lima D Jr, Scott IU. Vitreoretinal morphology in active ocular toxoplasmosis: a prospective study by optical coherence tomography. Br J Ophthalmol. 2007;91(6):773–80.
40. Silveira C, Belfort R Jr, Muccioli C, Holland GN, Victora CG, Horta BL, Yu F, Nussenblatt RB. The effect of long-term intermittent trimethoprim/sulfamethoxazole treatment on recurrences of toxoplasmic retinochoroiditis. Am J Ophthalmol. 2002;134(1):41–6.
41. Fernandes Felix JP, Cavalcanti Lira RP, Cosimo AB, Cardeal da Costa RL, Nascimento MA, Leite Arieta CE. Trimethoprim-sulfamethoxazole versus placebo in reducing the risk of toxoplasmic retinochoroiditis recurrences: a three-year follow-up. Am J Ophthalmol. 2016;170:176–82.
42. Bosch-Driessen LE, Berendschot TT, Ongkosuwito JV, Rothova A. Ocular toxoplasmosis: clinical features and prognosis of 154 patients. Ophthalmology. 2002;109(5):869–78.

Ocular Syphilis

Francesco Pichi and Thomas A. Albini

Syphilis remains an important cause of uveitis [1, 2]. After reaching a peak annual incidence in the United States of 20.3 cases per 100,000 population in 1990 [3], rates of primary and secondary syphilis declined over the ensuing decade to a record low of 2.1 cases per 100,000 population in 2000, an 89.7% decrease [3]. Despite efforts by the Centers for Disease Control to eradicate syphilis, there has been an increase in primary and secondary syphilis rates over the past decade [4], reaching 4.5 cases per 100,000 population in 2010 [5]. Reported syphilis diagnoses are on the rise, largely in young men who have sex with men (MSM) in the South and West of the United States. In 2014 (the last year with national data available), 63,450 total cases of syphilis were reported, which is a 12.3% increase from 2013, and the national syphilis rate increased to 6.3 cases per 100,000 population, the highest rate reported since 1994. The rate increase over time during 2000–2014 has been largely among MSM specifically [5].

Pathogenesis

Syphilis is a chronic bacterial infection caused by *Treponema pallidum*, subspecies *pallidum*, a long thin (6–15 μm), slowly growing bacterium that cannot be cultured for clinical purposes. With the exception of congenital syphilis, syphilis is spread

F. Pichi
Eye Institute, Cleveland Clinic Abu Dhabi, Abu Dhabi, UAE

Cleveland Clinic Lerner College of Medicine, Case Western Reserve University, Cleveland, OH, USA

T. A. Albini (✉)
Bascom Palmer Eye Institute, University of Miami Miller School, Department of Ophthalmology, Miami, FL, USA
e-mail: talbini@med.miami.edu

N. A. Rao et al. (eds.), *Posterior Uveitis*, Essentials in Ophthalmology,
https://doi.org/10.1007/978-3-030-03140-4_6

mainly through direct lesion contact. Because of the organism's slow growth, infection has a long incubation period, taking about 3 weeks from the time of inoculation to the appearance of initial (primary) lesions at the site of inoculation [6]. Without intervention, the organism then disseminates widely through the bloodstream and to the CNS where it might subsequently produce varying clinical manifestations.

The natural history of syphilis is one of a chronic infection that can cause a series of highly variable clinical manifestations during the first 2–3 years of infection, followed by a typically prolonged latent stage that can evolve into a clinically apparent tertiary infection stage years or even decades after initial infection [6].

Primary syphilis [6] refers to the presence of a primary or initial lesion at the site of inoculation of infection. In primary syphilis, the main clinical manifestation is the presence of a painless, usually solitary, indurated, clean-based ulcerative lesion that typically appears about 2–3 weeks after direct contact with another person's infectious lesion. The primary chancre can be accompanied by tender or non-tender regional lymphadenopathy. *T. pallidum* is present and might be demonstrable in specimens from the lesion base. Without treatment, after a period of 3–6 weeks, primary lesions spontaneously resolve without scarring. With treatment, lesions begin to resolve within a few days.

Secondary syphilis [6] results from hematogenous dissemination of infection. Although the classic manifestation of secondary syphilis is a painless, macular rash of 1–2 cm, reddish or copper colored, on the palms of the hands or soles of the feet (Fig. 1), symptoms such as malaise, myalgia, sore throat, headache, or low-grade fever are commonly detected. Without treatment, the lesions of secondary syphilis can spontaneously resolve without scarring. Resolution of untreated manifestations of secondary syphilis can typically take weeks to several months.

After resolution of secondary manifestations, untreated syphilis enters a latent stage in which clinical manifestations are absent, and the infection can only be detected through serological testing [6]. Latent syphilis [6] is further divided into early and late latent syphilis, a differentiation that affects treatment decisions. After a period of years, about a third of people with untreated latent syphilis will have further clinical manifestations as either late neurosyphilis (general paresis or tabes dorsalis), cardiovascular syphilis, or gummatous syphilis.

Neurosyphilis can occur at any time [6] during the course of infection. *T. pallidum* and cerebrospinal fluid (CSF) abnormalities can be detected in the CNS in a substantial proportion of patients with primary syphilis, many of whom do not have obvious neurological signs or symptoms. However, there is little evidence that the presence of CSF abnormalities affects therapeutic outcomes for patients with primary syphilis treated with long-acting penicillin. In later stages, CSF abnormalities in asymptomatic infected individuals are believed to identify those at increased risk for clinical neurosyphilis who require more intensive therapy.

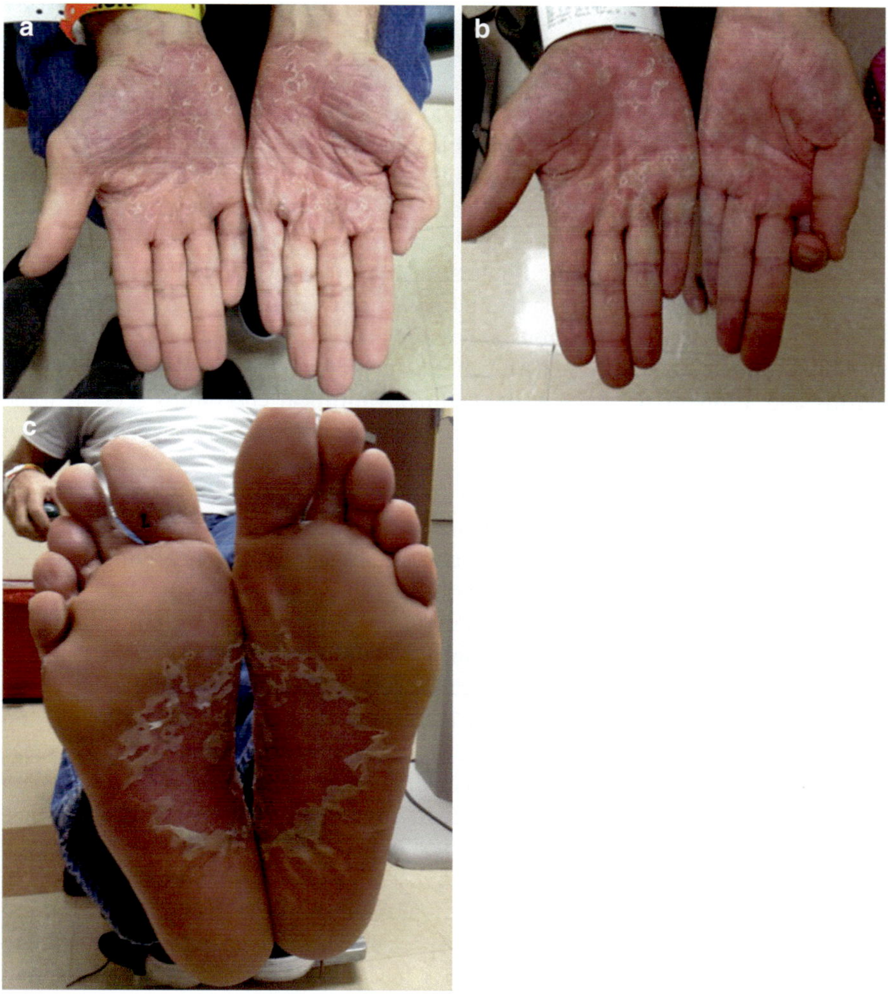

Fig. 1 A patient with secondary syphilis that presented with macular rash on the palms of the hands (**a**) that resolved after penicillin therapy (**b**). A similar rash can be seen on the soles of the feet (**c**)

Ocular Manifestations

Unlike other infectious agents that have a predilection either for the retina (cytomegalovirus) or for the choroid (*M. tuberculosis*), treponemas seem to be able to thrive in all the layers of the eye [7–9], resulting in a wide variety of clinical manifestations: anterior uveitis, focal/multifocal chorioretinitis, acute posterior placoid chorioretinitis, necrotizing retinitis, retinal vasculitis, intermediate uveitis, and panuveitis.

Syphilitic Posterior Uveitis

An important distinction is made between acute and chronic syphilitic posterior uveitis [10]. Acute syphilitic uveitic syndromes are usually florid, rapidly progressive, and associated with secondary syphilis and syphilitic meningitis [11]. Retinal involvement is a predominant feature and may lead to chorioretinitis, retinochoroiditis, neuroretinitis, and retinal necrosis [10–12]. Vitritis is prominent, and associated optic nerve swelling is seen in the majority of patients. Progressive visual loss is the rule [11], unless penicillin treatment is initiated that will clear inflammation in most patients. Chronic syphilitic posterior uveitis [10], a manifestation of tertiary syphilis, is often insidious and associated with subclinical neurosyphilis. Features common to all patients with chronic syphilitic posterior uveitis are a mild vitritis and a low-grade pigment epitheliitis. Multifocal choroiditis seen in some patients and mild retinal vasculitis observed in the majority are superimposed on this pattern.

1. *Syphilitic superficial retinal accumulations*: Preretinal accumulations [13–15], or precipitates even if nothing is actually "precipitating," overlying areas of active retinitis have been well described in the eyes with untreated syphilitic uveitis (Figs. 2, 3 and 4). Those unusual focal collections are probably white cells [13], as evidenced by the prominent concurrent vitritis and the fact that they quickly resolve after initiation of treatment [14]. They do not leave scars in the underlying retina. They are usually associated with retinal vasculitis [16] and mild, diffuse, adjacent retinal whitening. Retinal vasculitis tends to be vaso-occlusive [17] in nature and may affect all retinal vessels. Arteriolar involvement can take the form of occlusive arteriolitis, frosted branch angiitis, and/or Kyrieleis plaques. Small vessels are often involved in the form of cystoid macular edema. Retinal phlebitis [18] (Fig. 5) is the most frequent retinal vascular finding in posterior syphilis and may lead to angiographic changes consistent with central or branch vein occlusion. The clinical spectrum can range from vascular staining evident only on fluorescein angiography to increased vascular tortuosity, extensive perivascular exudation, and obliteration of vessels from an occlusive vasculitis [16–18].

   Fluorescein angiography and optical coherence tomography of these lesions have provided evidence for a focal accumulation of inflammatory material on the surface of the retina. On FA, the superficial retinal precipitates block fluorescence early and neither stain nor leak in late frames.
2. *Syphilitic multifocal retinitis*: Multiple reports have documented the occurrence of a distinctive multifocal retinitis in the eyes with syphilitic uveitis after administration of systemic or, more commonly, intravitreal corticosteroids in the absence of appropriate anti-treponemal therapy [19]. The intraretinal location of the foci of retinitis can be confirmed by SD-OCT and distinguishes these lesions from the previously described superficial retinal precipitates. The intraretinal location of these lesions may explain the limited recovery of vision in the eyes with macular involvement [19]. It is possible that corticosteroid exposure in the

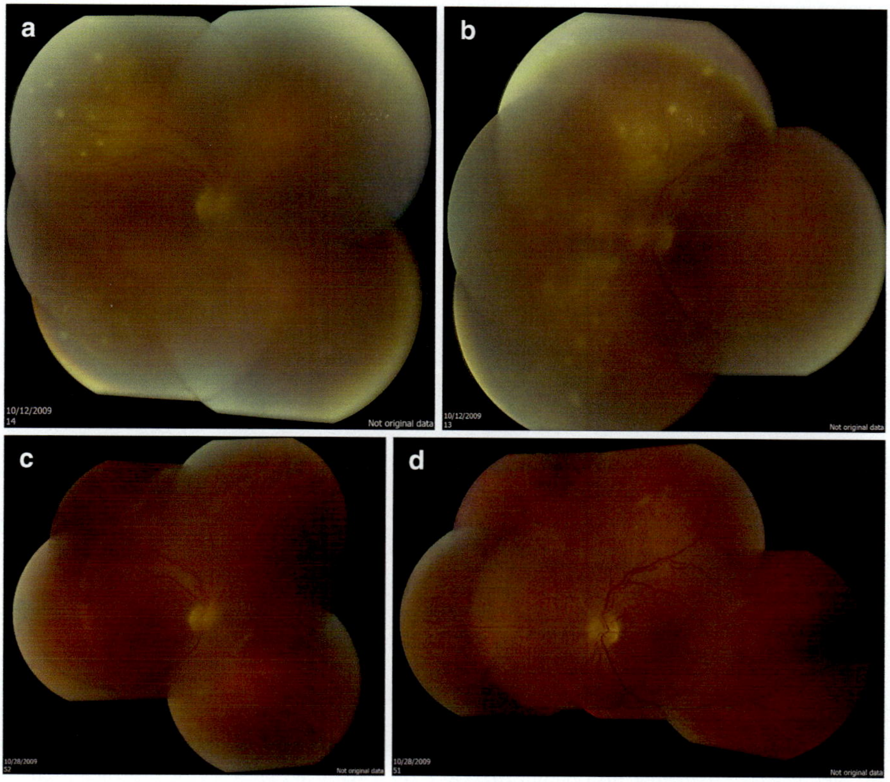

Fig. 2 Fundus photography (**a**) of the right eye and (**b**) of the left eye of a patient with superficial retinal accumulations. These findings resolve after penicillin therapy (**c**, **d**)

absence of antibiotic coverage can lead to treponemal infestation of the retina. Prompt penicillin therapy is essential to treat the retinal infection and limit permanent vision loss.

3. *Syphilitic retinochoroiditis*: There are two main forms of syphilitic chorioretinitis, confluent and placoid.
   - The confluent form presents with large, confluent areas of retinal whitening [20], which may resemble acute herpetic retinitis (Fig. 6) [21]. The confluent cases are typically "ground glass" in appearance, by which it is meant that the retinitis is not as densely necrotic as herpetic or toxoplasmic retinochoroiditis. There are, however, reports of denser, ARN- or toxo-like retinitis due to syphilis. Confluent retinochoroiditis is often in a triangular distribution and frequently associated with both vasculitis and overlying accumulations (Fig. 3a and b).
   - *Acute syphilitic posterior placoid chorioretinitis*. Gass et al. [22] coined the term ASPPC to describe a large, yellowish, circular, or oval placoid lesion at the level of the retinal pigment epithelium (RPE) in or near the macular (Fig. 7). This particular appearance, more common but not exclusive of HIV

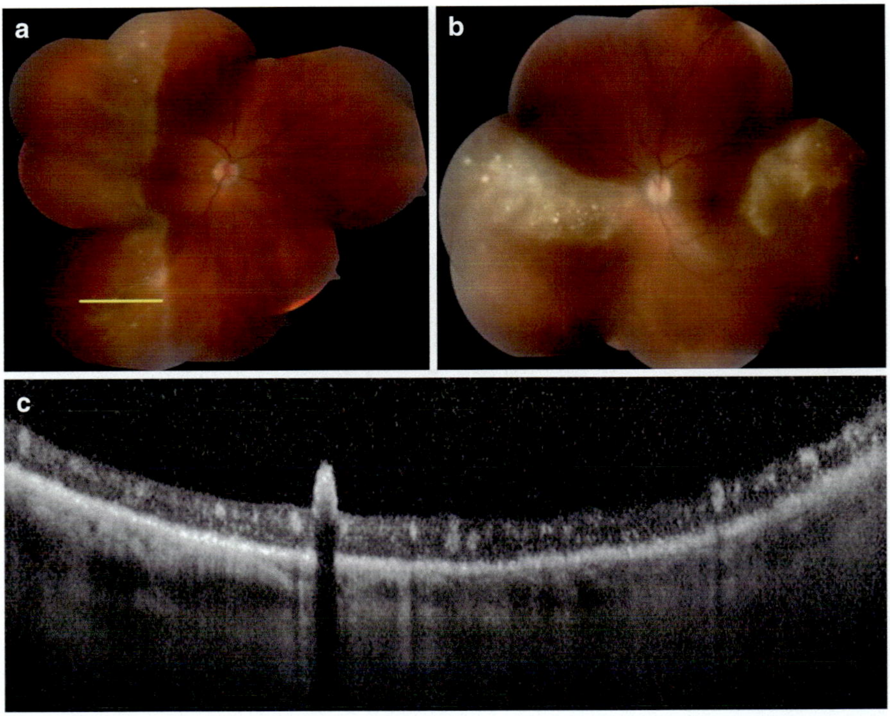

Fig. 3 A patient with bilateral syphilitic retinochoroiditis (**a**, **b**) with a ground-glass appearance (**a**) and a typical triangular distribution (**b**). OCT (**c**) reveals the presence of superficial retinal accumulations

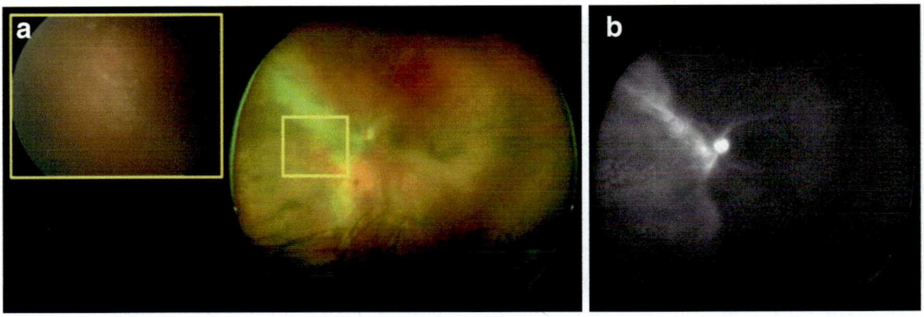

Fig. 4 An extensive focus of necrotic retinochoroiditis (**a**) with leakage of the margins in FA (**b**). On FA (**b**) multiple hypofluorescent spots correspond to superficial retinal accumulations (yellow square)

patients [23], is due to the fact that circulating *T. pallidum* organisms enter the choroidal circulation and gain access to the outer retina where the choroidal vascular supply is greatest—specifically the macula [24].

Fluorescein angiography shows early central hypofluorescence followed by progressive hyperfluorescence in the area of the lesion [24, 25]. This

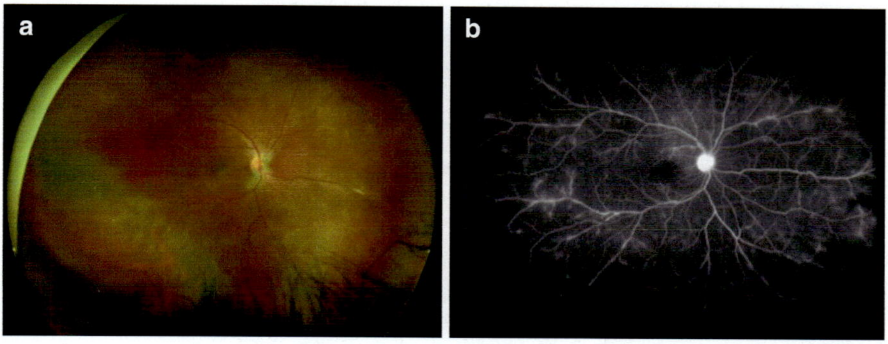

Fig. 5 Vasculitis in the right eye of a patient with syphilis uveitis. On color photography (**a**) Kyrieleis plaques are visible in the nasal periphery, but the diffuse extent of the vasculitis can be truly appreciated on FA (**b**)

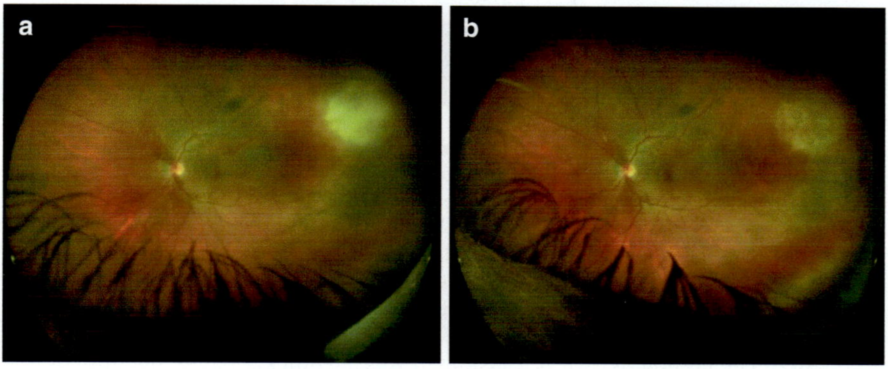

Fig. 6 A focus of necrotic retinochoroiditis (**a**) more "solid" in its appearance compared to Fig. 3. This aspect is less typical for syphilis and more common in acute retinal necrosis or toxoplasma retinitis. Following treatment there is resolution of inflammation (**b**)

hyperfluorescence may be associated with an active leading edge, identified angiographically as increased late leakage [25]. Occasionally a punctate hypofluorescence in a classic "leopard spot" pattern can be observed [25]. Indocyanine green angiography shows variable hypofluorescence in the area of the lesions suggesting either local choroidal hypoperfusion and/or blockage of the choroidal fluorescence by the overlying infected RPE [24].

On fundus autofluorescence, "geographic" hyperautofluorescence corresponding to the affected area can be noted, sometimes associated with punctate hyperautofluorescent spots suggestive of subretinal deposition of RPE-photoreceptor complex material and incomplete phagocytosis of outer segments [23, 26].

SD-OCT scans performed in the hyperacute phase (1–2 days) reveal [25] the uniform presence of a small amount of fluid under the fovea with no ELM disruption observed. Acute infection of the outer retina probably leads to disruption of the outer blood-ocular barrier producing variable amounts of

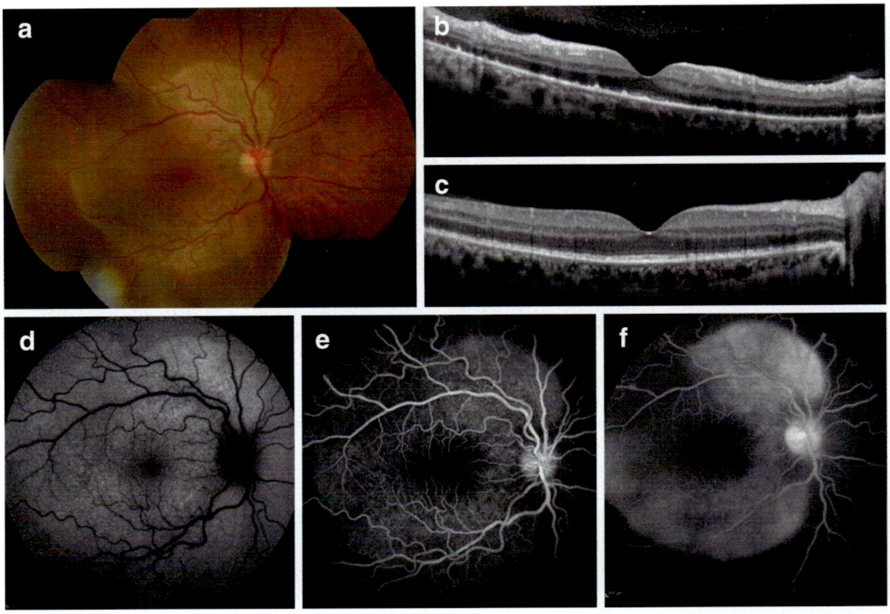

Fig. 7 Color photograph (**a**) of a patient with syphilitic placoid chorioretinitis showing an active, non-elevated, placoid yellowish outer retinal lesion involving the macula. SD-OCT shows an irregular thickening of the RPE layer with small nodular elevations along with a loss of the IS/OS junction and areas of punctate hyperreflectivity in the choroid (**b**). After therapy for neurosyphilis was completed, the SD-OCT showed complete restoration of the IS/OS junction and normalization of the contour of the RPE layer (**c**). Fundus autofluorescence (**d**) is punctate in the area of the lesion. Fluorescein angiography shows localized hyperfluorescence (**e**) with leakage from the area of the lesion (**f**)

SRF. The finding of SRF is transient, resolving quickly before the initiation of treatment. At 1 week after presentation, SD-OCT scans demonstrate an irregular hyperreflectivity with nodular elevations at the junction of the photoreceptors and the RPE. This is associated with segmental loss of the ellipsoid band. The irregularities of the RPE correspond to the hyperautofluorescent dots seen with FAF, suggesting the presence of lipofuscin accumulation or incomplete phagocytosis of outer segments. The ELM continues to appear intact at this time point. Spectral domain OCT scans taken at 1 month after therapy show complete resolution of the pathologic findings of the macula, with restoration of the ellipsoid zone and the RPE [25].

Syphilitic Optic Neuropathy

Although inflammatory conditions of the optic nerve are more common in the secondary stage, they may occur in tertiary syphilis as well [27].

Acute meningitis occurs in 1–2% of patients with secondary syphilis, and this can cause increased intracranial pressure and papilledema [28]. In pure papilledema,

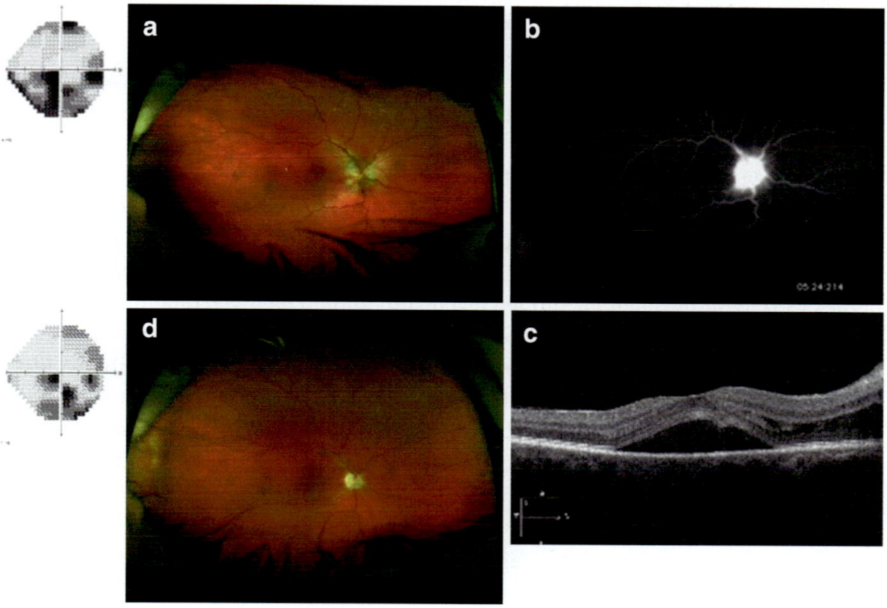

Fig. 8 Optic disc involvement in syphilitic uveitis (**a**) with papillitis presenting as centro-cecal scotoma. FA shows leakage from the swollen disc (**b**), and SD-OCT reveals subretinal fluid (**c**), confirming the diagnosis of neuroretinitis secondary to syphilis. Penicillin therapy resolves the inflammation of the nerve (**d**) with associated improvement of the visual field

there is enlargement of the blind spot but no signs of inflammatory cells in the vitreous. Papilledema should be differentiated from inflammatory optic disc edema due to optic neuritis, papillitis, or neuroretinitis. In papillitis [29], there is a swollen disc with intraretinal exudates and perivasculitis around it. When the inflammatory changes extend into the peripapillary retina resulting in hard exudates, the condition qualifies as neuroretinitis (Fig. 8).

The latter patients have marked loss of visual acuity and display central and cecocentral scotomas, or nerve fiber-bundle defects, and often have signs of vitreous inflammation.

Retrobulbar [30] syphilitic neuritis is associated with a funduscopically normal optic nerve or with minimal effacement of the edges.

Finally, syphilis can present as an optic perineuritis, which generally produces a concentric visual field defect and respects the visual acuity.

Laboratory Evaluation

Two different types of serologic tests are used [31], typically in sequence, one to identify individuals with possible infection and then a second unrelated confirmatory test to validate results and reduce false positives.

Traditional Algorithm Testing

So-called non-treponemal tests for syphilis are based on antigens extracted from normal mammalian tissues reacting with antibodies produced in response to *T. pallidum* infection [32]. Cardiolipin from beef heart allows the detection of anti-lipid IgG and IgM formed in the patient in response to lipoidal material released from cells damaged by the infection, as well as to lipids in the surface of *T. pallidum*. Prototypic non-treponemal tests include the rapid plasma reagin (RPR) and venereal disease research laboratory (VDRL) tests, which detect both IgG and IgM antibodies [33]. Non-treponemal antigen test results should be given quantitatively (i.e., titers, e.g., 1:16, 1:32). It should be emphasized that the titers of non-treponemal antigen tests correlate with the disease activity. Non-treponemal antibody titers decline as a result of treatment. A fourfold reduction in antibody titer of the same non-treponemal test is considered a significant response to treatment. Lack of expected reduction in titer or an increase in titer suggests treatment failure or reinfection [34].

Moreover, non-treponemal tests may be negative in as many as 30% of patients during the late latent or tertiary stages [32]. For this reason, if only one test can be obtained as an initial screening test for uveitis patients, a treponemal test is preferred. Ideally, a specific treponema antibody assay is obtained concurrently with the non-treponemal tests in all cases of suspected disease [33]; however, healthcare regulators and third-party payers are increasingly insisting on a single test for initial screening. Treponemal tests, which detect antibodies to treponemal antigens, include fluorescent treponemal antibody adsorbed (FTA-ABS) tests and *Treponema pallidum* particle agglutination (TPPA), but cheaper, easier to perform, and automatable treponemal tests such as enzyme immunoassays have become far more widely used. Irrespective, treponemal tests tend to be qualitative, rather than quantitative, but often remain positive for life, despite successful therapy and, therefore, are not helpful for evaluation of response to therapy.

Reverse Algorithm Testing

As the costs have decreased and the ease of treponemal tests has increased, so-called reverse algorithm testing has become more widely used in which a treponemal test is used as the initial screening test (typically IgG detection by EIA) [35]. It has been shown that in the general population, false-positive treponemal tests occur less frequently than false-positive non-treponemal tests, and starting with a treponemal test significantly reduces costs of the diagnostic procedure. Persons with a positive treponemal screening test should have a standard non-treponemal test performed (RPR). If the non-treponemal test is negative, then the laboratory should perform a different treponemal test (preferably one based on different antigens than the original test) to confirm the results of the initial test. If a second treponemal test is positive, persons with a history of previous treatment will require no further management (unless sexual history suggests likelihood of re-exposure). Those without a history of treatment for syphilis should be offered treatment. If the second treponemal test is negative, further evaluation or treatment is not indicated.

This reverse screening algorithm for syphilis testing strategy will identify both persons with previous treatment for syphilis and persons with untreated or incompletely treated syphilis, as well as some persons with false-positive results [36].

This approach has proven highly effective for screening low-prevalence populations, but a single head-to-head comparison of the reverse sequence algorithm with the traditional algorithm showed that the former would yield 6 false-positive results for each 1000 tests performed compared with none for the traditional algorithm [35, 36].

The CDC continues to recommend the use of the traditional RPR-based screening algorithm.

Cerebrospinal Fluid

Because neurosyphilis can be asymptomatic or present in many different ways, analysis of CSF is often helpful to confirm its presence. However, according to the CDC, only the following patients should have a lumbar puncture at diagnosis of syphilis [37]: those with neurologic, ophthalmic, or otologic signs or symptoms; evidence of active tertiary syphilitic disease; or treatment failure (defined as a sustained fourfold increase in VDRL or RPR or high (>1:32) RPR titer that does not decline 2 titers over 6–12 months in early syphilis or 12–24 months in latent syphilis). While a presumptive diagnosis of ocular syphilis can be made without a lumbar puncture, a lumbar puncture can confirm the diagnosis and provide guidance to the clinician in the case that the patient's symptoms do not resolve after treatment. The CDC recommends lumbar puncture in all patients with ocular syphilis to detect neurosyphilis, but there is debate whether this procedure is justified in patients with isolated anterior segment inflammation [37].

The standard serologic test for cerebrospinal fluid (CSF) is VDRL [31, 37]. Noteworthy, the other non-treponemal tests such as RPR and USR are not recommended for CSF. It is emphasized that the VDRL in CSF is highly specific. A positive result, in the absence of CSF contamination with blood, confirms the diagnosis. However, a negative result does not exclude neurosyphilis. CSF-VDRL may be negative in 30–70% of neurosyphilis cases. Both the IUSTI and CDC highlight that in the cases of the negative CSF-VDRL, other tests should be taken into consideration, such as treponemal assays, CSF cell count, and protein and glucose levels. Treponemal tests performed in CSF (TPHA, FTA-ABS, EIA) are highly sensitive but nonspecific for the neurosyphilis diagnosis. This means that the negative results exclude neurosyphilis, but the positive result does not confirm the diagnosis. The CSF white cell count cutoff values, which may suggest neurosyphilis, have been established on the ≥ 5 cells/mm^3 in immunocompetent patients with syphilis and ≥ 20 cells/mm^3 in HIV-positive patients. Neurosyphilis may be also associated with the CSF protein concentration higher than 45 mg/dl and the CSF glucose levels of less than 2.72 mmol/l.

Additionally, all patients with a new diagnosis of ocular syphilis should be tested for HIV infection as well as screening for other common STDs, especially gonorrhea and chlamydia. All patients with a new diagnosis of HIV should be screened for syphilis.

Treatment

Ocular syphilis is treated in exactly the same way as neurosyphilis [38]. Since benzathine penicillin does not penetrate the blood-ocular barrier, aqueous penicillin G or procaine penicillin G plus probenecid should be given [39]. For patients with neurosyphilis, recommended treatment is higher doses (18–24 million units per day in divided doses) of intravenous aqueous penicillin G administered every 4 h for 10–14 days, and some experts recommend two to three doses of benzathine benzylpenicillin after completion of intravenous therapy to mirror the duration of therapy for late infections [39].

Treatment of patients with syphilis who have a proven penicillin allergy can be challenging [40, 41]. Fluoroquinolone, sulfonamides, and aminoglycoside antibiotics are not effective. The data on doxycycline suggest that it is an acceptable alternate agent for early and late latent syphilis when penicillin therapy is not feasible [39–42]. Azithromycin as a single 2-g oral dose has been effective for treating early syphilis in some settings [40]. However, *T. pallidum* chromosomal mutations associated with azithromycin (and other macrolide) resistance and treatment failures have been documented in multiple geographical areas in the United States. Accordingly, azithromycin should be used with caution only when treatment with penicillin or doxycycline is not feasible. Azithromycin should not be used in MSM or pregnant women. Careful follow-up of patients receiving any alternative therapies is essential. There are no recommendations to modify therapy for pregnant women or for patients with HIV infection.

There is certainly a place for adjunctive corticosteroid therapy in the management of syphilitic eye disease. Topical steroids are of benefit as an adjunctive treatment in syphilitic keratitis, scleritis, and anterior uveitis. Systemic steroids always in combination with appropriate antibiotic therapy have a role in the treatment of posterior uveitis and optic nerve inflammation [38].

The current CDC guidelines recommend 6- and 12-month follow-up for HIV-uninfected persons and 3-, 6-, 9-, and 12-month follow-up visits for HIV-infected persons with early syphilis (to maximize the probability of follow-up at some time) [39].

After syphilis treatment, 30–50% of treated patients have a Jarisch-Herxheimer reaction, an acute febrile illness with headache, myalgia, chills, and rigors that occur within 24 h of the initiation of treatment for ocular syphilis, probably as a result of endotoxin release and cytokine elevation [41]. Typically, patients have been described as having a rapid loss of vision after the first adequate dose of penicillin. Systemic steroids may dampen but not completely prevent the Jarisch-Herxheimer reaction. Antitumor necrosis factor antibodies seem to be more effective than steroids.

Response to therapy is indicated by a two fold or greater dilution decline in nontreponemal serological test titers or, if initial titers are positive at a 1:1 or 1:2 dilution, by becoming nonreactive [39, 42]. A meaningful serological response to therapy is more likely if patients are younger, have earlier stages of disease, have higher serological test titers at the time of diagnosis, or experience a Jarisch-Herxheimer reaction.

Monitoring of response to therapy in neurosyphilis can be challenging, and there have been few formal studies of its efficacy because of difficulties in getting follow-up lumbar punctures. A serological response to therapy using the rapid plasma reagin test is highly predictive of resolution of both neurological and CSF abnormalities. The CDC recommends repeating a lumbar puncture if CSF pleocytosis was present initially (and recommends considering repeating an LP if the CSF-VDRL or CSF protein evaluations were abnormal) every 6 months until the cell count has normalized. If the cell count has not decreased after 6 months, or CSF cell count or protein has not normalized after 6 months, retreatment should be considered. When follow-up CSF studies are available, the white blood cell count is the earliest variable to respond, whereas a reactive CSF-VDRL test can take years to change and additionally could be slower in individuals with HIV. CSF protein determination in individuals with neurosyphilis is both nonspecific and can be slow to resolve.

Compliance with Ethical Requirements Francesco Pichi and Thomas A. Albini declare that they have no conflict of interest. No human or animal studies were carried out by the authors for this chapter.

References

1. Rothschild BM. History of syphilis. Clin Infect Dis. 2005;40(10):1454–63. https://doi.org/10.1086/429626.
2. Fracastorius H. Syphilis Sive Morbus Gallicus (Venice, 1530) Hieronymus Fracastor's Syphilis [anonymous translation]. St. Louis: Philmar; 1911. p. 24.
3. Hook EW, Peeling RW. Syphilis control—a continuing challenge. N Engl J Med. 2004;351(2):122–4. https://doi.org/10.1056/NEJMp048126.
4. Centers for Disease Control and Prevention. Sexually transmitted disease surveillance 2015. Atlanta: U.S. Department of Health and Human Services; 2016.
5. Fonollosa A, Giralt J, Pelegrín L, Sánchez-Dalmau B, Segura A, García- Arumí J, Adan A. Ocular syphilis—back again: understanding recent increases in the incidence of ocular syphilitic disease. Ocul Immunol Inflamm. 2009;17(3):207–12.
6. Anderson J, Mindel A, Tovey SJ, Williams P. Primary and secondary syphilis, 20 years' experience. 3: diagnosis, treatment, and follow up. Genitourin Med. 1989;65(4):239–43.
7. Aldave AJ, King JA, Cunningham ET. Ocular syphilis. Curr Opin Ophthalmol. 2001;12(6):433–41. https://doi.org/10.1097/00055735-200112000-00008.
8. Davis JL. Ocular syphilis. Curr Opin Ophthalmol. 2014;25(6):513–8. https://doi.org/10.1097/ICU.0000000000000099.
9. Tamesis RR, Foster CS. Ocular syphilis. Ophthalmology. 1990;97(10):1281–7.
10. Villanueva AV, Sahouri MJ, Ormerod LD, Puklin JE, Reyes MP. Posterior uveitis in patients with positive serology for syphilis. Clin Infect Dis. 2000;30(3):479–85. https://doi.org/10.1086/313689.

11. Ormerod LD, Puklin JE, Sobel JD. Syphilitic posterior uveitis: correlative findings and significance. Clin Infect Dis. 2001;32(12):1661–73. https://doi.org/10.1086/320766.
12. Kuo A, Ziaee SM, Hosseini H, et al. The great imitator: ocular syphilis presenting as posterior uveitis. Am J Case Rep. 2015;16:434–7. https://doi.org/10.12659/AJCR.893907.
13. Fu EX, Geraets RL, Dodds EM, et al. Superficial retinal precipitates in patients with syphilitic retinitis. Retina. 2010;30(7):1135–43.
14. Rodrigues RAM, Nascimento HM d, Muccioli C, Rodrigues RAM, do NHM, Muccioli C. Yellowish dots in the retina: a finding of ocular syphilis? Arq Bras Oftalmol. 2014;77(5):324–6.
15. Reddy S, Cunningham ET, Spaide RF. Syphilitic retinitis with focal inflammatory accumulations. Ophthalmic surgery, lasers imaging. Off J Int Soc Imaging Eye. 2006;37(5):429–31.
16. Crouch ER, Goldberg MF. Retinal periarteritis secondary to syphilis. Arch Ophthalmol (Chicago, Ill 1960). 1975;93(5):384–7.
17. Yokoi M, Kase M. Retinal vasculitis due to secondary syphilis. Jpn J Ophthalmol. 2004;48(1):65–7. https://doi.org/10.1007/s10384-003-0011-5.
18. Lobes LA, Folk JC. Syphilitic phlebitis simulating branch vein occlusion. Ann Ophthalmol. 1981;13(7):825–7.
19. Curi AL, Sarraf D, Cunningham ET Jr. Multimodal imaging of syphilitic multifocal retinitis. Retin Cases Brief Rep. 2015;9(4):277–80.
20. Lima BR, Mandelcorn ED, Bakshi N, Nussenblatt RB, Sen HN. Syphilitic outer retinopathy. Ocul Immunol Inflamm. 2014;22(1):4–8.
21. Mendelsohn AD, Jampol LM. Syphilitic retinitis. A cause of necrotizing retinitis. Retina. 1984;4(4):221–4.
22. Gass JD, Braunstein RA, Chenoweth RG. Acute syphilitic posterior placoid chorioretinitis. Ophthalmology. 1990;97(10):1288–97.
23. Meira-Freitas D, Farah ME, Höfling-Lima AL, Aggio FB. Optical coherence tomography and indocyanine green angiography findings in acute syphilitic posterior placoid choroidopathy: case report. Arq Bras Oftalmol. 2009;72:832–5.
24. Eandi CM, Neri P, Adelman RA, et al. Acute syphilitic posterior placoid chorioretinitis: report of a case series and comprehensive review of the literature. Retina. 2012;32:1915–41.
25. Pichi F, Ciardella AP, Cunningham ET Jr, Morara M, Veronese C, Jumper JM, Albini TA, Sarraf D, McCannel C, Voleti V, Choudhry N, Bertelli E, Giuliari GP, Souied E, Amer R, Regine F, Ricci F, Neri P, Nucci P. Spectral domain optical coherence tomography findings in patients with acute syphilitic posterior placoid chorioretinopathy. Retina. 2014;34(2):373–84.
26. Cunningham ET Jr, Eandi CM, Pichi F. Syphilitic uveitis. Ocul Immunol Inflamm. 2014 Feb;22(1):2–3.
27. Smith GT. Neurosyphilis with optic neuritis: an update. Postgrad Med J. 2006;82(963):36–9.
28. Currie JN, Coppeto JR, Lessell S. Chronic syphilitic meningitis resulting in superior orbital fissure syndrome and posterior fossa gumma. A report of two cases followed for 20 years. J Clin Neuroophthalmol. 1988;8(3):145–59.
29. Weinstein JM, Lexow SS, Ho P, Spickards A. Acute syphilitic optic neuritis. Arch Ophthalmol. 1981;99(8):1392–5.
30. Folk JC, Weingeist TA, Corbett JJ, Lobes LA, Watzke RC. Syphilitic neuroretinitis. Am J Ophthalmol. 1983;95(4):480–6.
31. Hart G. Syphilis tests in diagnostic and therapeutic decision making. Ann Intern Med. 1986;104(3):368–76.
32. Majumder PD, Sudharshan S, Biswas J. Laboratory support in the diagnosis of uveitis. Indian J Ophthalmol. 2013;61(6):269–76.
33. Morshed MG. Current trend on syphilis diagnosis: issues and challenges. Adv Exp Med Biol. 2014;808:51–64.
34. Tsang RS, Morshed M, Chernesky MA, Jayaraman GC, Kadkhoda K. Canadian Public Health Laboratory Network laboratory guidelines for the use of direct tests to detect syphilis in Canada. Can J Infect Dis Med Microbiol. 2015;26(Suppl A):13A–7A.

35. Centers for Disease Control and Prevention. Discordant results from reverse sequence syphilis screening- five laboratories, United States, 2006–2010. MMWR Morbid Mortal Wkly Rep. 2011;60:133–7.
36. Centers for Disease Control and Prevention. Syphilis testing algorithms using treponemal tests for initial screening- four laboratories, New York City, 2005–2006. MMWR Morbid Mortal Wkly Rep. 2008;57:872–5.
37. Guarner J, Jost H, Pillay A, et al. Evaluation of treponemal serum tests performed on cerebrospinal fluid for diagnosis of neurosyphilis. Am J Clin Pathol. 2015;143(4):479–84.
38. Jay CA. Treatment of neurosyphilis. Curr Treat Options Neurol. 2006;8(3):185–92.
39. Browning DJD. Posterior segment manifestations of active ocular syphilis, their response to a neurosyphilis regimen of penicillin therapy, and the influence of human immunodeficiency virus status on response. Ophthalmology. 2000;107(0):2015–23.
40. Lukehart SA, Godornes C, Molini BJ, et al. Macrolide resistance in Treponema pallidum in the United States and Ireland. N Engl J Med. 2004;351(2):154–8.
41. Martin IE, Tsang RSW, Sutherland K, et al. Molecular characterization of syphilis in patients in Canada: azithromycin resistance and detection of Treponema pallidum DNA in whole-blood samples versus ulcerative swabs. J Clin Microbiol. 2009;47(6):1668–73.
42. Rolfs RT, Joesoef MR, Hendershot EF, et al. A randomized trial of enhanced therapy for early syphilis in patients with and without human immunodeficiency virus infection. The Syphilis and HIV Study Group. N Engl J Med. 1997;337(5):307–14.

Ocular Tuberculosis

Soumyava Basu

Introduction, Clinical Features, Differential Diagnosis, and Treatment

Mycobacterium tuberculosis has been associated with a wide variety of intraocular inflammation, especially in tuberculosis (TB)-endemic countries [1]. Even in non-endemic countries with significant migrant populations [2], it remains one of the important differentials for a variety of uveitis presentations. The disease is diagnosed on the basis of suggestive clinical signs; presence of ancillary evidence of TB such as tuberculin skin test (TST), interferon gamma release assays (IGRA), or radiological signs of TB; and exclusion of non-TB entities. Microbiological evidence of *M. tuberculosis* is rarely found in ocular fluid samples.

Clinical features of intraocular TB can manifest in any tissue of the eye, except the crystalline lens. However, isolated anterior uveitis (granulomatous or non-granulomatous) or intermediate uveitis are relatively uncommon in intraocular TB. The disease more commonly manifests in the posterior segment of the eye. The "classic" posterior segment manifestations such as choroidal tubercles, choroidal or optic nerve tuberculoma, and subretinal abscess are generally associated with systemic TB, relatively easy to diagnose but rare in ophthalmology practice. More commonly, patients present with retinal vasculitis (with or without focal chorioretinitis overlying blood vessels), multifocal choroiditis, or serpiginous-like choroiditis [3]. Here ocular imaging plays a crucial role in identification of specific patterns that have been associated with intraocular TB. These include fundus photography, fluorescein and indocyanine green angiography, autofluorescence, optical coherence tomography (OCT) and OCT-angiography, or multimodal imaging involving several of the above techniques [4]. *Ancillary tests* such as TST, IGRA, and chest

S. Basu (✉)
Retina and Uveitis Service, L V Prasad Eye Institute, Bhubaneswar, India
e-mail: basu@lvpei.org

N. A. Rao et al. (eds.), *Posterior Uveitis*, Essentials in Ophthalmology,
https://doi.org/10.1007/978-3-030-03140-4_7

radiography provide evidence for systemic mycobacterial infection, but neither are they positive confirmatory tests for intraocular TB, nor do negative tests completely rule out the condition. In addition to the above ancillary tests, patients often require specific laboratory investigations for exclusion of different infectious and noninfectious etiologies.

Differential diagnosis of intraocular TB depends on the clinical presentation of the disease. Thus, for anterior uveitis, it could vary from sarcoidosis to HLA-B27-associated uveitis, while for serpiginous-like choroiditis, it could be autoimmune serpiginous choroidopathy or one of the several infections that can cause a similar clinical appearance. Conversely, TB should be ruled out in any form of uveitis in case there is no conclusive evidence of a specific etiological diagnosis and there is history of exposure to TB-endemic populations.

The *treatment* of intraocular TB requires a combination of anti-TB therapy and corticosteroid therapy. The World Health Organization (WHO) guidelines for anti-TB therapy (ATT) are summarized in Table 1. While there are no specific WHO guidelines for intraocular TB, generally anti-TB therapy is initiated with 4-drug therapy for 2 months and followed with 2-drug therapy for 4–7 months [5]. Concomitant corticosteroid therapy can be given topically, locally, or systemically depending on the degree and primary location of inflammation. Paradoxical worsening of ocular inflammatory lesions can be seen after initiation of ATT – these are

Table 1 World Health Organization (WHO) recommendations for first-line treatment of tuberculosis (2010, 4th ed.)

Drug	Daily dosage (mg/kg body weight)	Side effects (*common*)
Rifampicin (R)	5 (4–6), maximum 300 mg	Gastrointestinal upset, drug interactions, hepatitis, flu-like symptoms
Isoniazid (H)	10 (8–12), maximum 600 mg	Rash, hepatitis, peripheral neuropathy
Pyrazinamide (Z)	25 (20–30)	Hepatitis, rash, gastrointestinal upset, hyperuricemia
Ethambutol (E)	15 (15–20)	Optic neuritis, rash
Standard regimen	2 months of HRZE and 4 months of HR (there is no recommendation yet on duration for ocular TB, although longer duration has been advised for central nervous system, bone, and joint TB). WHO *no longer* recommends omission of ethambutol during the intensive phase of treatment for patients with non-cavitary, smear-negative PTB or EPTB who are known to be HIV-negative	
Treatment of latent TB	Recommended in the following groups: people living with HIV, adult and child contacts of pulmonary TB cases, patients initiating anti-TNF treatment, patients receiving dialysis, patients preparing for organ or hematologic transplantation, and patients with silicosis. Various regimens have been suggested, most commonly isoniazid monotherapy for 6–9 months	

PTB pulmonary tuberculosis, *EPTB* extrapulmonary tuberculosis, *HIV* human immunodeficiency virus, *TNF* tumor necrosis factor usually managed by increasing corticosteroid dosage while continuing ATT. Since microbiological evidence of *M. tuberculosis* infection is lacking in nearly all cases of intraocular TB, serial ocular imaging is critical during the follow-up period to evaluate efficacy of treatment and possible recurrences.

Widefield Color Fundus Photo, Fluorescein Angiography, and ICG Angiography

Fundus photography helps in accurately documenting chorioretinal lesions in posterior and panuveitis. Serial fundus photographs during the course of treatment can help in documenting resolution or progression of existing lesions or the appearance of new lesions (Fig. 1). Recently, widefield and ultra-widefield photography has been applied for acquiring images of the peripheral fundus that are usually missed by conventional imaging [6]. It also has the advantage of rapidly imaging the entire fundus with minimal discomfort to the patient.

Fluorescein angiography has two important applications in intraocular TB: demonstration of specific patterns in different posterior segment presentations and detection of post-inflammatory complications. Thus, choroidal lesions such as serpiginous-like choroiditis or choroidal granuloma would reveal early hypo- and late hyperfluorescence, at the active sites (Fig. 2a–c). Tubercular retinal vasculitis is typically associated with large areas of capillary non-perfusion, which is generally not seen in sarcoidosis. At a later stage, such retinal ischemia can lead to neovascularization of the retina or disc. Rarely, healed or even active choroiditis lesions may

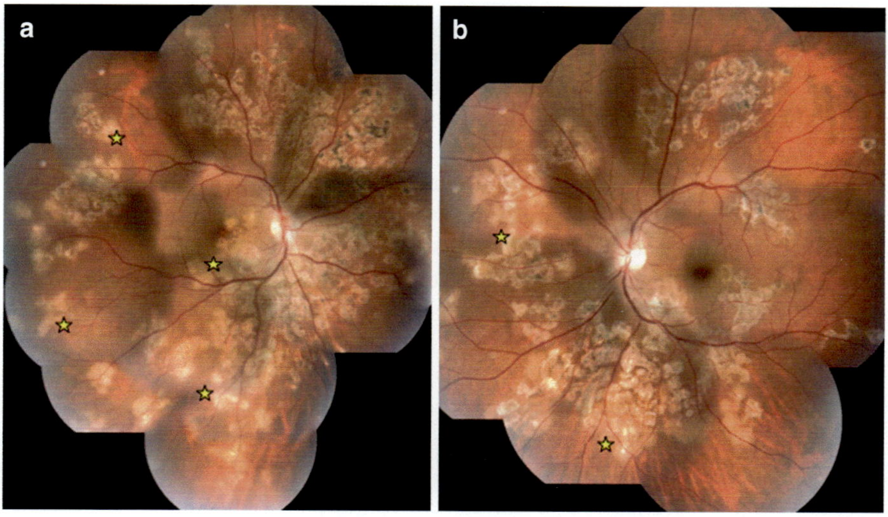

Fig. 1 (**a**, **b**) Color montage photograph of right and left fundus, respectively, of a 22-year-old female, with multifocal areas of confluent, serpigenoid choroiditis. Active lesions appear as bright yellow (stars), while healing lesions have various degrees of pigmentation

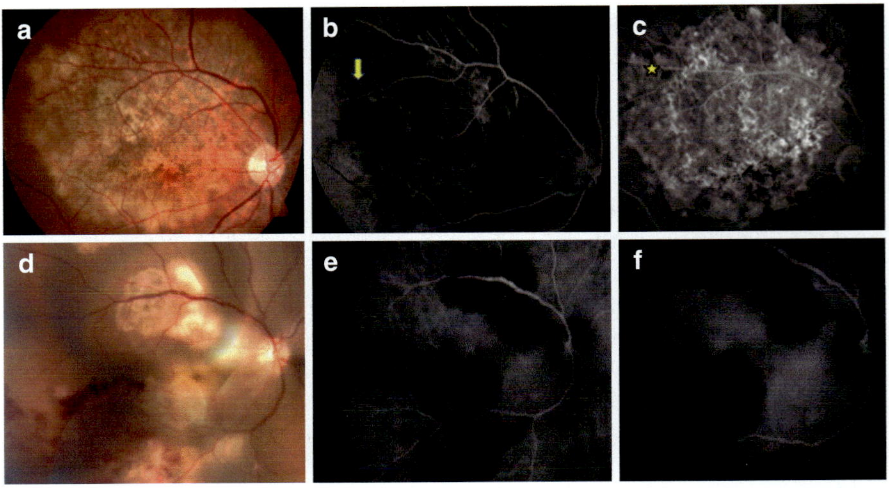

Fig. 2 (**a**) Color fundus photograph of the right eye of a 32-year-old female with TB-associated serpiginous-like choroiditis. (**b**, **c**) Fluorescein angiogram of the same eye with hypofluorescence corresponding to active lesions that later became hyperfluorescent due to staining of lesions. (**d**) Color fundus photograph of the right eye of a 28-year-old male, with serpiginous-like choroiditis involving the superior vascular arcade. (**e**, **f**) Indocyanine green angiogram of the above patient showing hypocyanescence in the early stage that persists in the late stage

be associated with choroidal neovascularization, which needs to be differentiated from choroidal inflammation, for initiation of anti-angiogenic therapy. Widefield and ultra-widefield fluorescein angiography can reveal additional information on extent of vasculitis or choroiditis lesions, simultaneously imaging both central and peripheral fundus [7, 8].

ICG angiography has a special role in diagnosis of intraocular TB, as a large number of lesions originate either in the outer retina-choriocapillaris complex (serpiginous-like choroiditis) or entirely within the choroid (choroidal tubercle). Serpiginous-like choroiditis is associated with multifocal areas of choriocapillaris occlusion [9, 10]. These appear hypocyanescent in the initial frames of the ICG angiogram and remain so even in the late stages, unlike in fluorescein angiography where active lesions become hyperfluorescent due to staining in late stages (Fig. 2d–f). Purely choroidal lesions are also hypocyanescent in the early stages. However, partial-thickness lesions become isocyanescent in the later stages, while full-thickness lesions remain hypocyanescent, due to the mass effect.

Autofluorescence

Fundus autofluorescence is a noninvasive technique for delineating chorioretinal lesions in posterior and panuveitis. The autofluorescence is derived from lipofuscin accumulated in the cytosol of retinal pigment epithelium (RPE). Experimental models have revealed mitochondrial oxidative damage to photoreceptors following

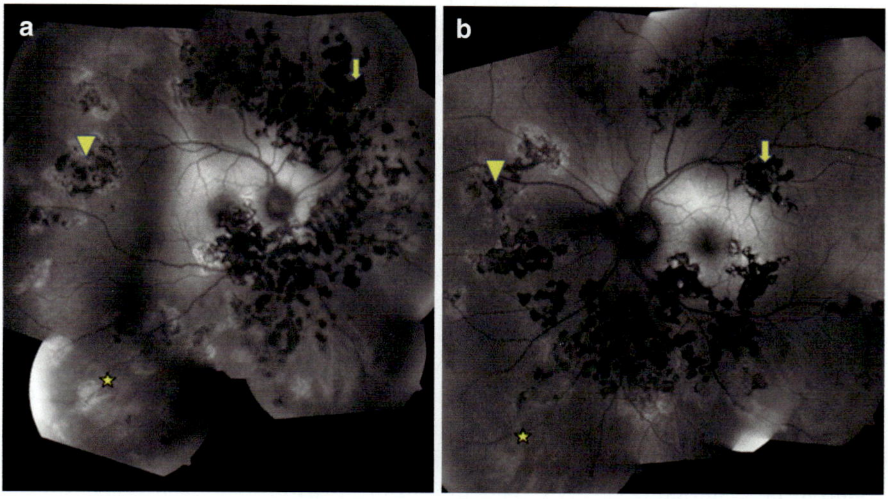

Fig. 3 (**a**, **b**) Fundus autofluorescence photographs of the left and right eyes of a patient in Fig. 1, showing varying degrees of activity. New, active lesions (mostly in the periphery) show diffuse hyperautofluorescence (star). As the lesions heal, they develop gradual increase in mottling (initially hyper- and later hypoautofluorescence mottling) till they become uniformly hypoautofluorescent

inflammatory stimulus, leading to the accumulation of lipofuscin in RPE [11]. This happens before infiltration of inflammatory cells into the retina/choroid and probably represents the earliest clinical sign of inflammation. Fundus autofluorescence is most commonly used for studying the pattern, progression, and response to treatment in serpiginous-like choroiditis [12–14]. Active inflammation appears as hyperautofluorescence, while complete resolution typically leads to hypoautofluorescence (Fig. 3). Intermediate stages of resolution appear as increasing dots of hypoautofluorescence within earlier areas of hyperautofluorescence [13]. The few remaining punctate areas of hyperautofluorescence tend to persist for up to 3 months during the chronic phase of the disease. Thus, autofluorescence could be one of the earliest signs of disease activity and also one of the last to disappear, following initiation of therapy.

OCT

OCT has been used for evaluation of various retinal layers including the RPE, as well as the choroid. It has applications in identification of disease pattern, progression as well as various complications of intraocular TB (Fig. 4). The outer retina – RPE – choriocapillaris complex is typically imaged in serpiginous-like choroiditis, where hyper-reflective bumps are seen corresponding to the areas of hyperautofluorescence [4, 12]. The histological basis of these OCT features was recently revealed in a patient with serpiginous-like choroiditis, in whom chorioretinal biopsy of the lesions was performed following poor response to treatment [15]. The biopsy showed granulomatous inflammation with caseous necrosis of the inner choroid that was accompanied by photoreceptor disruption, focal loss, and necrosis of the RPE.

As lesions heal and hypoautofluorescence gradually appears, these hyper-reflective bumps on OCT are replaced by thinning of the outer retina. Rarely, anatomical restoration of the outer retina is seen instead of atrophy. The choroid also regains normal thickness in these rare cases.

Enhanced depth imaging OCT (EDI-OCT) is used for visualization of the choroid and inner sclera. Choroidal imaging is vital as it is central to the pathogenesis of intraocular TB, either as the primary site of infection or from being contiguous to infection originating in the RPE and retina. EDI-OCT can be used for anatomical localization of the lesions as well as assessing changes in choroidal thickness after initiation of treatment. Recent studies have shown that choroidal thickness is significantly increased in active disease and decreases with resolution of inflammation, with or without atrophy of the choriocapillaris [16]. Interestingly, similar thickening is seen in ocular sarcoidosis as well, but here the medium vessel Sattler's layer is found to be disproportionately enlarged. EDI-OCT also provides insights into the morphological changes in the choroid, corresponding to the focal lesions seen in intraocular TB [17]. The active chorioretinitis lesions that appear as choriocapillaris hypoperfusion on ICG have been associated with areas of increased choroidal

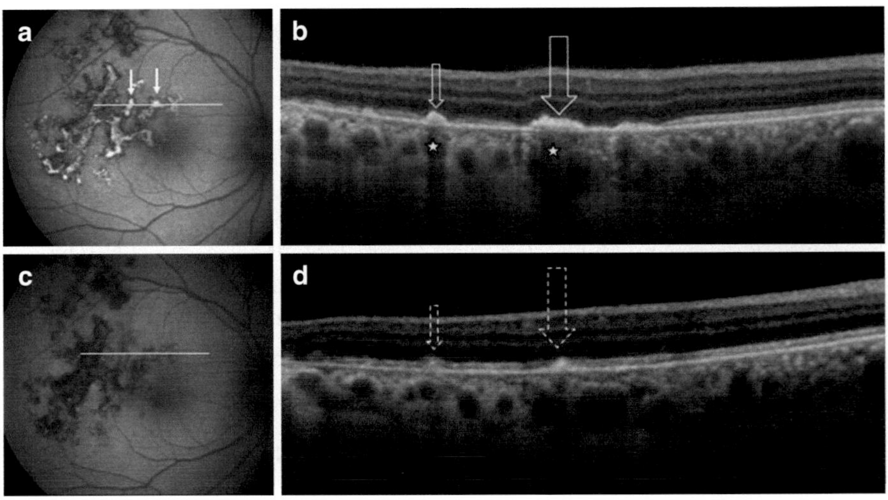

Fig. 4 (**a**, **b**) Fundus autofluorescence photograph of a patient with serpiginous-like choroiditis, and the corresponding EDI-OCT scan showing hyper-reflective bumps in the outer retina (block arrows) through areas of hyperautofluorescence (arrows). The underlying choroid is thickened and shows areas of increased choroidal homogeneity (stars) that are hypodense and suggestive of a granuloma. However, increased choroidal transmittance through the lesions, as reported earlier, was not seen in the scan. Greater transmittance is seen through the adjacent luminal structures that represent choroidal vessels. (**c**, **d**) Healed lesions in the same patient showing hypoautofluorescence and disappearance of outer retinal hyper-reflectivity in the corresponding EDI-OCT scan (dashed arrows). The choroidal thickness also appears to have reduced, and the homogenous areas reduced in size

homogeneity on EDI-OCT that could be hypo- or isodense, representative of a tubercular granuloma (Fig. 4b, d). These homogenous areas can be differentiated from large choroidal vessels by increased transmittance through the lesion. They regain the normal heterogenous pattern on resolution of inflammation.

Evolving Imaging Modalities

New treatment modalities have emerged in the last few years that provide valuable insight into morphology and likely patho-mechanisms of intraocular TB. Prominent among these is *OCT-angiography* (OCT-A) – a noninvasive imaging tool for vascular networks in the retina and choroid. The OCT-A features in serpiginous-like choroiditis have been well characterized (Fig. 5). During active inflammation, flow void areas are seen in the choriocapillaris layer that correspond to hypoperfusion seen on ICG angiography and hyperautofluorescence [4]. As the lesions heal, the flow void areas are gradually replaced by an irregular meshwork of choriocapillaris that persist even after the lesions have healed completely. OCT-A changes appear to occur earlier that that seen on autofluorescence and correspond better to subjective improvement reported by patients [18]. OCT-A can also be useful in demonstration of choroidal neovascularization and non-neovascular tufts in the choriocapillaris layer and capillary non-perfusion in the retinal vasculature in eyes with retinal vasculitis.

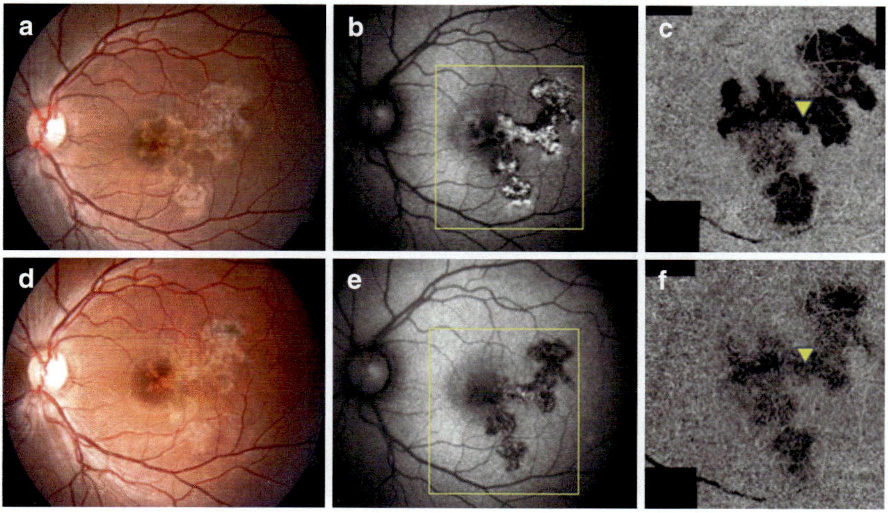

Fig. 5 (**a–c**) Active serpiginous-like choroiditis (inset) in the left eye, showing "flow void areas" in the choriocapillaris layer on OCT-angiography, corresponding to areas of hyperautofluorescence. (**d–f**) As the lesions heal, the flow void areas are replaced by a tangled meshwork of vessels, whose arrangement is different from the surrounding choriocapillaris. This change may appear even though parts of the lesion continue to be hyperautofluorescent

Table 2 Imaging characteristics of TB-associated serpiginous-like choroiditis in active and healed stages

	Active	Healed
FAF	Diffuse hyperautofluorescence	Gradual mottling during healing, finally leading to complete hypoautofluorescence
EDI-OCT	"Bumpy" hyper-reflectivity in outer retina and retinal pigment epithelium (RPE)	Atrophy of outer retina and RPE – disruption of ellipsoid, myoid layers, and external limiting membrane
FFA	Early hypofluorescence and late hyperfluorescence	Early and late hyperfluorescence due to RPE transmission defect
ICGA	Hypocyancescence in early phase, which persists in late phases	Same as in active stage

FAF fundus autofluorescence, *EDI-OCT* enhanced depth imaging-optical coherence tomography, *FFA* fundus fluorescein angiography, *ICGA* indocyanine green angiography

Retromode imaging is another noninvasive imaging technique that uses confocal scanning laser ophthalmoscopy to create shadows for pseudo-three-dimensional imaging of the outer retina and RPE. This technique has been successfully used in other uveitis entities such as Vogt-Koyanagi-Harada disease [19] and should be useful in intraocular TB as well, especially serpiginous-like choroiditis.

Multimodal imaging collates all the above imaging techniques to provide information on the following: anatomical location of lesion, disease activity, response to treatment, and post-inflammatory complications [4]. Thus, for example, autofluorescence, OCT-A, and EDI-OCT can provide complimentary information regarding disease activity, location, and treatment response in a patient with serpiginous-like choroiditis, without the need for invasive techniques such as FFA and ICG angiography. The multimodal imaging characteristics of TB-associated serpiginous-like choroiditis are summarized in Table 2.

Response to Treatment Imaging

Imaging has a critical role after initiation of treatment for intraocular TB. As mentioned above, microbiological evidence of *M. tuberculosis* infection is rarely found in ocular samples, and serial imaging becomes vital in documentation of resolution of inflammation. Second, intraocular TB, particularly serpiginous-like choroiditis, is often associated with paradoxical worsening after initiating anti-TB therapy [20]. This is best diagnosed on serial imaging, especially extrafoveal increase in size of lesions that is asymptomatic and can be missed on clinical examination. Finally, complications such as retinal or choroidal neovascularization, epiretinal membranes, or cystoid macular edema can also develop during course of treatment and are best detected by an appropriate imaging technique.

Acknowledgment The author would like to acknowledge Krushna Gopal Panda, optometrist at L V Prasad Eye Institute, Bhubaneswar, for painstakingly acquiring and preparing all the images.

Compliance with Ethical Requirements Soumyava Basu declares no conflict of interest. No human or animal studies were carried out by the authors for this article.

References

1. Gupta V, Gupta A, Rao NA. Intraocular tuberculosis—an update. Surv Ophthalmol. 2007;52(6):561–87.
2. Hong BK, Khanamiri HN, Bababeygy SR, Rao NA. The utility of routine tuberculosis screening in county hospital patients with uveitis. Br J Ophthalmol. 2014;98(8):1091–5.
3. Balne PK, Modi RR, Choudhury N, Mohan N, Barik MR, Padhi TR, Sharma S, Panigrahi SR, Basu S. Factors influencing polymerase chain reaction outcomes in patients with clinically suspected ocular tuberculosis. J Ophthalmic Inflamm Infect. 2014;4(1):10.
4. Agarwal A, Mahajan S, Khairallah M, Mahendradas P, Gupta A, Gupta V. Multimodal imaging in ocular tuberculosis. Ocul Immunol Inflamm. 2016;11:1–12.
5. Kee AR, Gonzalez-Lopez JJ, Al-Hity A, Gupta B, Lee CS, Gunasekeran DV, Jayabalan N, Grant R, Kon OM, Gupta V, Westcott M. Anti-tubercular therapy for intraocular tuberculosis: a systematic review and meta-analysis. Surv Ophthalmol. 2016;61(5):628–53.
6. Aggarwal K, Mulkutkar S, Mahajan S, Singh R, Sharma A, Bansal R, Gupta V, Gupta A. Role of ultra-wide field imaging in the management of tubercular posterior uveitis. Ocul Immunol Inflamm. 2016;6:1–6.
7. Kaines A, Tsui I, Sarraf D, Schwartz S. The use of ultra widefield fluorescein angiography in evaluation and management of uveitis. Semin Ophthalmol. 2009;24(1):19–24.
8. Nicholson BP, Nigam D, Miller D, Agron E, Dalal M, Jacobs-El N, et al. Comparison of wide-field fluorescein angiography and 9-field montage angiography in uveitis. Am J Ophthalmol. 2014;157(3):673–7.
9. Herbort CP. Indocyanine green angiography. In: Gupta A, Gupta V, Herbort CP, Khairallah M, editors. Uveitis: text and Imaging. New Delhi: Jaypee Brothers; 2009. p. 88–144.
10. Bansal R, Gupta A, Gupta V. Imaging in the diagnosis and management of serpiginous choroiditis. Int Ophthalmol Clin. 2012;52:229–36.
11. Rajendran R, Saraswathy S, Rao NA. Photoreceptor mitochondrial oxidative stress in early experimental autoimmune uveitis. Br J Ophthalmol. 2007;91:531–7.
12. Bansal R, Kulkarni P, Gupta A, Gupta V, Dogra MR. High-resolution spectral domain optical coherence tomography and fundus autofluorescence correlation in tuberculosis in tubercular serpiginous like choroiditis. J Ophthalmic Inflamm Infect. 2011;4:157–63.
13. Gupta A, Bansal R, Gupta V, Sharma A. Fundus autofluorescence in serpiginous-like choroiditis. Retina. 2012;32:814–25.
14. Khanamiri HN, Rao NA. Serpiginous choroiditis and infectious multifocal serpiginoid choroiditis. Surv Ophthalmol. 2013;58:203–32.
15. Kawali A, Emerson GG, Naik NK, Sharma K, Mahendradas P, Rao NA. Clinicopathologic features of tuberculous serpiginous-like choroiditis. JAMA Ophthalmol. 2018;136(2):219–21.
16. Mehta H, Sim DA, Keane PA, Zarranz-Ventura J, Gallagher K, Egan CA, Westcott M, Lee RW4, Tufail A, Pavesio CE. Structural changes of the choroid in sarcoid- and tuberculosis-related granulomatous uveitis. Eye (Lond). 2015;29(8):1060–8.
17. Invernizzi A1, Mapelli C, Viola F, Cigada M, Cimino L, Ratiglia R, Staurenghi G, Gupta A. Choroidal granulomas visualized by enhanced depth imaging optical coherence tomography. Retina. 2015;35(3):525–31.
18. Jain L, Panda KG, Basu S. Clinical outcomes of adjunctive sustained-release intravitreal dexamethasone implants in tuberculosis-associated multifocal serpigenoid choroiditis. Ocul Immunol Inflamm. 2018;26(6):877–83.

19. Kinoshita T, Imaizumi H, Miyamoto H, Katome T, Mitamura Y. Detection of choroidal folds in patients with Vogt–Koyanagi–Harada disease by retromode scanning laser ophthalmoscopy. Retin Cases Brief Rep. 2016;10(2):160–4.
20. Basu S, Nayak S, Padhi TR, Das T. Progressive ocular inflammation following anti-tubercular therapy for presumed ocular tuberculosis in a high-endemic setting. Eye. 2013;27(5):657–62.

Viral Retinitis

Dana Yousef Darwish, Mei Zhou, and Ann-Marie Lobo

Necrotizing Herpetic Retinitis

Necrotizing herpetic retinitis defines a spectrum of disease secondary to herpes viruses, specifically herpes simplex virus 1 and 2 (HSV-1 and HSV-2), varicella zoster virus (VZV), and cytomegalovirus (CMV).

Acute Retinal Necrosis

Background

Acute retinal necrosis (ARN) is an ocular inflammatory syndrome typically seen in immunocompetent patients. Urayama first reported a constellation of findings including acute necrotizing retinitis, retinal arteritis, and subsequent retinal detachment [65]. The association of herpes viruses with ARN was first confirmed with the isolation of VZV, HSV-1, and HSV-2 from tissue cultures of vitreous and aqueous specimens and immunocytology [13, 14, 55]. Although ARN is a clinical syndrome, polymerase chain reaction (PCR) of the vitreous and aqueous specimens is sensitive and specific for confirming the causative viral agent.

Clinical Features and Diagnostic Criteria

Patients typically present with findings of ocular pain, photophobia, redness, blurred vision, and floaters [59]. The 1994 American Uveitis Society guidelines specify the

D. Y. Darwish · M. Zhou · A.-M. Lobo (✉)
Illinois Eye and Ear Infirmary, University of Illinois at Chicago, Department of Ophthalmology and Visual Sciences, Chicago, IL, USA
e-mail: alobo2@uic.edu

N. A. Rao et al. (eds.), *Posterior Uveitis*, Essentials in Ophthalmology,
https://doi.org/10.1007/978-3-030-03140-4_8

following five clinical features for the diagnosis of ARN: (1) focal well-demarcated area of retinal necrosis in peripheral retina, (2) rapid progression of disease without antiviral therapy, (3) circumferential progression of necrosis, (4) occlusive vasculopathy, and (5) prominent inflammatory reaction in vitreous and anterior chamber [28]. There is a slight predilection to males, and it typically affects patients aged 20–60 [15, 16]. Anterior segment findings include conjunctival injection, fine or granulomatous keratic precipitates, and anterior chamber and vitreous cells. Posterior segment findings include vitreous cell and haze, areas of retinal whitening/necrosis, arteriole narrowing and sheathing of large retinal vessels, and scattered hemorrhages [15, 16]. The disease tends to progress rapidly within days to weeks from the periphery to the macula. The affected areas become thin and atrophic, frequently complicated by full thickness retinal holes. Expectedly, rates of retinal detachment are as high as 80% in some studies and are both rhegmatogenous and tractional in nature [41].

Progressive Outer Retinal Necrosis

Progressive outer retinal necrosis (PORN) is characterized by deep, multifocal, white/yellow retinal lesions which progress rapidly [18, 20]. The condition is exclusively seen in immunocompromised patients, particularly those with HIV/AIDS and CD4 counts less than 50 cells/uL. VZV antigen has been isolated from chorioretinal and vitreous specimens of patients affected with PORN [46]. The etiology is similar to ARN, involving reactivation of a latent herpes infection, but there are distinguishing clinical features.

Clinical Features

Patients initially present with painless disturbance in peripheral vision. On examination, intraocular inflammation is typically absent. Fundus exam shows areas of multifocal retinal necrosis with opacification in the outer retina [20]. Without therapy, the necrosis rapidly progresses to involve the entire retina in a circumferential fashion. Resolution during this process may present with perivenous clearing within areas of retinal whitening with a “cracked mud appearance” [18]. Retinal detachments frequently occur secondary to thin necrotic retina.

PORN Versus ARN

ARN and PORN represent a spectrum of herpetic retinitis (Table 1). ARN is associated with an exuberant inflammatory response, whereas in PORN, there is little intraocular inflammation. In PORN, macular involvement tends to be earlier, with rapid progression starting centrally and spreading in a nonspecific pattern in direct contrast to ARN’s circumferential spread from the periphery. Furthermore, PORN

Table 1 Clinical features of necrotizing herpetic retinitis

	ARN	PORN	CMVR
Symptoms	Eye pain Redness Decreased peripheral vision Floaters Photophobia	Painless Decreased peripheral vision	Painless Decreased peripheral or central vision May be asymptomatic
Clinical features	Peripheral retinal whitening Vasculitis Vitritis	Multifocal deep retinal white lesions that become confluent Early posterior pole involvement	Perivascular retinitis Hemorrhages Granular borders
Immune status	Immunocompetent	Immunocompromised	Immunocompromised
Focus	Multifocal	Multifocal	Single focus
Vasculitis	Yes	No	Variable
Vitritis	Common	Uncommon	Less common
Progression	Rapid	Rapid	Slow
Pattern of progression	Circumferential from periphery	Central and nonspecific	Perivascular
Management	Systemic antiviral Intravitreal antiviral Prednisone	Systemic antiviral Intravitreal antiviral HAART	Systemic antiviral Intravitreal antiviral HAART

tends to be a multifocal disease without granular borders, whereas ARN tends to have discrete borders [18].

Differential Diagnoses

The differential for necrotizing herpetic retinitis should include any diseases that cause retinal whitening. Infectious possibilities include CMV retinitis, toxoplasma chorioretinitis, and ocular syphilis. Autoimmune diseases include Behcet's disease, acute multifocal hemorrhagic retinal vasculitis, and sarcoidosis. Neoplastic and vascular etiologies include intraocular lymphoma, retinal artery occlusion, and retinoblastoma [16].

Imaging

Fluorescein Angiography/Indocyanine Green Angiography

Fluorescein (FA) and indocyanine green (ICG) angiography is not necessary for diagnosis of acute retinal necrosis, and has limited utility in cases with severe vitritis, but can be helpful in delineating the extent of disease (Table 2). During active disease, capillary non-perfusion is noted in affected areas as well as leakage of the few perfused

Table 2 Imaging features in viral retinitis

	FA	ICG	OCT	FAF
ARN: active disease	Capillary non-perfusion and leakage of major vessels Vascular occlusion Abrupt demarcation in perfusion Late optic disc staining	Limited leakage of retinal vessels	Inner retina hyperreflectivity Macula edema/exudates Retinal traction	Hyperfluorescent border
ARN: treated	Window defects		Retinal thinning/atrophy Loss of ellipsoid in macula disease	
PORN: active disease	Early blockage/late staining Retinal leakage in areas of retinal whitening		Outer retinal thickening and hyporeflectivity	Hypoautofluorescence
PORN: treated	Widespread late leakage of choriocapillaris		Retinal thinning/atrophy RPE irregularity	Stippled hyperfluorescence with retinal atrophy
CMVR: active disease	Microaneurysms Blocking in areas of hemorrhage Leaking or non-perfusion of vessels in affected areas	Hypocyanescence in areas of retinal edema/inflammation	Full thickness retinal edema Foveal and parafoveal inner retina reflectivity	Hyperautofluorescence of active borders Hypofluorescence in areas of full thickness retinitis
CMVR: treated	Staining due to window defects	Staining due to window defects	Retinal thinning, choroid hyperreflectivity Cystoid macula edema from immune-recovery uveitis Epiretinal membrane/vitreoretinal traction	Mottled hyper and hypoautofluorescence in healing

major vessels [71]. Obstruction of the central retinal artery or one of its branches has been reported [16]. Areas of acute retinitis show an abrupt demarcation in perfusion of both arteries and veins (Fig. 1) [16]. Other findings include late staining of the optic disc during the recirculation phase and perifoveal leakage [16]. After disease resolution, window defects may be seen in previously affected areas due to RPE abnormalities [16]. ICG leakage from retinal vessels was much more limited [63].

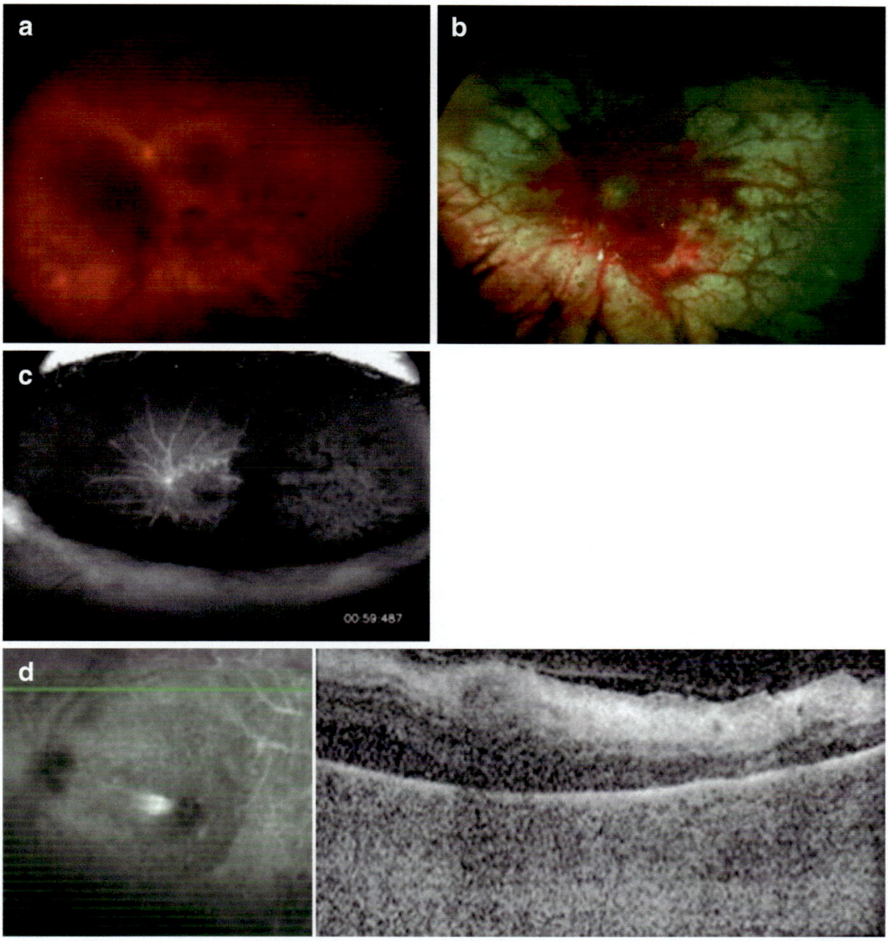

Fig. 1 Acute retinal necrosis. (**a**) Acute retinal necrosis with significant vitritis, peripheral areas of hemorrhage, and retinitis. (**b**) Follow up image after pars plana vitrectomy with 360 degrees of retinitis and hemorrhage. (**c**) Fluorescein angiogram showing extensive retinal ischemia and blockage from hemorrhages. (**d**) SD-OCT with inner retinal hyperreflectivity. (Figures courtesy of Dr. William Mieler)

In progressive outer retinal necrosis, FA has provided insights into disease evolution. Early in the course of disease, the multifocal peripheral lesions display early blockage and late staining [20, 46]. Beyond these areas of punctate retinal whitening, however, extensive retinal microvascular alterations (capillary loss and microaneurysms) of the equatorial and peripheral retina have also been noted [67]. Larger more confluent areas of retinal whitening displayed retinal leakage. Despite treatment with parenteral antivirals, the disease can progress with extensive damage to the RPE manifesting as widespread late leakage of the choriocapillaris on fluorescein angiography. As the disease reactivates, a "brush-fire" pattern of leakage from the choriocapillaris at the border of normal and affected retina appears [67].

Optical Coherence Tomography

Optical coherence tomography (OCT) is an imaging technique that provides visualization of optical cross-sectional images of the ocular tissues using low coherence interferometry [32]. Suzuki et al. described time domain OCT findings in seven eyes in seven patients with ARN [62]. Acutely, in areas of retinal whitening, OCT showed highly reflective inner retina lesions and obscuration of the retinal architecture. This has also been noted in spectral domain (SD) and swept source (SS) OCT [51]. Macular edema and exudates have also been noted in the acute phase [50]. SD-OCT has also been used outside of the macula to image areas of peripheral retinitis with findings of full thickness retinal hyperreflectivity and intraretinal and subretinal cysts [40]. With initiation of antiviral treatment and normalization of the retina appearance clinically, OCT shows marked retinal thinning and atrophy [50, 51, 62]. In patients with macular disease at presentation, the ellipsoid layer did not recover despite disease regression and visual acuity remained poor [51]. With worsening of intraocular inflammation, SD-OCT findings of inflammatory retinal traction and eventual development of combination tractional/rhegmatogenous detachment have been reported [40].

Time domain OCT of HIV-positive patients with VZV-related PORN show acute findings of outer retina thickening and hyporeflectivity [3, 7, 11]. After treatment, the areas which appear atrophic on clinical exam demonstrate thinning, loss of identifiable retinal structures, and RPE irregularity on OCT (Fig. 2) [3, 11]. Several months after treatment, OCT demonstrated full thickness neurosensory atrophy of the central macula [7]. The authors feel that the disease presents as an outer retinal disease but will eventually involve the full thickness of the retina [7]. This notion

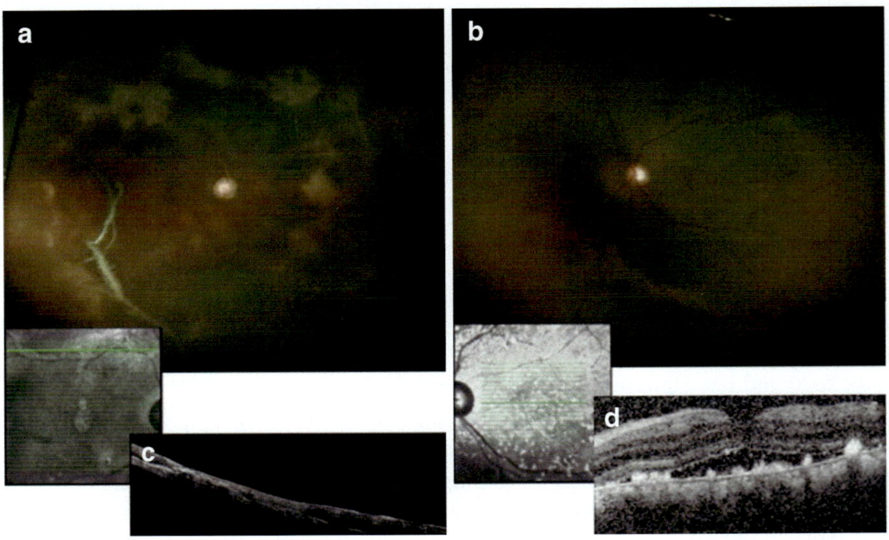

Fig. 2 Progressive outer retinal necrosis. (**a**) Right eye and. (**b**) Left eye showing multifocal, deep retinal lesions in the periphery and perivascular whitening. (**c**) SD-OCT macula of right eye with retinal hyperreflectivity and thinning in areas of retinitis. (**d**) SD-OCT macula of left eye with subretinal deposits, full thickness retinal hyperreflectivity. (Figures courtesy of Dr. Felix Chau)

has recently been debated as histological studies of early PORN show relative sparing of the outer retina [45]. Others have proposed that PORN begins with deep capillary ischemia [72]. Further imaging studies with high-resolution OCT and OCT angiography may provide more insights into the disease process.

Fundus Autofluorescence

Fundus autofluorescence (FAF) imaging allows for a topographic map of lipofuscin accumulation in the RPE, and autofluorescence is thought to precede frank photoreceptor degeneration. Patients with PORN acutely show areas of hypofluorescence due to obscuration by retinal opacification which later become stippled with hyperfluorescence as these opacified areas atrophy on funduscopy [11]. FAF changes in progressive outer retinal necrosis are delayed compared to clinical findings and appear subsequent to lipofuscin accumulation in areas of retinal inflammation. FAF offers higher contrast delineation of ARN lesions with a hyperfluorescent border which may assist in monitoring of disease progression [68].

Treatment

Systemic antiviral therapy was first shown to be effective for the treatment of herpetic retinitis in the 1980s with intravenous acyclovir [8, 27]. Since then, newer antiviral agents such as valacyclovir (acyclovir prodrug) and famciclovir (prodrug of penciclovir) which can achieve systemic levels similar to that of intravenous acyclovir obviated the need for patients to be hospitalized [1, 5, 17]. Additionally, oral antivirals were shown to be beneficial for preventing fellow eye involvement [52].

Adjunctive Therapy with Intravitreal Antiviral Injections

The addition of intravitreal antiviral agents was first shown to be effective in HIV-positive patients with PORN [57]. Subsequently, successful results with adjunctive therapy with intravitreal antivirals in patients with ARN were described in several series [38, 44, 64]. Combination systemic and intravitreal antiviral therapy is now considered the standard of care for necrotizing herpetic retinitis. Patients receiving combination systemic and intravitreal antiviral therapy are more likely to have improvement in visual acuity and lower incidence of retinal detachment than those treated with systemic therapy alone [19].

Laser

Prophylactic laser to uninvolved retina adjacent to diseased retina can decrease the rates of progression to retinal detachment, although this remains controversial [25, 61]. More severe cases tend to be treated with laser but also have higher rates of retinal detachment [53].

Role of Surgery

Retinal breaks and rhegmatogenous retinal detachment are a frequent complication of herpetic retinitis, in up to 50–80% of cases [12, 24, 41]. Although retinal detachment repair with pars plana vitrectomy, scleral buckle, long-acting gas, or silicone oil tamponade has been successful, many patients require more than one surgery, and visual acuity may remain poor after surgery despite successful reattachment [2, 12, 48, 60]. Early or prophylactic vitrectomy by removing inflammation and preventing detachment has been explored but remains controversial [6, 33, 43].

CMV Retinitis

Cytomegalovirus (CMV) retinitis is seen exclusively in immunocompromised patients, particularly in HIV/AIDS, or as a result of congenital infection. Risk factors for CMV retinitis include CD4 T cell counts <50 cells/uL and presence of one or more opportunistic infections [39]. However, CMV retinitis may also occur after solid organ or allogeneic bone marrow transplantation especially in the case of CMV-negative patients and CMV-positive donors [34].

Clinical Findings

Unlike necrotizing retinopathies caused by HSV and VZV, CMV retinitis is a more slowly progressive disease [29–31]. Patients may be asymptomatic or present with decreased visual acuity. Vitritis is usually absent. There are variations in presentation of CMV retinitis, including (1) hemorrhagic retinitis within the posterior pole distributed along retinal vasculature; (2) a granular, indolent form with active retinitis at borders of the lesion; and (3) a perivascular or frosted branch angiitis [10, 21].

Imaging

Ultrawide-field fundus imaging (UWF) which captures approximately 200° of the retina has been used to monitor disease progression in CMV retinitis (Fig. 3). In one study comparing UWF imaging with the Optos system to standard montage fundus photography, UWF imaging captured 40% more CMV affected areas compared to standard photography [49]. UWF provides improved monitoring of peripheral lesions and response to treatment.

Fluorescein angiography highlights vascular abnormalities such as enlarged foveal avascular zone, microaneurysms, hypofluorescence in areas of retinal edema and inflammation, as well as marked vascular leakage [22].

SD-OCT findings in three patients with active CMV retinitis showed full thickness retinal edema and disruption of retinal architecture in affected areas of retina (Fig. 4) [40]. As the lesions healed with treatment with antivirals, retina thinning

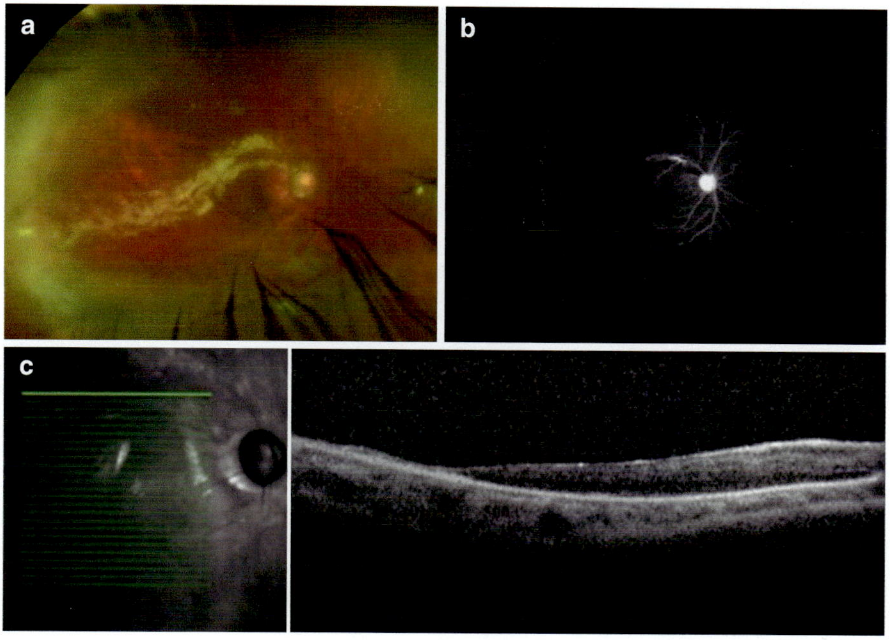

Fig. 3 CMV retinitis. (**a**) Ultrawide-field image demonstrating perivascular distribution of fluffy white retinal infiltration and small areas of hemorrhage along superior arcade. (**b**) Fluorescein angiogram demonstrating extensive retinal ischemia. (**c**) SD-OCT macula showing loss of retinal tissue in areas of retinal whitening. (Figures courtesy of Dr. Lawrence Ulanski)

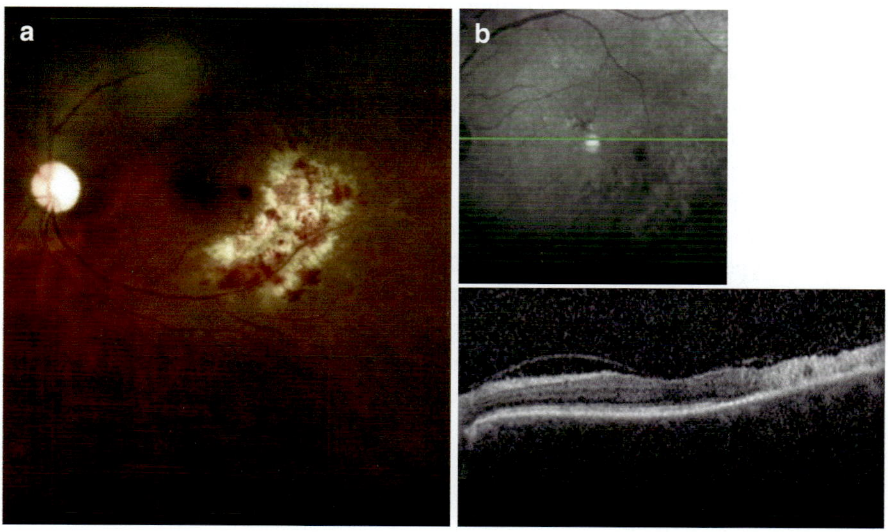

Fig. 4 CMV retinitis. (**a**) Focal area of hemorrhage and perivascular infiltrate. (**b**) SD-OCT showing disruption of retinal architecture and full thickness retinal hyperreflectivity in affected area. (Figures courtesy of Dr. Felix Chau)

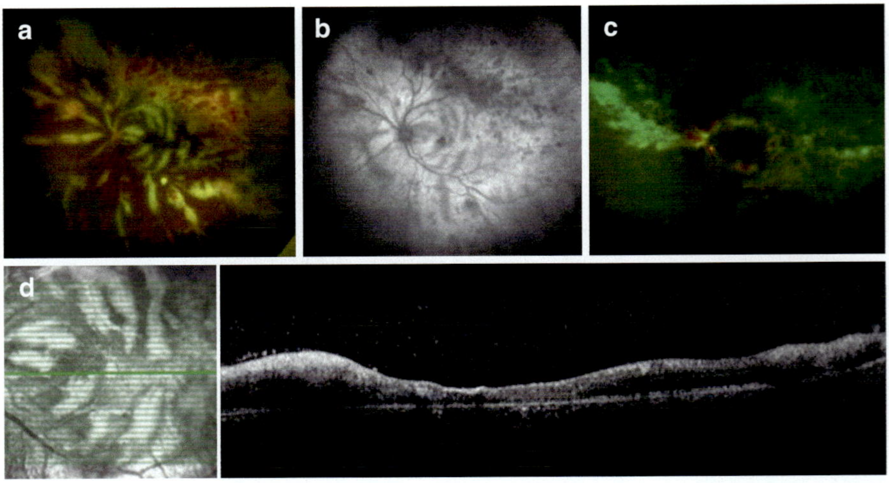

Fig. 5 CMV retinitis. (**a**) Frosted branch angiitis with extensive perivascular infiltrates and hemorrhage. (**b**) Autofluorescence image with hypoautofluorescence in areas of perivascular infiltrates. (**c**) Resolving perivascular infiltrates and hemorrhages. (**d**) SD-OCT showing inner retina hyperreflectivity and retinal edema in area of active retinitis and atrophy, loss of retinal architecture in inactive or resolving areas. (Figures courtesy of Dr. Yannek Leiderman)

and choroid hyperreflectivity secondary to RPE atrophy were apparent on OCT [40]. An additional finding is that of cystoid macular edema, thought to be secondary to immune-recovery uveitis. SD-OCT can help distinguish retinitis from a cotton wool spot which can also be seen in patients with HIV and only affects the inner retina [40]. Inner retinal hyperreflectivity, corresponding to areas of retinal ischemia on FA, has also been seen. With treatment, there is reduction in retinal thickness [4].

SD-OCT has also been used to study the vitreoretinal interface. In 42 eyes from 21 patients with healed CMV retinitis scars, a majority had abnormalities including epiretinal membrane and vitreoretinal gliosis, which may provide further explanation for high rates of retinal detachment in patients with CMV retinitis [9].

FAF imaging in active CMV retinitis demonstrates hyperautofluorescence at the active borders of affected areas, while areas of full thickness retinitis in the posterior pole were hypoautofluorescent (Fig. 5) [70]. Mottled regions of hyper- and hypoautofluorescence corresponded to either RPE atrophy or various stages of healing. In this series, FAF was particularly helpful for patients with subtle findings of disease activity on clinical exam by highlighting disease recurrence with hyperautofluorescence at the active borders in patients previously affected by CMV on chronic antiviral therapy [70]. With treatment of CMV retinitis, the hyperautofluorescent borders seemed to decrease.

Treatment

The use of highly active antiretroviral therapy (HAART) significantly reduced the incidence and severity of a number of opportunistic infections in HIV/AIDS patients, including CMV retinitis. Anti-CMV therapy, however, still plays a critical role for treatment of CMV retinitis in the HAART era. Intravenous antiviral treatment options include ganciclovir, foscarnet, and cidofovir. Oral antivirals include valganciclovir, a prodrug of ganciclovir. Intraocular agents include intravitreal ganciclovir and foscarnet and a long-acting ganciclovir implant. Systemic antiviral therapy prevents dissemination of the virus either to the second eye or elsewhere in the body. Anti-CMV therapy improved mortality for HIV-infected patients, even with the widespread use of HAART therapy [35]. Combination systemic and intravitreal therapy, as well as treatment of HIV with HAART, is considered to be the standard approach for treatment of HIV-positive CMV retinitis patients [35].

Epstein-Barr Virus and Ebola Virus

Epstein-Barr virus (EBV) has been implicated in cases of bilateral uveitis, keratitis, conjunctivitis, and ARN following viral reactivation [47, 69]. However, EBV is present ubiquitously in mucosal tissue, and the pathogenesis of EBV in viral retinitis is unclear. Most cases that have isolated EBV in diseased eyes reported coinfection with VZV [26, 41], and therefore its role as a causative agent in ocular pathology is difficult to discern. Two recent case studies have reported EBV as a sole causative agent of ARN by immunohistopathologic confirmation of positive EBV titers [23, 56].

The recent outbreak of Ebola has led to reports of Ebola-related ocular disease. Although the pathogenesis of Ebola-related uveitis is unclear, anterior uveitis and panuveitis have developed during the convalescent stage in Ebola survivor patients [66]. 21 out of 96 Ebola survivors developed an Ebola virus disease-related uveitis [58]. Patients present with eye pain, photophobia, and visual loss [42] with clinical findings of keratic precipitates, vitritis, peripheral chorioretinal scars, and elevated intraocular pressure as the uveitis progresses [58]. Ebola virus has been found within the ocular fluid even after clearance of viremia [66]. Whether the uveitis is caused by active viral replication, viral persistence in the eye, or immunological reaction to the virus is unclear and needs further investigation.

Imaging

One case report of EBV-associated retinitis described the use of FA, which highlighted disc leakage and retinal vasculitis at disease onset. With 4 weeks of antiviral therapy, disc edema and phlebitis improved. By 3 months of treatment, these findings had resolved [36].

Treatment

EBV lacks a virus-specific thymidine kinase; however, acyclovir has 100 times more affinity for EBV DNA polymerase than that of the human host [37]. In a meta-analysis of 45 immunocompetent patients with manifestations of infectious mononucleosis, acyclovir was the most commonly prescribed antiviral although the role of antivirals in what is a typically self-limited viral disease has been questioned [54]. In ocular disease, the use of systemic and topical acyclovir has been described [23, 69]. Early diagnostic vitrectomy, focal panretinal photocoagulation in areas of retinal ischemia, and intravitreal antivirals have also been used as treatment in EBV-associated ocular infection [36, 56].

The treatment of Ebola-related uveitis is largely experimental. Intraocular inflammation is treated with topical, periocular, and systemic steroids [66]. Use of favipiravir, an experimental antiviral drug, has also been employed.

Conflict of Interest Ann-Marie Lobo, Mei Zhou, and Dana Darwish declare that they have no conflict of interest.

Informed Consent No human or animal studies were carried out by the authors for this article.

References

1. Aizman A, Johnson MW, Elner SG. Treatment of acute retinal necrosis syndrome with oral antiviral medications. Ophthalmology. 2007;114(2):307–12. https://doi.org/10.1016/j.ophtha.2006.06.058.
2. Almeida DR, Chin EK, Tarantola RM, Tegins EO, Lopez CA, Boldt HC, Gehrs KM, Sohn EH, Russell SR, Folk JC. Long-term outcomes in patients undergoing vitrectomy for retinal detachment due to viral retinitis. Clin Ophthalmol. 2015;9:1307.
3. Almony A, Dhalla MS, Feiner L, Shah GK. Macular optical coherence tomography findings in progressive outer retinal necrosis. Can J Ophthalmol. 2007;42(6):881.
4. Arevalo JF, Garcia RA, Arevalo FA, Fernandez CF. Unilateral ischemic maculopathy associated with cytomegalovirus retinitis in patients with AIDS: optical coherence tomography findings. J Ophthalmic Vis Res. 2015;10(4):487.
5. Aslanides IM, De Souza S, Wong DT, Giavedoni LR, Altomare F, Detorakis ET, Kymionis GD, Pallikaris IG. Oral valacyclovir in the treatment of acute retinal necrosis syndrome. Retina. 2002;22(3):352–4.
6. Berker N, Ozdal P, Batman C, Soykan E. Prophylactic vitrectomy in acute retinal necrosis syndrome. Eye. 2007;21(1):104–6.
7. Blair MP, Goldstein DA, Shapiro MJ. Optical coherence tomography of progressive outer retinal necrosis. Retina. 2007;27(9):1313–4.
8. Blumenkranz MS, Culbertson WW, Clarkson JG, Dix R. Treatment of the acute retinal necrosis syndrome with intravenous acyclovir. Ophthalmology. 1986;93(3):296–300.
9. Brar M, Kozak I, Freeman WR, Oster SF, Mojana F, Yuson RM. Vitreoretinal interface abnormalities in healed cytomegalovirus retinitis. Retina. 2010;30(8):1262–6.
10. Carmichael A. Cytomegalovirus and the eye. Eye. 2012;26(2):237–40.
11. Chew EY, Weichel ED, Lew JC, Nussenblatt RB, Yeh S, Wong WT. Fundus autofluorescence and OCT in the management of progressive outer retinal necrosis. Ophthalmic Surg Lasers Imaging. 2010;9:1–4.
12. Clarkson JG, Blumenkranz MS, Culbertson WW, Flynn HW, Lewis ML. Retinal detachment following the acute retinal necrosis syndrome. Ophthalmology. 1984;91(12):1665–8.
13. Culbertson WW, Blumenkranz MS, Haines H, Gass JDM, Mitchell KB, Norton EW. The acute retinal necrosis syndrome: part 2: histopathology and etiology. Ophthalmology. 1982;89(12):1317–25.

14. Culbertson WW, Blumenkranz MS, Pepose JS, Stewart JA, Curtin VT. Varicella zoster virus is a cause of the acute retinal necrosis syndrome. Ophthalmology. 1986;93(5):559–69.
15. Duker JS, Blumenkranz MS. Diagnosis and management of the acute retinal necrosis (ARN) syndrome. Surv Ophthalmol. 1991;35(5):327–43.
16. Duker JS, Nielsen JC, Eagle RC, Bosley TM, Granadier R, Benson WE. Rapidly progressive acute retinal necrosis secondary to herpes simplex virus, type 1. Ophthalmology. 1990;97(12):1638–43.
17. Emerson GG, Smith JR, Wilson DJ, Rosenbaum JT, Flaxel CJ. Primary treatment of acute retinal necrosis with oral antiviral therapy. Ophthalmology. 2006;113(12):2259–61.
18. Engstrom RE, Holland GN, Margolis TP, Muccioli C, Lindley JI, Belfort R, Holland SP, Johnston WH, Wolitz RA, Kreiger AE. The progressive outer retinal necrosis syndrome: a variant of necrotizing herpetic retinopathy in patients with AIDS. Ophthalmology. 1994;101(9):1488–502.
19. Flaxel CJ, Yeh S, Lauer AK. Combination systemic and intravitreal antiviral therapy in the management of acute retinal necrosis syndrome (an American ophthalmological society thesis). Trans Am Ophthalmol Soc. 2013;111:133–44.
20. Forster DJ, Dugel PU, Frangieh GT, Liggett PE, Rao NA. Rapidly progressive outer retinal necrosis in the acquired immunodeficiency syndrome. Am J Ophthalmol. 1990;110(4): 341–8.
21. Freeman WR, Lerner CW, Mines JA, Lash RS, Nadel AJ, Starr MB, Tapper ML. A prospective study of the ophthalmologic findings in the acquired immune deficiency syndrome. Am J Ophthalmol. 1984;97(2):133–42.
22. Friedman A, Orellana J, Freeman W, Luntz M, Starr M, Tapper M, Spigland I, Roterdam H, Tejada RM, Braunhut S. Cytomegalovirus retinitis: a manifestation of the acquired immune deficiency syndrome (AIDS). Br J Ophthalmol. 1983;67(6):372–80.
23. Gallego-Pinazo R, Harto M, Garcia-Medina JJ, Serra I, España E, Pinazo-Duran MD. Epstein-Barr virus and acute retinal necrosis in a 5-year-old immunocompetent child. Clin Ophthalmol. 2008;2(2):451–5.
24. Gore DM, Gore SK, Visser L. Progressive outer retinal necrosis: outcomes in the intravitreal era. Arch Ophthalmol. 2012;130(6):700–6.
25. Han DP, Lewis H, Williams GA, Mieler WF, Abrams GW, Aaberg TM. Laser photocoagulation in the acute retinal necrosis syndrome. Arch Ophthalmol. 1987;105(8):1051–4.
26. Hillenkamp J, Nölle B, Bruns C, Rautenberg P, Fickenscher H, Roider J. Acute retinal necrosis: clinical features, early vitrectomy, and outcomes. Ophthalmology. 2009;116(10):1971–5. e1972
27. Hirst L, Beyer T, Waters D, Fleischman J. Successful management of acute retinal necrosis with intravenous acyclovir. Ann Ophthalmol. 1987;19(12):445–8.
28. Holland GN. Standard diagnostic criteria for the acute retinal necrosis syndrome. Executive Committee of the American Uveitis Society. Am J Ophthalmol. 1994;117(5):663–7.
29. Holland GN, Gottlieb MS, Yee RD, Schanker HM, Pettit TH. Ocular disorders associated with a new severe acquired cellular immunodeficiency syndrome. Am J Ophthalmol. 1982;93(4):393–402.
30. Holland GN, Vaudaux JD, Jeng SM, Yu F, Goldenberg DT, Folz I-C, Cumberland WG, McCannel CA, Helm CJ, Hardy WD. Characteristics of untreated AIDS-related cytomegalovirus retinitis. I. Findings before the era of highly active antiretroviral therapy (1988 to 1994). Am J Ophthalmol. 2008a;145(1):5–11. e10
31. Holland GN, Vaudaux JD, Shiramizu KM, Yu F, Goldenberg DT, Gupta A, Carlson M, Read RW, Novack RD, Kuppermann BD. Characteristics of untreated AIDS-related cytomegalovirus retinitis. II. Findings in the era of highly active antiretroviral therapy (1997 to 2000). Am J Ophthalmol. 2008b;145(1):12–22. e10
32. Huang D, Swanson EA, Lin CP, Schuman JS, Stinson WG, Chang W, Hee MR, Flotte T, Gregory K, Puliafito CA. Optical coherence tomography. Science. 1991;254(5035):1178.
33. Ishida T, Sugamoto Y, Sugita S, Mochizuki M. Prophylactic vitrectomy for acute retinal necrosis. Jpn J Ophthalmol. 2009;53(5):486–9.

34. Iu LP, Fan MC, Lau JK, Chan TS, Kwong Y-L, Wong IY. Long-term follow-up of cytomegalovirus retinitis in non-HIV immunocompromised patients: clinical features and visual prognosis. Am J Ophthalmol. 2016;165:145–53.
35. Jabs DA, Ahuja A, Van Natta M, Dunn J, Yeh S, Group SotOCoAR. Comparison of treatment regimens for cytomegalovirus retinitis in patients with AIDS in the era of highly active antiretroviral therapy. Ophthalmology. 2013;120(6):1262–70.
36. Keorochana N. A case report of Epstein-Barr virus-associated retinal vasculitis: successful treatment using only acyclovir therapy. Int Med Case Rep J. 2016;9:213–8. https://doi.org/10.2147/IMCRJ.S107089.
37. Kim SJ, Barañano DE, Grossniklaus HE, Martin DF. Epstein-Barr infection of the retina: case report and review of the literature. Ret Cases Brief Rep. 2011;5(1):1–5.
38. King J, Chung M, DiLoreto DA Jr. A 9 year-old girl with herpes simplex virus type 2 acute retinal necrosis treated with intravitreal foscarnet. Ocul Immunol Inflamm. 2007;15(5):395–8.
39. Kuppermann BD, Petty JG, Richman DD, Mathews WC, Fullerton SC, Rickman LS, Freeman WR. Correlation between CD4+ counts and prevalence of cytomegalovirus retinitis and human immunodeficiency virus--related noninfectious retinal vasculopathy in patients with acquired immunodeficiency syndrome. Am J Ophthalmol. 1993;115(5):575–82.
40. Kurup SP, Khan S, Gill MK. Spectral domain optical coherence tomography in the evaluation and management of infectious retinitis. Retina. 2014;34(11):2233–41.
41. Lau CH, Missotten T, Salzmann J, Lightman SL. Acute retinal necrosis features, management, and outcomes. Ophthalmology. 2007;114(4):756–62. https://doi.org/10.1016/j.ophtha.2006.08.037.
42. Lin P. Infectious uveitis. Curr Ophthalmol Rep. 2015;3(3):170–83.
43. Luo Y-H, Duan X-C, Chen B-H, Tang L-S, Guo X-J. Efficacy and necessity of prophylactic vitrectomy for acute retinal necrosis syndrome. Int J Ophthalmol. 2012;5(4):482.
44. Luu KK, Scott IU, Chaudhry NA, Verm A, Davis JL. Intravitreal antiviral injections as adjunctive therapy in the management of immunocompetent patients with necrotizing herpetic retinopathy. Am J Ophthalmol. 2000;129(6):811–3.
45. Margo CE, Friedman SM. Progressive outer retinal necrosis (PORN): a catchy acronym but is the anatomy correct? The salient observation of Lorenz E. Zimmerman, MD. JAMA Ophthalmol. 2014;132(5):651–2.
46. Margolis TP, Lowder CY, Holland GN, Spaide RF, Logan AG, Weissman SS, Irvine AR, Josephberg R, Meisler DM, O'Donnell JJ. Varicella-zoster virus retinitis in patients with the acquired immunodeficiency syndrome. Am J Ophthalmol. 1991;112(2):119–31.
47. Matoba AY. Ocular disease associated with Epstein-Barr virus infection. Surv Ophthalmol. 1990;35(2):145–50.
48. Matsuo T. CASE REPORT vitrectomy and silicone oil tamponade as an initial surgery for retinal detachment after acute retinal necrosis syndrome. Ocul Immunol Inflamm. 2005;13(1):91–4.
49. Mudvari SS, Virasch VV, Singa RM, MacCumber MW. Ultra-wide-field imaging for cytomegalovirus retinitis. Ophthalmic Surg Lasers Imaging. 2010;41(3):311–5.
50. Murata K, Yamada W, Nishida T, Murase H, Ishida K, Mochizuki K, Sugita S. Sequential optical coherence tomography images of early macular necrosis caused by acute retinal necrosis in non-human immunodeficiency virus patients. Retina. 2016;36(7):e55–7.
51. Ohtake-Matsumoto A, Keino H, Koto T, Okada AA. Spectral domain and swept source optical coherence tomography findings in acute retinal necrosis. Graefes Arch Clin Exp Ophthalmol. 2015;253(11):2049–51.
52. Palay DA, Sternberg P, Davis J, Lewis H, Holland GN, Mieler WF, Jabs DA, Drews C. Decrease in the risk of bilateral acute retinal necrosis by acyclovir therapy. Am J Ophthalmol. 1991;112(3):250–5.
53. Park JJ, Pavesio C. Prophylactic laser photocoagulation for acute retinal necrosis. Does it raise more questions than answers? Br J Ophthalmol. 2008;92(9):1161–2.
54. Rafailidis PI, Mavros MN, Kapaskelis A, Falagas ME. Antiviral treatment for severe EBV infections in apparently immunocompetent patients. J Clin Virol. 2010;49(3):151–7.

55. Rahhal FM, Siegel LM, Russak V, Wiley CA, Tedder DG, Weinberg A, Rickman L, Freeman WR. Clinicopathologic correlations in acute retinal necrosis caused by herpes simplex virus type 2. Arch Ophthalmol. 1996;114(11):1416–9.
56. Schaal S, Kagan A, Wang Y, Chan C-C, Kaplan HJ. Acute retinal necrosis associated with Epstein-Barr virus: immunohistopathologic confirmation. JAMA Ophthalmol. 2014;132(7):881–2.
57. Scott IU, Luu KM, Davis JL. Intravitreal antivirals in the management of patients with acquired immunodeficiency syndrome with progressive outer retinal necrosis. Arch Ophthalmol. 2002;120(9):1219–22.
58. Shantha JG, Crozier I, Hayek BR, Bruce BB, Gargu C, Brown J, Fankhauser J, Yeh S (2016) Ophthalmic manifestations and causes of vision impairment in Ebola virus disease survivors in Monrovia, Liberia. Ophthalmology. 2017;124(2):170–7.
59. Sims JL, Yeoh J, Stawell RJ. Acute retinal necrosis: a case series with clinical features and treatment outcomes. Clin Exp Ophthalmol. 2009;37(5):473–7.
60. Spaide RF, Martin DF, Teich SA, Katz A, Toth I. Successful treatment of progressive outer retinal necrosis syndrome. Retina. 1996;16(6):479–87.
61. Sternberg P, Han DP, Yeo JH, Barr CC, Lewis H, Williams GA, Mieler WF. Photocoagulation to prevent retinal detachment in acute retinal necrosis. Ophthalmology. 1988;95(10):1389–93.
62. Suzuki J, Goto H, Minoda H, Iwasaki T, Sakai J, Usui M. Analysis of retinal findings of acute retinal necrosis using optical coherence tomography. Ocul Immunol Inflamm. 2006;14(3):165–70.
63. Takei H, Ohno-Matsui K, Hayano M, Mochizuki M. Indocyanine green angiographic findings in acute retinal necrosis. Jpn J Ophthalmol. 2002;46(3):330–5.
64. Tran THC, Cassoux N, Bodaghi B, Lehoang P. Successful treatment with combination of systemic antiviral drugs and intravitreal ganciclovir injections in the management of severe necrotizing herpetic retinitis. Ocul Immunol Inflamm. 2003;11(2):141–4.
65. Urayama A, Yamada N, Sasaki T, Nishiyama Y, Watanabe H, Wakusawa S, Satoh Y, Takahashi K, Takei Y. Unilateral acute uveitis with retinal periarteritis and detachment. Jpn J Clin Ophthalmol. 1971;25(3):607–19.
66. Varkey JB, Shantha JG, Crozier I, Kraft CS, Lyon GM, Mehta AK, Kumar G, Smith JR, Kainulainen MH, Whitmer S. Persistence of Ebola virus in ocular fluid during convalescence. N Engl J Med. 2015;372(25):2423–7.
67. Walton RC, Byrnes GA, Chan CC, Nussenblatt RB. Fluorescein angiography in the progressive outer retinal necrosis syndrome. Retina. 1996;16(5):393–8.
68. Ward TS, Reddy AK. Fundus autofluorescence in the diagnosis and monitoring of acute retinal necrosis. J Ophthalmic Inflamm Infect. 2015;5(1):1.
69. Wong KW, D'Amico DJ, Hedges TR, Soong HK, Schooley RT, Kenyon KR. Ocular involvement associated with chronic Epstein-Barr virus disease. Arch Ophthalmol. 1987;106(6):788–92.
70. Yeh S, Forooghian F, Faia LJ, Weichel ED, Wong WT, Sen HN, Chan-Kai B, Witherspoon SR, Lauer AK, Chew EY. Fundus autofluorescence changes in cytomegalovirus retinitis. Retina. 2010;30(1):42.
71. Young NJ, Bird AC. Bilateral acute retinal necrosis. Br J Ophthalmol. 1978;62(9):581–90.
72. Yu S, Freund KB. Could progressive outer retinal necrosis begin with retinal deep capillary ischemia? JAMA Ophthalmol. 2015;133(1):110–1.

Intraocular Lymphoma: A Posterior Uveitis Masquerade Syndrome

Brian K. Do, Jesse L. Berry, and Damien C. Rodger

Types of Ocular Lymphoma

Ocular and adnexal lymphomas are rare and have varied presentations and significantly different prognoses. They can be classified by site of origin/involvement and whether the disease is primarily in the eye or secondary to systemic lymphoma. The nomenclature can be as varied as the diagnoses, and there are many overlapping terms. Ocular lymphoma can be classified as primary intraocular lymphoma (PIOL) (also known as primary vitreoretinal lymphoma (PVRL)), primary uveal lymphoma, primary ocular adnexal lymphoma which has overlap with uveal lymphoma, and secondary lymphoma from systemic disease. PVRL/PIOL is the most aggressive of the subtypes.

B. K. Do
USC Roski Eye Institute, Keck School of Medicine of the University of Southern California, Department of Ophthalmology, Los Angeles, CA, USA

J. L. Berry
USC Roski Eye Institute, Keck School of Medicine of the University of Southern California, Department of Ophthalmology, Los Angeles, CA, USA

Children's Hospital Los Angeles, Keck School of Medicine of the University of Southern California, Los Angeles, CA, USA

D. C. Rodger (✉)
Department of Ophthalmology, Kaiser Permanente Los Angeles Medical Center, Los Angeles, CA, USA

N. A. Rao et al. (eds.), *Posterior Uveitis*, Essentials in Ophthalmology,
https://doi.org/10.1007/978-3-030-03140-4_9

Primary Intraocular/Vitreoretinal Lymphoma

Primary intraocular lymphoma (PIOL) is thought to be a subset of primary central nervous system lymphoma (PCNSL) [1]; this is because PCNSL has a predilection for brain, leptomeningeal, and ocular tissues. CNS disease may occur prior to, concurrently with, or subsequent to the diagnosis of ocular disease or sometimes not at all. Bilateral involvement is seen 80% of the time. Approximately 25% of patients with PCNSL will have PVRL and upwards of 80% of patients with present with PIOL or PVRL will go on to develop CNS disease [2]. This is considered the most aggressive of the ocular lymphomas. It is a non-Hodgkin, diffuse large B-cell lymphoma (DLBCL). The vitreoretinal type is differentiated from the uveal type, which is an extremely rare uveal reactive hyperproliferation of essentially normal B-cells thought to correspond to a very low-grade malignancy, and these are further differentiated from a secondary process from systemic lymphoma [3]. Primary intraocular lymphoma simulates a chronic uveitis, and as such, its diagnosis is often very elusive. However, the difference is that the disorder is not primarily inflammatory; rather, inflammation is secondary to neoplastic, degenerative retinal change, or from ocular ischemia from B-cell hyperproliferation. As such, vitreous aspirates will be an admixture of both the primary neoplastic cells and the inflammatory cells resultant to the primary process.

Diagnosis

PIOL is known as a "masquerade syndrome" precisely because it simulates many other causes of uveitis and a delay in diagnosis is common with this disease entity. On clinical examination there are generally fine vitreous cells, vitreous haze, and subretinal pigmented epithelium (sub-RPE) deposits that may be focal or diffuse and may involve the choroid (see Fig. 1). The classic teaching is to consider PIOL in cases of idiopathic uveitis (usually intermediate [4] or posterior) that do not respond well to steroids. There can sometimes be an initial improvement; however the inflammation usually will then worsen even without a corticosteroid taper. While the secondary inflammatory component may respond modestly, the primary neoplastic process is usually unremitting in the face of steroids. As a result, this remains one of the most important considerations in helping to make the diagnosis. Of course, ocular imaging studies can provide clues as to the possibility of PIOL and should help key one in to the diagnosis. The most important diagnostic study once PIOL/PVRL is on the differential diagnosis is to investigate for other CNS involvement. Usually, this consists of brain imaging with magnetic resonance imaging (MRI) with gadolinium, looking for lesions that enhance with contrast typically in contact with subarachnoid cerebrospinal fluid spaces [5] or leptomeningeal enhancement. A lumbar puncture is also typically performed to acquire CSF for cytology, immunophenotyping, as well as gene rearrangement studies. Immunophenotyping helps

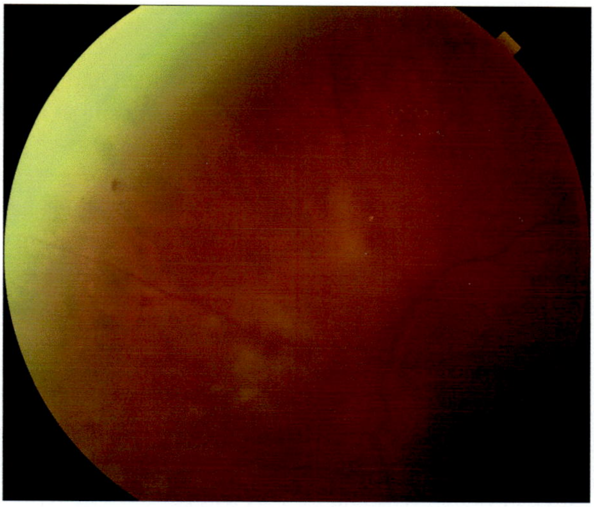

Fig. 1 Color fundus photograph demonstrating hazy media and retinal infiltrates in the setting of active PIOL/PVRL

to identify the cluster designation (CD) of cells and establish whether there exists a clonal population of CD20-positive B-cells in a sample with identical kappa or lambda light chains. Gene rearrangement heavy chain and kappa light chain PCR studies can also be performed to identify clonality. These CSF tests can be very helpful as oncologists usually desire a tissue diagnosis prior to initiating treatment. If all of these studies still remain negative, the patient should undergo typically staged vitreoretinal surgical procedures where first a standard vitrectomy is performed and the fluid sent for the same types of studies as for the CSF [4, 6] as well as for the IL-10 to IL-6 ratio which should be >1 in PIOL and PCNSL and < 1 in cases of uveitis [7–10]. If these studies are not revealing, and suspicion is still high, the last step is the more aggressive chorioretinal biopsy that is sent for pathologic analysis for cell morphology, immunofluorescence, and immunohistochemistry to determine a diagnosis [11, 12].

Treatment and Prognosis

The treatment paradigms for PIOL and PCNSL are beyond the scope of this chapter. In general, high-dose intravenous methotrexate is given for PCNSL. If there is ocular involvement, intravitreal injections of methotrexate or rituximab or external beam radiotherapy are usually employed in the disease [13]. Needless to say, when and if intraocular lymphoma is diagnosed, it is critically important to rule out CNS or systemic involvement, as this changes the necessary treatment. Unfortunately, PIOL carries with it a guarded prognosis, as the likelihood of eventual CNS involvement is upwards of 80% and portends a poor outcome [13].

Uveal Lymphoma

As expected, uveal lymphoma can be divided into choroidal, iridal, and ciliary body lymphoma. The choroid is the most frequent site of involvement. The most common histopathologic subtype is also a non-Hodgkin B-cell lymphoma but generally is a low-grade, extranodal marginal zone (EMZL) variety with a fairly indolent course, although more aggressive B-cell and T-cell origins have been described. Reactive lymphoid hyperplasia also falls into the spectrum of uveal lymphoma and is no longer considered a benign process but rather a low-grade B-cell lymphoma [14].

Diagnosis

As with PVRL, primary uveal lymphoma is also known to masquerade and may even do so more frequently – but is discussed less often – due in part both to the rarity of the disease and its indolent nature. This type of ocular lymphoma classically presents in patients between 50 and 70 years of age with a slow decrease in vision. Clinical exam reveals scattered creamy, yellow subretinal and choroidal infiltrates (see Fig. 2). These tend to be less focal and less "punched-out" than what is seen in PVRL, and while there may be associated exudative retinal detachment, there is minimal to no inflammation. As the disease progresses, there will be diffuse swaths of choroidal thickening which may extend extraocularly and, if anteriorly, will present with a "salmon patch" which can easily be biopsied to confirm the diagnosis; if this is not present, there may be posterior extrascleral lesions, or a chorioretinal biopsy may be required. Rarely, ciliary body and iris involvement in advanced uveal disease may lead to secondary angle-closure glaucoma, with associated pain and severe vision loss [15].

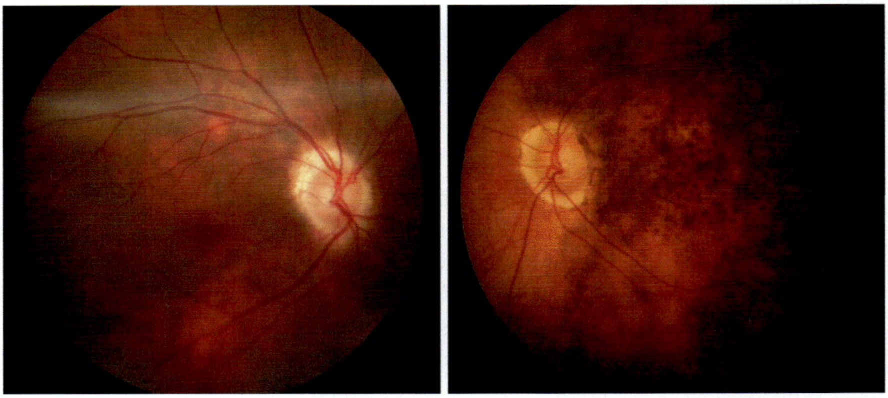

Fig. 2 Color fundus photographs of both the right and left eye in an individual with bilateral uveal lymphoma with choroidal involvement. Note the creamy, yellow-orange choroidal infiltrates in both eyes, as well as pigmentary changes in the left eye

Treatment and Prognosis

The treatment for uveal lymphoma, like other lymphomas, depends most critically on the level of systemic involvement. A work-up with PET CT scan should be done and primary therapy targeted to systemic disease. Ocular involvement may respond to systemic therapy, particularly monoclonal antibody therapy (e.g., rituximab); uveal lymphoma is otherwise typically radiosensitive. Uveal lymphoma is often localized to the eye, and given its indolent nature, it responds very well to external beam radiotherapy (EBRT). In fact, while the classic teaching is that a dose in the range of 24 Gy is needed, de-escalation studies such as the FORT trial have shown non-inferiority, and the authors of this chapter have seen impressive response to significantly lower doses of radiation therapy [16].

Ocular Adnexal Lymphoma

By definition, primary ocular adnexal lymphoma (OAL) involves the eyelids, conjunctiva, lacrimal gland, and orbit in the absence of systemic disease (see Fig. 3). OAL accounts for 1% of lymphomas [17]. It also has overlap with primary uveal lymphoma [18].

Diagnosis

Diagnosis of OAL is varied by site. Classically the patient will present with a slow-growing, painless, orange-red "salmon patch" mass lesion which is a collection of lymphoproliferative cells (see Fig. 3); however presentation with an orbitopathy is also a hallmark of disease when the orbit is primarily involved. Tissue diagnosis is key. Histopathologically, OAL is of the low-grade non-Hodgkins B-cell EMZL/MALT subtype. However, more aggressive forms like follicular, mantle, lymphoplasmocytic, and DLBCL variants are known. Rarely, OAL may arise from T cells or NK cells.

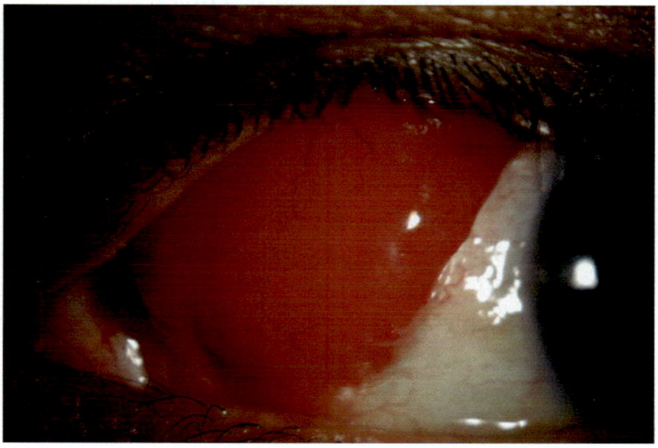

Fig. 3 External color photograph exhibiting conjunctival involvement (note the salmon patch lesion) in a patient with ocular adnexal lymphoma

Treatment and Prognosis

As OAL and uveal lymphoma are considered overlapping entities, the treatment modalities are the same. It should be noted that even for rare localized conjunctival disease, this is not considered an entity that is managed by simple surgical excision, and other systemic modalities or radiotherapy are key. Prognosis in OAL varies more widely simply based on cell type; 80% that are MALT lymphomas tend to respond, while the more rare and aggressive subtypes, such as DLBCL, have a poorer prognosis.

Ophthalmic Imaging in Ocular Lymphoma

Slit Lamp Photography

In the setting of active PIOL/PVRL, keratic precipitates, anterior chamber cells, and flare, and, in rare circumstances, a pseudohypopyon may be visible at the slit lamp and photographable [19]. Rates at which iritis and keratic precipitates are seen vary widely, ranging from 25% in a study by the Japanese collaborative group [20], vs. 75% of a cohort of 53 French patients with PIOL [21]. Additionally, when attempting to differentiate lymphoma from non-lymphoma patients, anterior chamber flare and posterior synechiae are reportedly found with significantly lower frequency in those with lymphoma [21].

An astute clinician may also be able to detect subtle iris nodules [22]. These findings, as well as the retinal and choroidal findings documented below, are nonspecific, are nondiagnostic, and may be present in various other infectious and noninfectious inflammatory conditions of the eye.

In uveal lymphoma, the anterior chamber and vitreous tend to remain clear and absent of cellular infiltration, unlike in PIOL. In the exceedingly rare iridal lymphoma secondary to systemic non-Hodgkin lymphoma, however, iris nodules may be present on examination and photography [23]. Extraocular, transscleral epibulbar extensions of uveal lymphoma may be seen anteriorly and manifest as a visible subconjunctival, sub-Tenon's pink "salmon patch" mass. Present in as many as 34% of cases [24], these anterior extensions of uveal disease may be an important clue to the correct diagnosis [25–32].

Fundus Photography

While fundus photography may have some interference from generally hazy media, the retinal findings visible on color fundus imaging or wide-field fundus imaging are important clues as to the diagnosis of PIOL and are important to document treatment and must be looked for carefully.

The presence of vitreous cells is the hallmark of PIOL/PVRL, although yellowish retinal and subretinal infiltrates are also characteristic. Less commonly, vascular sheathing, exudates, retinal hemorrhages, thickened-appearing retina with a gray-white color, and optic nerve edema can also be seen [33]. Multifocal "punched-out" lesions at the level of the retinal pigment epithelium (RPE) [34] and optic atrophy [35] have also been described in certain cases. Infiltration of tumor cells into the retina can cause areas of focal whitening of the retina as well [36]. Over time, exudative retinal detachments can rarely occur and would be most easily imaged on wide-field photography. These lesions can be photographed over time to assess for improvement with treatment.

Especially in the setting of retinal infiltrates, perivasculitis, retinal hemorrhages, and significant vitreous cells, PIOL/PVRL can masquerade as acute retinal necrosis (ARN) syndrome, a rapidly progressive necrotizing retinitis caused by the herpesvirus family that tends to affect the retinal periphery in immunocompetent patients (see Fig. 4). Certain diffuse forms of retinochoroidal toxoplasmosis, which occur largely in immunocompromised patients, may be difficult to differentiate from PIOL; this is especially true in the presence of RPE alterations, which may mimic toxoplasmosis scars [37, 38].

In uveal lymphoma, multifocal creamy-yellow choroidal patches are likely the most helpful funduscopic feature in establishing the diagnosis and may be seen in approximately half of the eyes [24]. Similar lesions may be seen in PIOL/PVRL, although these lesions are located between the RPE and Bruch's membrane [39]. The use of additional testing modalities to determine the location of these infiltrates will be discussed in subsequent sections. Other clinical features of uveal lymphoma that may be present and visible on fundus photography include subretinal fluid, which has been reported to be present in as many as 48% of affected eyes [24], and obscuration of choroidal vessels by diffuse choroidal infiltrates [25, 40]. Less common findings include choroidal folds [25, 32, 41, 42], lipofuscin clumps (which manifest as orange pigment), and optic disc swelling [24].

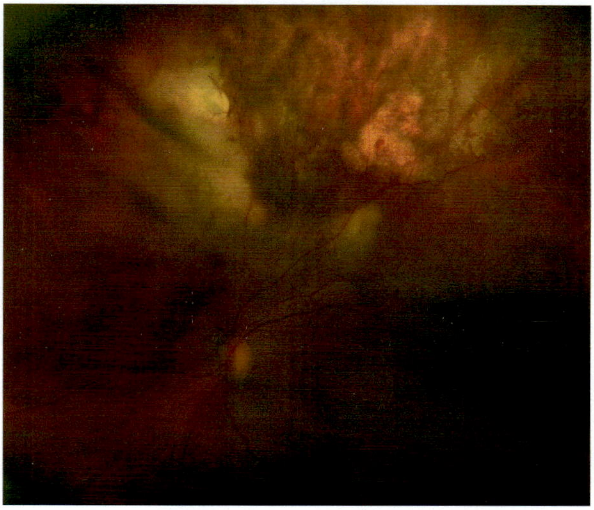

Fig. 4 Wide-field color fundus photograph of an eye with PIOL/PVRL previously and incorrectly diagnosed with acute retinal necrosis. Note the hazy media, patches of retinal whitening/infiltrates, and retinal hemorrhages

Fluorescein Angiography

Fluorescein angiography (FA) will likely give additional clues as to the diagnosis of PIOL. Classically described as a leopard spot, granular pattern of hyperfluorescence [43, 44], the findings on FA can be variable, with some authors describing hypofluorescent spots persistent from early to late frames of the angiogram [19, 21]. This is thought to be due to the fact that the collections of active tumor cells which accumulate between Bruch's membrane and the RPE have a cytoplasm that can not absorb fluorescein dye due to an intact overlying cell membrane [45]. The clusters of small, round, hypofluorescent lesions have been reported to be present in as many as 45% of PIOL/PVRL patients in a study by Fardeau et al. [21]; on the other hand, they were present in only 2% of non-lymphoma cases included in the same study. These spots were found to correlate with small, white punctate lesions observed clinically on ophthalmoscopy.

Confusing the matter, hyperfluorescent window defects can also be present if the overlying RPE is damaged and lead to the overarching granular pattern (see Fig. 5). Staining of the infiltrates can also occur if the cells die and enable dye accumulation [19]. Large blocking lesions can also stain in later phases of the angiogram [46]. Pigment epithelial detachments found in the disease can show early hyperfluorescence and show progressive pooling in late stages of the angiogram if mostly serous in nature or alternatively can block underlying choroidal fluorescence if densely packed with tumor cells and show relative hypofluorescence [44]. Further, in areas of tumor infiltration into the retina, bright and uniform hyperfluorescence with occasional mild leakage can be seen. This finding is thought to be the result of exudates or fluid within the retina around the diffuse invasion of tumor cells above the RPE [47].

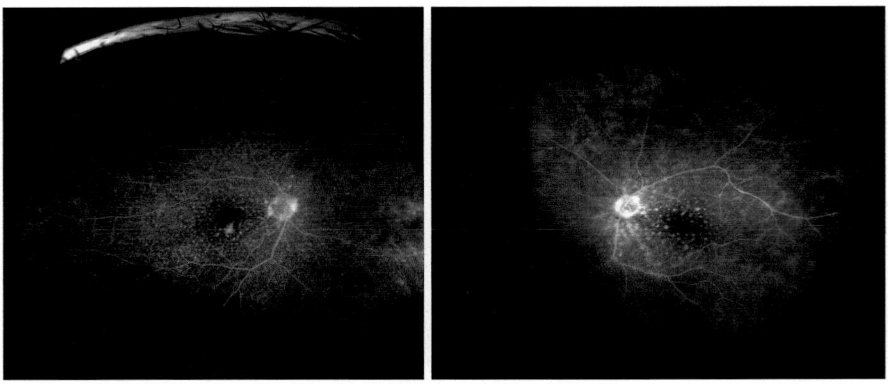

Fig. 5 Wide-field fluorescein angiography of the right and left eyes demonstrating findings in a patient with bilateral PIOL/PVRL. Of note are disc leakage notable in the left eye, numerous hyperfluorescent spots within the posterior poles of both eyes (window defects in areas of RPE atrophy following regression of sub-RPE lesions in the affected areas), and mild late vascular leakage

Finally, although less common, other inflammatory stigmata may also be present, including optic disc hyperfluorescence, macular leakage, and vascular leakage [19]. However, commonly the FA may not reveal any significant abnormalities in PIOL/PVRL, leading to the need for other testing modalities or an overall high index of suspicion.

In eyes with uveal lymphoma, the fluorescein findings can be contradictory and variable between patients. Fluorescein angiography may demonstrate early hypofluorescence with multiple foci of hyperfluorescence and staining in the late phase [15]. However, another study conducted by Aronow et al. described high rates of early hyperfluorescence (78.6%), as well as choroidal folds and hypofluorescent spots [48]. As is the case with PIOL/PVRL, there is no "classic" presentation of uveal lymphoma on fluorescein angiography, the manifestations of which can vary broadly depending on the extent of disease.

Indocyanine Green Angiography (ICG)

On ICG angiography, the classic finding in PIOL/PVRL, if any, is the prevalence of hypocyanescent spots that fade in the later phases of the angiogram [21]. These lesions appear to be less numerous than the lesions seen on FA. This likely corresponds to blockage from the tumor cells, which then is overcome due to the widespread choroidal filling later in the angiogram. If there are large choroidal or sub-RPE infiltrates, these may block throughout the entire angiogram. It has also been suggested that the lesions seen on ICG may represent a lymphocytic response within the choroid [49, 50]. Fardeau et al. noted that these hypocyanescent lesions were observed in 26% of individuals with PIOL/PVRL, compared with only 9% of those with nonlymphomatous cases [21].

Especially in cases of suspected primary uveal lymphoma with choroidal involvement or secondary choroidal lymphoma in the setting of systemic lymphoma, ICG angiography provides superior characterization of the choroidal vasculature in comparison to fluorescein angiography. Multiple, round, hypocyanescent lesions are typically present, and correspond to areas of nonperfusion secondary to space-occupying choroidal infiltrates. These lesions have been reported in up to 100% of cases of choroidal lymphoma, even more so when wide-field angiography is employed [48].

Fundus Autofluorescence

Fundus autofluorescence (FAF) is a noninvasive way to visualize RPE function. Damaged or deranged RPE typically causes a hyperautofluorescent signal due to accumulation of lipofuscin, whereas areas of RPE loss or destruction and corresponding photoreceptor death demonstrate hypoautofluorescence [51]. FAF is not routinely used in the diagnosis of PIOL/PVRL, but may highlight several clinical features, and helps somewhat to explain the pathophysiologic mechanisms behind them.

The autofluorescence findings in PIOL depend on the level of the tumor cells in the retina [52]. Malignant cells in their normal location, between Bruch's membrane and the RPE, cause overlying RPE derangement, resulting in hyperautofluorescence. In a small series of five eyes, sub-RPE infiltrates demonstrated weak hyperautofluorescence, whereas the brown clumps of pigment on the surface of these lesions exhibited brighter autofluorescence [47]. However, if the tumor cells find a way through the RPE, they can rest subretinally or intraretinally and block the normal autofluorescence of the RPE and result in spots of hypoautofluorescence [53]. Finally, when the RPE dies and the overlying photoreceptors are also destroyed, the result is another type of hypoautofluorescent lesion [43, 47, 53] (See Fig. 6). As such, authors generally describe an "inversion" of findings on FAF from the FA findings, where lesions that are hypofluorescent on FA may demonstrate hyperautofluorescence on FAF. However, this is far from universal.

Unfortunately, no significant consensus on the FAF findings in either primary or secondary choroidal lymphoma exist at this time.

Optical Coherence Tomography (OCT)

OCT is the imaging modality which provides the highest resolution of microanatomical retinal details [54]. The advent of enhanced-depth imaging (EDI) OCT, along with other developments to improve resolution and analysis of choroidal and scleral anatomy, has made it possible to visualize deeper structures at a submillimeter level [55]. The resolution of modern iterations of this technology has been reported to be as high as 4 μm [56]. As is the case with other ophthalmic imaging modalities, however, OCT findings in both PIOL/PVRL and choroidal lymphoma (whether primary or secondary) are nondiagnostic. They may provide, though, clues to diagnosis and help differentiate these entities from other uveitic conditions. Additionally, EDI-OCT may provide additional information on the effects of these lesions on overlying retina, visual outcome, and tumor behavior [57–60].

In one series, hyperreflective, nodular RPE lesions were reported in 42% of patients with PIOL/PVRL, in comparison to 15% of those with nonlymphomatous conditions [21]. These OCT findings, which have been described in other series [47], are compatible with histopathologic examination of autopsy of the eyes from patients with PIOL/PVRL, which has demonstrated clusters of malignant cells in the space between the RPE and Bruch's membrane [61–63] (See Fig. 7).

OCT of the macula in PIOL/PVRL eyes also typically reveals a near-normal macular thickness (mean: 231 μm, SD: 45 μm), as opposed to the increased foveal thickness (mean: 327 μm, SD: 114 μm) seen in uveitic processes, a difference which is presumably secondary to the presence of inflammatory edema in nonlymphomatous cases [21]. A small series of patients with PIOL/PVRL demonstrated small pigment epithelial detachments (PEDs) and exudates above the RPE, which may be difficult, if not impossible, to detect on clinical examination or with other imaging modalities [47].

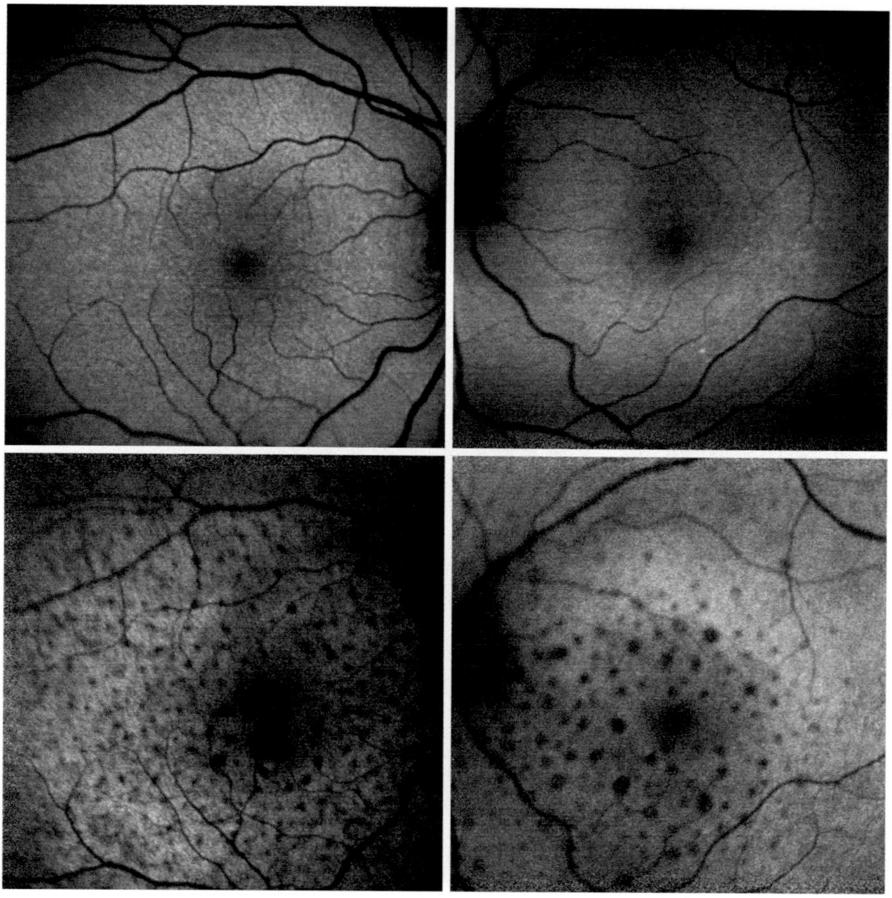

Fig. 6 Fundus autofluorescence early (top) and later within the clinical course (bottom) of a patient with bilateral PIOL/PVRL. The bottom photos were taken on the same visit as the fluorescein angiogram depicted in Fig. 5. Note a mild speckling of the autofluorescence pattern in the upper photos, in contrast to the multiple hypoautofluorescent lesions seen in both eyes in the lower photos

Several cases of secondary intraocular/vitreoretinal lymphoma in the setting of systemic lymphoma have also been reported, in which OCT demonstrated irregularities at the level of the RPE, as well as retinal and subretinal infiltrates [3].

With regard to OCT findings in uveal lymphoma, a case series describing clinical and imaging data from 14 eyes of 13 patients described by Shields and colleagues showed evidence of tumor infiltration on EDI-OCT that varied with the extent of choroidal involvement [54]. Tumors were classified as demonstrating smooth, rippled, or undulating inner choroidal surfaces on OCT, with the thickest and most diffuse tumors being associated with the most irregular choroidal contours on OCT, and with chorioretinal folds clinically [54] (See Fig. 8).

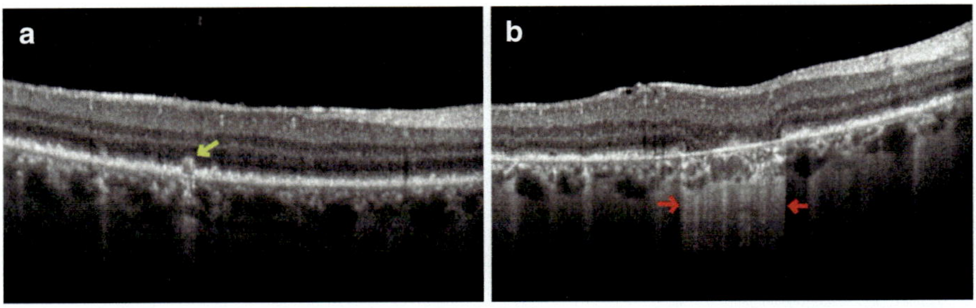

Fig. 7 Spectral-domain ocular coherence tomography (SD-OCT) of the macula in a patient with PIOL/PVRL. (**a**) Sub-RPE infiltrate (yellow arrow) and irregularities at the level of the RPE. (**b**) After regression of the lesions, note the resultant transmission defect (red arrows)

Fig. 8 Spectral-domain ocular coherence tomography (SD-OCT) of the macula in a patient with uveal lymphoma, with choroidal involvement. Note the undulating appearance of the inner choroidal contour, as well as serous subretinal fluid

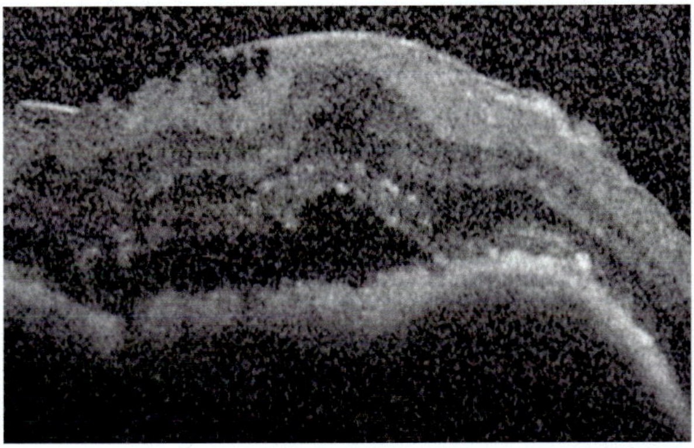

Not surprisingly, in eyes in which choroidal thickness was measurable (9 of 14 eyes), subfoveal choroidal thickness in affected eyes (484 μm) measured 81% greater than that in unaffected eyes (267 μm). Mean choroidal thickness in the affected eyes of 8 individuals in whom maximum tumor thickness was available (602 μm) was 2.17 times greater than a mean choroidal thickness of 278 μm in the unaffected fellow eyes [54].

One notable limitation of EDI-OCT in the imaging of these tumors is an inability to resolve sclerochoroidal details beyond a choroidal/tumor thickness of 2 mm. Ultrasonography is capable of measuring tumor thickness in these situations but may significantly overestimate values when compared to EDI-OCT; in eyes with choroidal lymphoma in which ultrasonography and EDI-OCT were both performed, ultrasonography measured mean tumor thickness as 1762 μm, compared to 602 μm by OCT [54].

B-Scan Ultrasonography

While ultrasonography likely has little utility in the diagnosis and monitoring of treatment response in PIOL/PVRL save for if significant vitritis precludes view to the retina, this technology can provide valuable diagnostic information when uveal

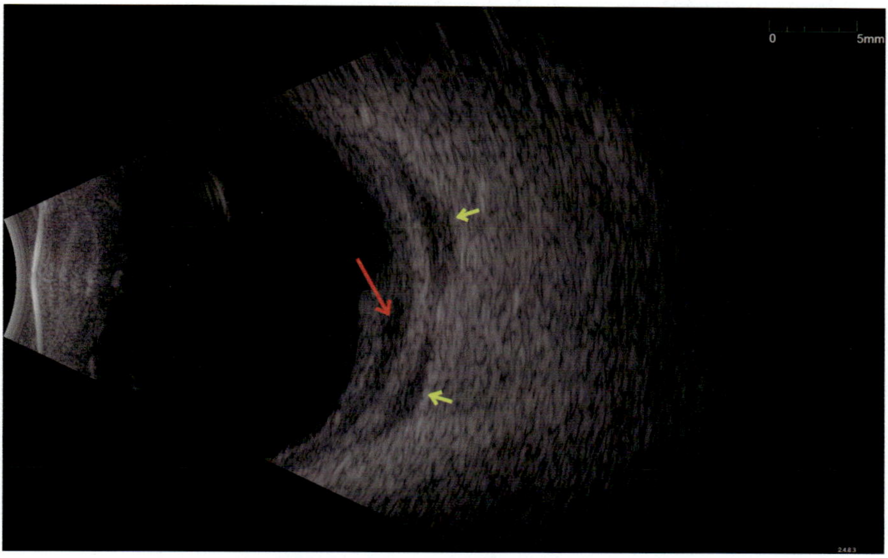

Fig. 9 B-scan ultrasonography of an eye with uveal lymphoma, demonstrating acoustically hollow extrascleral extension (yellow arrows), as well as significant choroidal thickening (red arrow)

lymphoma is suspected. This is especially true when one may have limited access to EDI-OCT or dye-based angiography.

B-scan ultrasonography of eyes with uveal lymphoma will typically reveal marked uveal thickening with low echogenicity [15]. Additionally, examination may reveal acoustically hollow extrascleral extension posteriorly in anywhere from 50% to 76% of eyes with evidence of disease, providing further clues in the diagnosis of choroidal/uveal lymphoma [24, 48]. Subretinal fluid may also be seen ultrasonographically in a small percentage of eyes with choroidal involvement [48] (See Fig. 9).

Conclusions

The difficulty and delay in diagnosing these syndromes often lie in the clinical course seen in these subtypes of lymphoma. Therefore, a practitioner's suspicion should be raised in the setting of an incomplete response or rebound inflammation following corticosteroid therapy, especially with characteristic chorioretinal lesions and/or vitritis without other evidence of inflammatory sequelae. The findings seen with the types of ophthalmic imaging described in this chapter may provide ophthalmologists with additional information, which may help to arrive at the correct diagnosis.

Ultimately, while various types of ophthalmic imaging may provide some aid in the diagnosis of masquerade syndromes, diagnosis and treatment must be guided by adequate clinical suspicion and the appropriate testing. The diagnosis of both vitreoretinal and uveal forms of lymphoma requires a cellular specimen and, once confirmed, should prompt the practitioner to initiate or continue further work-up for extraocular disease.

Compliance with Ethical Requirements Brian K. Do, Jesse L. Berry, and Damien C. Rodger declare that they have no financial conflicts of interest pertaining to the material presented here. No human or animal studies were carried out by the authors for this chapter for the material presented herein.

References

1. Fend F, Ferreri AJ, Coupland SE. How we diagnose and treat vitreoretinal lymphoma. Br J Haematol. 2016;173(5):680–92.
2. Karimi M, Soheilian M, Kanavi MR. Bilateral primary intraocular lymphoma. J Ophthalmic Vis Res. 2011;6(4):344–7.
3. Salomão DR, Pulido JS, Johnston PB, et al. Vitreoretinal presentation of secondary large B-cell lymphoma in patients with systemic lymphoma. JAMA Ophthalmol. 2013;131(9):1151–8.
4. Verbraeken HE, Hanssens M, Priem H, et al. Ocular non-Hodgkin's lymphoma: a clinical study of nine cases. Br J Ophthalmol. 1997;81(1):31–6.
5. Kuker W, Nagele T, Korfel A, et al. Primary central nervous system lymphomas (PCNSL): MRI features at presentation in 100 patients. J Neuro-Oncol. 2005;72(2):169–77.
6. Coupland SE, Bechrakis NE, Anastassiou G, et al. Evaluation of vitrectomy specimens and chorioretinal biopsies in the diagnosis of primary intraocular lymphoma in patients with masquerade syndrome. Graefes Arch Clin Exp Ophthalmol. 2003;241(10):860–70.
7. Whitcup SM, Stark-Vancs V, Wittes RE, et al. Association of interleukin 10 in the vitreous and cerebrospinal fluid and primary central nervous system lymphoma. Arch Ophthalmol. 1997;115(9):1157–60.
8. Chan CC, Whitcup SM, Solomon D, Nussenblatt RB. Interleukin-10 in the vitreous of patients with primary intraocular lymphoma. Am J Ophthalmol. 1995;120(5):671–3.
9. Buggage RR, Velez G, Myers-Powell B, et al. Primary intraocular lymphoma with a low interleukin 10 to interleukin 6 ratio and heterogeneous IgH gene rearrangement. Arch Ophthalmol. 1999;117(9):1239–42.
10. Kuo DE, Wei MM, Armbrust KR, et al. Gradient boosted decision tree classification of endophthalmitis versus uveitis and lymphoma from aqueous and vitreous IL-6 and IL-10 levels. J Ocul Pharmacol Ther. 2017;33(4):319–24.
11. Eliott D, Rao PK. Surgical management of intraocular inflammation and infection. London: JP Medical; 2013.
12. Cassoux N, Charlotte F, Rao NA, et al. Endoretinal biopsy in establishing the diagnosis of uveitis: a clinicopathologic report of three cases. Ocul Immunol Inflamm. 2005;13(1):79–83.
13. Jahnke K, Thiel E, Abrey LE, et al. Diagnosis and management of primary intraocular lymphoma: an update. Clin Ophthalmol. 2007;1(3):247–58.
14. Cockerham GC, Hidayat AA, Bijwaard KE, Sheng ZM. Re-evaluation of "reactive lymphoid hyperplasia of the uvea": an immunohistochemical and molecular analysis of 10 cases. Ophthalmology. 2000;107(1):151–8.
15. Aronow ME, Singh AD. The use of imaging in the diagnosis and management of intraocular lymphoma. Int Ophthalmol Clin. 2012;52(4):199–208.
16. Hoskin PJ, Kirkwood AA, Popova B, et al. 4 Gy versus 24 Gy radiotherapy for patients with indolent lymphoma (FORT): a randomised phase 3 non-inferiority trial. Lancet Oncol. 2014;15(4):457–63.
17. Verdijk RM. Lymphoproliferative tumors of the ocular adnexa. Asia Pac J Ophthalmol (Phila). 2017;6(2):132–42.
18. Fuller ML, Sweetenham J, Schoenfield L, Singh AD. Uveal lymphoma: a variant of ocular adnexal lymphoma. Leuk Lymphoma. 2008;49(12):2393–7.
19. Cassoux N, Merle-Beral H, Leblond V, et al. Ocular and central nervous system lymphoma: clinical features and diagnosis. Ocul Immunol Inflamm. 2000;8(4):243–50.

20. Kimura K, Usui Y, Goto H. Japanese intraocular lymphoma study G. clinical features and diagnostic significance of the intraocular fluid of 217 patients with intraocular lymphoma. Jpn J Ophthalmol. 2012;56(4):383–9.
21. Fardeau C, Lee CP, Merle-Beral H, et al. Retinal fluorescein, indocyanine green angiography, and optic coherence tomography in non-Hodgkin primary intraocular lymphoma. Am J Ophthalmol. 2009;147(5):886–94. 94 e1.
22. Chan C-C, Gonzales JA. Primary intraocular lymphoma. Hackensack: World Scientific; 2007. xv, 284 p.
23. Coupland S. Uveal lymphoproliferative tumors. In: Singh AD, Damato B, Peer J, et al., editors. Clinical ophthalmic oncology. Philadelphia: Elsevier Inc.; 2007.
24. Mashayekhi A, Shukla SY, Shields JA, Shields CL. Choroidal lymphoma: clinical features and association with systemic lymphoma. Ophthalmology. 2014;121(1):342–51.
25. Ciulla TA, Bains RA, Jakobiec FA, et al. Uveal lymphoid neoplasia: a clinical-pathologic correlation and review of the early form. Surv Ophthalmol. 1997;41(6):467–76.
26. Coupland SE, Foss HD, Bechrakis NE, et al. Secondary ocular involvement in systemic "memory" B-cell lymphocytic leukemia. Ophthalmology. 2001;108(7):1289–95.
27. Grossniklaus HE, Martin DF, Avery R, et al. Uveal lymphoid infiltration. Report of four cases and clinicopathologic review. Ophthalmology. 1998;105(7):1265–73.
28. Hoang-Xuan T, Bodaghi B, Toublanc M, et al. Scleritis and mucosal-associated lymphoid tissue lymphoma: a new masquerade syndrome. Ophthalmology. 1996;103(4):631–5.
29. Jakobiec FA, Sacks E, Kronish JW, et al. Multifocal static creamy choroidal infiltrates. An early sign of lymphoid neoplasia. Ophthalmology. 1987;94(4):397–406.
30. Ryan SJ, Zimmerman LE, King FM. Reactive lymphoid hyperplasia. An unusual form of intraocular pseudotumor. Trans Am Acad Ophthalmol Otolaryngol. 1972;76(3):652–71.
31. Saga T, Ohno S, Matsuda H, et al. Ocular involvement by a peripheral T-cell lymphoma. Arch Ophthalmol. 1984;102(3):399–402.
32. Sarraf D, Jain A, Dubovy S, et al. Mucosa-associated lymphoid tissue lymphoma with intraocular involvement. Retina. 2005;25(1):94–8.
33. Ridley ME, McDonald HR, Sternberg P Jr, et al. Retinal manifestations of ocular lymphoma (reticulum cell sarcoma). Ophthalmology. 1992;99(7):1153–60. discussion 60-1.
34. Lang GK, Surer JL, Green WR, et al. Ocular reticulum cell sarcoma. Clinicopathologic correlation of a case with multifocal lesions. Retina. 1985;5(2):79–86.
35. Purvin V, Van Dyk HJ. Primary reticulum cell sarcoma of the brain presenting as steroid-responsive optic neuropathy. J Clin Neuroophthalmol. 1984;4(1):15–23.
36. Shields CL, Bianciotto C, Pirondini C, et al. Autofluorescence of choroidal melanoma in 51 cases. Br J Ophthalmol. 2008;92(5):617–22.
37. Ryan ME, Shantha JG, Grossniklaus HE, Yeh S. Secondary vitreoretinal lymphoma masquerading as acute retinal necrosis. Ophthalmic Surg Lasers Imaging Retina. 2015;46(10):1048–50.
38. Sen HN, Bodaghi B, Hoang PL, Nussenblatt R. Primary intraocular lymphoma: diagnosis and differential diagnosis. Ocul Immunol Inflamm. 2009;17(3):133–41.
39. Akpek EK, Ahmed I, Hochberg FH, et al. Intraocular-central nervous system lymphoma: clinical features, diagnosis, and outcomes. Ophthalmology. 1999;106(9):1805–10.
40. Desroches G, Abrams GW, Gass JD. Reactive lymphoid hyperplasia of the uvea. A case with ultrasonographic and computed tomographic studies. Arch Ophthalmol. 1983;101(5):725–8.
41. Cheung MK, Martin DF, Chan CC, et al. Diagnosis of reactive lymphoid hyperplasia by chorioretinal biopsy. Am J Ophthalmol. 1994;118(4):457–62.
42. Holz FG, Boehmer HV, Mechtersheimer G, et al. Uveal non-Hodgkin's lymphoma with epibulbar extension simulating choroidal effusion syndrome. Retina. 1999;19(4):343–6.
43. Casady M, Faia L, Nazemzadeh M, et al. Fundus autofluorescence patterns in primary intraocular lymphoma. Retina. 2014;34(2):366–72.
44. Velez G, Chan CC, Csaky KG. Fluorescein angiographic findings in primary intraocular lymphoma. Retina. 2002;22(1):37–43.
45. Gass JD. Fluorescein angiography. An aid in the differential diagnosis of intraocular tumors. Int Ophthalmol Clin. 1972;12(1):85–120.

46. Kirmani MH, Thomas EL, Rao NA, Laborde RP. Intraocular reticulum cell sarcoma: diagnosis by choroidal biopsy. Br J Ophthalmol. 1987;71(10):748–52.
47. Ishida T, Ohno-Matsui K, Kaneko Y, et al. Fundus autofluorescence patterns in eyes with primary intraocular lymphoma. Retina. 2010;30(1):23–32.
48. Aronow ME, Portell CA, Sweetenham JW, Singh AD. Uveal lymphoma: clinical features, diagnostic studies, treatment selection, and outcomes. Ophthalmology. 2014;121(1):334–41.
49. Chan CC, Sauer TC. Ocular imaging in primary retinal lymphoma. Am J Ophthalmol. 2009;147(5):764–5.
50. Lopez JS, Chan CC, Burnier M, et al. Immunohistochemistry findings in primary intraocular lymphoma. Am J Ophthalmol. 1991;112(4):472–4.
51. Meleth AD, Sen HN. Use of fundus autofluorescence in the diagnosis and management of uveitis. Int Ophthalmol Clin. 2012;52(4):45–54.
52. Davis JL. Intraocular lymphoma: a clinical perspective. Eye (Lond). 2013;27(2):153–62.
53. Egawa M, Mitamura Y, Hayashi Y, et al. Changes of fundus autofluorescence and spectral-domain optical coherence tomographic findings after treatment of primary intraocular lymphoma. J Ophthalmic Inflamm Infect. 2014;4(1):7.
54. Shields CL, Arepalli S, Pellegrini M, et al. Choroidal lymphoma shows calm, rippled, or undulating topography on enhanced depth imaging optical coherence tomography in 14 eyes. Retina. 2014;34(7):1347–53.
55. Spaide RF, Koizumi H, Pozzoni MC. Enhanced depth imaging spectral-domain optical coherence tomography. Am J Ophthalmol. 2008;146(4):496–500.
56. Kiernan DF, Mieler WF, Hariprasad SM. Spectral-domain optical coherence tomography: a comparison of modern high-resolution retinal imaging systems. Am J Ophthalmol. 2010;149(1):18–31.
57. Say EA, Shah SU, Ferenczy S, Shields CL. Optical coherence tomography of retinal and choroidal tumors. J Ophthalmol. 2012;2012:385058.
58. Shah SU, Kaliki S, Shields CL, et al. Enhanced depth imaging optical coherence tomography of choroidal nevus in 104 cases. Ophthalmology. 2012;119(5):1066–72.
59. Shields CL, Kaliki S, Rojanaporn D, et al. Enhanced depth imaging optical coherence tomography of small choroidal melanoma: comparison with choroidal nevus. Arch Ophthalmol. 2012;130(7):850–6.
60. Shields CL, Materin MA, Shields JA. Review of optical coherence tomography for intraocular tumors. Curr Opin Ophthalmol. 2005;16(3):141–54.
61. Corriveau C, Easterbrook M, Payne D. Lymphoma simulating uveitis (masquerade syndrome). Can J Ophthalmol. 1986;21(4):144–9.
62. Grimm SA, McCannel CA, Omuro AM, et al. Primary CNS lymphoma with intraocular involvement: international PCNSL collaborative group report. Neurology. 2008;71(17):1355–60.
63. Whitcup SM, de Smet MD, Rubin BI, et al. Intraocular lymphoma. Clinical and histopathologic diagnosis. Ophthalmology. 1993;100(9):1399–406.

Part IV

Non-Infectious Uveitis: Treatment Options

Noninfectious Uveitis: Systemic and Local Corticosteroids

Ashleigh Laurin Levison

Corticosteroids, specifically glucocorticoids, are both a natural compound made by the adrenal glands and synthetic exogenous medications that serve as an important form of immunosuppression to treat inflammatory disease. Corticosteroids serve as an essential and necessary component to the treatment of patients with uveitis and uveitis-associated cystoid macular edema (CME). They are able to improve inflammation by inhibiting important steps in the inflammatory cascade [1]. Corticosteroids act through the glucocorticoid receptor where its actions allow for the upregulation of anti-inflammatory proteins and downregulation of the expression of pro-inflammatory proteins [1–3]. Corticosteroids improve inflammation by suppressing cellular infiltration, reducing capillary dilation, reducing proliferation of fibroblasts, and limiting collagen deposition. These activities are responsible for corticosteroid's powerful immunosuppressive effect. Corticosteroids are used broadly in medicine to treat inflammatory conditions other than uveitis as well [4–6].

For the treatment of uveitis, corticosteroids can be given both systemically and locally. Local treatment includes topical therapy, periocular and intravitreal injectable steroids and injectable implants, as well as surgically placed steroid implants. The spectrum of available local steroid therapy has diversified over the recent years. The various options available provide us with opportunities to treat with different durations of action and potency.

The glucocorticoid receptor is involved in many signaling pathways, and therefore long-term exposure or high doses of corticosteroids can lead to side effects unrelated to resolution or reduction of inflammation [1]. There can be both local ocular side effects from systemic and local corticosteroids and significant systemic side effects from oral or intravenous corticosteroids. One of the well-known local side effects of corticosteroids is elevation of intraocular pressure. Studies have shown that the mechanism of intraocular pressure rise is due to effects of

A. L. Levison (✉)
Colorado Retina Associates, Denver, CO, USA
e-mail: alevison@retinacolorado.com

N. A. Rao et al. (eds.), *Posterior Uveitis*, Essentials in Ophthalmology,
https://doi.org/10.1007/978-3-030-03140-4_10

glucocorticoids on the trabecular meshwork and myocilin gene expression. Aqueous humor outflow is reduced by increasing extracellular matrix in the trabecular meshwork as well as by limiting extracellular matrix degradation [7]. In addition there may be cross-linking of actin fibers in the trabecular meshwork [7]. Corticosteroids can also lead to cataract formation. This is thought to occur due to effects they have on changing protein structure of lens proteins [1].

This chapter will discuss both systemic and local steroids, including topical steroids, periocular injections, intravitreal steroid injections and implants, as well as surgical steroid implants for the treatment of uveitis and cystoid macular edema secondary to uveitis.

Systemic Corticosteroids

Oral corticosteroids are a widely used treatment for an initial or subsequent flare of noninfectious intermediate, posterior, and panuveitis. In certain cases of severe anterior uveitis that do not respond to topical therapy, especially HLA-B27-associated anterior uveitis, oral corticosteroids are often an important adjunctive therapy. Oral steroids are also used in the setting of some forms of infectious uveitis but only in the setting of concurrent treatment of the infectious etiology. While some patients may remain on long-term low-dose oral steroids, high-dose oral steroids are not an accepted long-term therapy due to systemic side effects, and instead other steroid-sparing immunosuppressive agents or local therapies are used [8].

Prednisone is the most commonly prescribed oral steroid. Other options are available including prednisolone for those patients with liver dysfunction. Methylprednisolone dose packs are not typically used for the treatment of uveitis due to their low dose and short duration of treatment. When used, oral prednisone is typically initially prescribed at 1 mg/kg/day. In the setting of severe vision-threatening diseases that require higher doses of systemic steroids, intravenous methylprednisolone sodium (SOLU-MEDROL, Pfizer, New York City, New York) can be given. Commonly intravenous methylprednisolone is dosed at 1 gram daily for 3 consecutive days followed by oral prednisone [8]. There are no widely accepted rules to how corticosteroids are to be tapered, but expert panels have recommended that high-dose steroids are not to be used for more than 1 month. Oral steroids are then tapered over a period of time, depending on severity of disease and risk of vision loss. Because corticosteroids suppress the hypothalamic-pituitary-adrenal axis, patients are at risk of Addison's crisis if tapered too quickly [6]. If patients require long-term prednisone therapy, the accepted goal is to keep that dose below 10 mg daily [8].

While beneficial in treating uveitis and helping to bring resolution of a flare, oral steroids have both significant short-term and long-term side effects [8]. Long-term systemic corticosteroid use is associated with diabetes, hypertension, hypercholesterolemia, myopathy, and osteoporosis [9]. Given the significant impact prednisone can have on bone density, often vitamin D and calcium are recommended in conjunction with steroids. The use of corticosteroids is associated with weight gain,

Cushingoid changes, acne, and mood changes as well [9]. Patients can easily bruise and have poor wound healing with use of steroids. In addition, due to gastric side effects of prednisone, some physicians recommend to take an antacid such as a proton pump inhibitor along with use of prednisone. Previous publications however have suggested this may not be necessary [8]. Ocular side effects include glaucoma and cataracts; however, oral steroids typically have less ocular side effects relative to local therapy.

Topical Steroids

Topical steroids are most commonly used to treat anterior chamber inflammation [6]. They are not typically used for the treatment of intermediate or posterior uveitis [9]. Topical corticosteroids reduce inflammation and scarring by reducing inflammatory cell infiltration, fibroblast proliferation, and collagen deposition [6]. Topical steroids successfully improve the redness, photophobia, and pain associated with anterior chamber inflammation [10].

The most commonly used topical steroids for the treatment of uveitis are prednisolone acetate 1% and difluprednate 0.05%. Prednisolone acetate is prescribed as Pred Forte® (Allergan Pharmaceuticals, Irvine, CA) or as generic prednisolone acetate 1% [11]. Difluprednate ophthalmic emulsion 0.05% (Durezol; Alcon Research, Ltd., Fort Worth, TX) became FDA approved in 2008 [12, 13]. Difluprednate has increased corticosteroid potency and better penetration, therefore increasing the anti-inflammatory effect [14]. Difluprednate 0.05% can therefore be dosed less frequently than prednisolone acetate 1%. While prednisolone acetate treats anterior chamber inflammation, difluprednate has greater penetration, and a study has shown radioactive-labeled difluprednate penetration into posterior retina and choroid [15].

A phase 3 randomized control trial was performed comparing prednisolone acetate 1% to difluprednate 0.05% for noninfectious anterior uveitis. Patients in the prednisolone acetate 1% group were treated eight times a day, while the difluprednate 0.05% group was treated four times a day. The study found that difluprednate 0.05% four times daily was non-inferior to prednisolone acetate 1% eight times daily for the treatment of anterior uveitis [14]. Improvement in anterior chamber cell grade occurred in both groups in the study. Less frequent need for drops would likely increase compliance of medication with patients. An important concern with difluprednate is rise in intraocular pressure; however, infrequently in the study did intraocular pressure rise above 21 [14]. There was no difference between the two groups regarding IOP rise. Cataracts were not discussed [16].

Due to difluprednate's increase potency compared to prednisolone acetate, it has been used for treatment of some cases of intermediate and posterior uveitis. Case reports of serous detachments from Vogt-Koyanagi-Harada disease resolving with difluprednate have been published [17, 18]. A case report with use of difluprednate in the treatment of pars planitis has been published as well [19]. While this is not standard of care, use of difluprednate might be beneficial in some cases of uveitis other than isolated anterior uveitis. More studies are needed however to better understand its role in the treatment of intermediate, posterior, and panuveitis.

Loteprednol etabonate 0.5% (Lotemax; Bausch & Lomb, Rochester, NY), a weaker steroid, is an ester corticosteroid that has good anti-inflammatory effect with an improved safety over other available corticosteroids. It is much less likely to induce elevation in IOP compared to other available corticosteroids such as prednisolone acetate [20]. Two randomized controlled trials were performed comparing prednisolone acetate 1% to loteprednol etabonate 0.5% at reducing the ocular signs and symptoms associated with anterior uveitis. Both treatments successfully decreased cell, flare, pain, and photophobia after 28 days of treatment. In the first study, however, more patients in the prednisolone group reached zero active inflammation. While both corticosteroids in the study were effective, prednisolone acetate was more effective overall, but loteprednol etabonate did have a lower side effect profile [10]. Loteprednol is therefore less commonly used in the treatment of uveitis. Another weak steroid, fluorometholone 0.1% (FML; Allergan, Parsippany, NJ) while used in other ophthalmic conditions, is also not typically used in the treatment of uveitis.

A vision-threatening complication of uveitis is cystoid macular edema [21]. Depending on the anatomic location of the inflammation that led to the macular edema, it can be treated in various ways. If the macular edema is secondary to anterior uveitis, often resolution of anterior inflammation leads to resolution of the CME. The effect of topical corticosteroids in the treatment of cystoid macular edema depends on their ability to penetrate to the macula. Difluprednate 0.05% has higher potency than other topical steroids available, and therefore studies have shown difluprednate has the potency to treat uveitic macular edema as well as macular edema from other causes such as pseudophakic cystoid macular edema [21–23].

Topical steroids can have local side effects, most commonly rise in IOP and progression of cataracts. Topical steroids are more likely to cause elevation of IOP than systemic steroids [24]. Difluprednate must be used with caution as it has more local side effects than prednisolone acetate; however these are much greater in pediatric patients than adult patients. In a study of 3488 adult patients who were on difluprednate postoperatively for cataract surgery, the mean IOP increase over baseline was within ±2 mmHg and reduced back to baseline 3–6 weeks after surgery. The odds ratio of IOP ≥21 mmHg or ≥10 mmHg from baseline 5 to 10 days after surgery in those receiving difluprednate was 1.84 [25]. Slabaugh et al. published a retrospective case series regarding the use of difluprednate 0.5% in pediatric patients with uveitis and cystoid macular edema. While very successful at treating inflammation and reducing cystoid macular edema, there was a severe IOP response in this pediatric population. An IOP response >10mmgHg above baseline and IOP >24 were seen in 50% of the eyes. Three of 26 eyes required glaucoma surgery. There was a high rate of cataract development as well, as 10 of 26 eyes developed a visually significant cataract and 5 of the 26 eyes underwent cataract surgery [26]. If used, difluprednate must be used with extreme caution in children.

Regional/Periocular

Many methods of periocular injection have been described. Triamcinolone acetonide (Kenalog-40, Bristol-Myers Squibb, New York City, New York) is the drug most often used for periocular injections [9]. Overall, compared to intravitreal injections, periocular injections are less effective due to decreased penetration through the sclera and the choroid but can have great benefit and utility in the treatment of uveitis [27].

Steroids can be injected into the subconjunctival space; however this method is not used for the treatment of uveitis. Instead, subconjunctival injections are most commonly used after intraocular surgery to deliver the short-acting steroid, dexamethasone. Posterior subtenon's injections, trans-tenon's retrobulbar injections, and orbital floor injections have been described as well [28]. Moorfields Eye Hospital performed a study that compared injection of posterior subtenon's triamcinolone to orbital floor methylprednisolone. Both methods were found to be beneficial in treating vitritis and uveitic cystoid macular edema. No difference was found between the two in percentage of eyes that achieved ≥2 lines of improvement [29]. Another study found no difference between posterior subtenon's corticosteroid from retrobulbar corticosteroid [30]. Posterior subtenon's has however been adopted as the most frequently performed periocular injection.

While performing posterior subtenon's injections, the drug is most commonly injected superotemporally. A study with ultrasound found that superotemporal injections were more likely to result in placement of the drug into the subtenon's space. In addition, gravity helps the drug move over the macula, an important site for it to be delivered in the treatment of cystoid macular edema [31].

After a posterior subtenon's triamcinolone injection, it is possible to see an improvement in inflammation within days to weeks with improvement in macular edema following. Sen et al. published the largest study to date looking at patients who had received at least one periocular injection for uveitis. Included were 914 patients and 1192 eyes. Within 6 months of injection 72.7% of eyes had complete resolution of their inflammation. The eyes that responded best were those with anterior uveitis. In those with anterior uveitis, 88.29% were controlled at 6 months, 66.9% with intermediate uveitis had resolution of activity, and 63.6% of patients with posterior or panuveitis were fully controlled [32]. Resolution of macular edema was similar regardless if the patient had anterior, intermediate, pan-, or posterior uveitis. This is likely due to placement of steroid into space near the macula which is independent of where the inflammation originates [32]. Factors that led to lower likelihood of response were duration of uveitis with a 3% decrease in odds of improvement for each additional year since the patient was diagnosed with uveitis [32].

Regarding duration of action, Tanner et al. published a paper of a series of 28 posterior subtenon's Kenalog injections in 13 patients with intermediate uveitis. None of the patients in the study required a second injection before 3 months, and all patients decreased or stopped their immunosuppression after their posterior subtenon's triamcinolone injection [24]. In clinical practice, injections typically need to be repeated every 2–4 months for the treatment of uveitis [9].

Not all studies published of posterior subtenon's corticosteroids have had as successful results as Sen's and Tanner's publications. Helm et al. showed a 67% response rate to a single subtenon's triamcinolone injection with 78% response with one or two injections with improvement of at least two Snellen lines on visual acuity testing [33]. Salek et al. published a retrospective study of 109 eyes in 81 patients who underwent periocular corticosteroid injections for the treatment of uveitis. Only 36% had resolution of inflammation at 1 month and 48% at 3 months. Overall 18% of eyes needed more than one injection to bring inflammation under control [34]. Approximately one third of eyes had halving of visual angle which is lower than reported in some other studies [34].

In addition to using posterior subtenon's steroids for the treatment of the inflammation associated with uveitis, they are often used for the treatment of cystoid macular edema secondary to uveitis. Leder et al. published a retrospective study evaluating 156 eyes of 126 patients who underwent periocular steroid injections for the treatment of cystoid macular edema secondary to uveitis. Following the first injection, at 1 month 53% of patients had resolution of their CME, and at 3 months 57% had resolution. Of those who had resolution at 1 month, none had recurrence of their CME at 3 months. The 40 eyes that had CME remaining at 1 month underwent repeat injections with some patients receiving greater than 2 additional injections. Higher resolution of CME was seen with greater number of injections. If resolved after first injection, median time to resolution was 3.7 weeks [35]. Of eyes that had resolution of their CME, 53% had recurrence of their edema at 1 year. The mean time to recurrence was 20.2 weeks from resolution. Therefore while beneficial for treating CME, near half the time patients required multiple injections to reach resolution [35].

Posterior subtenon's steroid injections carry the risk of intraocular pressure rise as do other forms of steroid therapy for uveitis [32]. Posterior subtenon's injections are however less associated with glaucoma than anterior subtenon's injection likely due to proximity of the drug to the trabecular meshwork [33]. Not many studies are published on this topic, and therefore rates of IOP rise vary significantly. Like with topical difluprednate, young age has been shown to be associated with higher risk of IOP elevation [36]. Patients receiving more injections are likely to be more at risk of intraocular pressure-related issues as well [33]. In a 1972 study, Nozik et al. reported only 3 of 175 patients with uveitis had an intraocular pressure rise with periocular steroid injections [37]. In the Sen et al. publication of 914 patients, at 12 months 34.0% of patients had an IOP $\geq$ 24 mmHg, and 15.0% had $\geq$30 mmHg. Only 2.4% of patients had glaucoma surgery by month 12 [32]. A French study evaluated 61 patients who received 1 or more subtenon's injections of triamcinolone acetonide for uveitis. Thirteen of 61 patients (21.3%) experienced a rise in IOP. They were unable to control intraocular pressure in 3 of the 13 patients. Instead of glaucoma surgery, however, they performed surgical excision of the steroid which was successful in lowering intraocular pressure [38].

Iwao et al. published a study of 115 patients who underwent posterior subtenon's triamcinolone injections and had a slow increase in mean IOP from the time of injection reaching its peak at 2 months. After 2 months the IOP decreased slowly, and the minimum IOP was seen at 12 months. The mean number of intraocular pressure lowering drops given during the follow-up period was 1.5. The study found if injections were repeated within 6 months, then the IOP with second injection was statistically significantly higher than with the first, but this was not the case if they were not within 6 months of each other [36].

The Iwao study showed 15% risk of cataract development with posterior subtenon's triamcinolone injections [36]. Sen et al. found that within 12 months, of phakic eyes that were initially 20/40 or better, the rate of reduction in visual acuity to less than 20/40 due to cataract was 20.2%. At 12 months 13.8% of phakic eyes had undergone cataract surgery [32]. Besides direct effects of steroids creating cataract and intraocular pressure rise, periocular injections carry risks associated with the injection themselves including globe perforation, ptosis, cutaneous hypopigmentation, orbital fat atrophy, and very rarely vascular occlusion [39–43].

While beneficial in treating uveitis and macular edema in children, a study showed 21% of their patients had posterior subcapsular cataract formation and underwent cataract surgery [44]. Cataracts can induce amblyopia in children and therefore can be of significant consequence. Cataract surgery creates loss of accommodation which is of great consequence in children. The impact of cataracts and cataract surgery need to be considered strongly before proceeding with periocular injections in children [44].

Intravitreal Triamcinolone

Both triamcinolone in the form of Kenalog-40 (Bristol-Myers Squibb, New York City, New York) and TRIESENCE (Alcon, Fort Worth, TX, USA) have been used for the treatment of uveitis and cystoid macular edema associated with uveitis. While TRIESENCE is preservative-free, the preservative present in Kenalog-40 is 0.99% benzyl alcohol. There is debate regarding the intraocular toxicity of triamcinolone acetonide containing preservatives [24]. Present on the packaging of Kenalog-40 is now a label reporting the drug is not for intraocular use [45]. The FDA-approved drug for the treatment of uveitis is TRIESENCE® (triamcinolone acetonide injectable suspension) 40 mg/mL. It was approved by the FDA in 2007 for treatment of sympathetic ophthalmia, temporal arteritis, uveitis, and ocular inflammatory conditions unresponsive to topical corticosteroids [46]. Since triamcinolone was initially FDA approved in 1957, TRIESENCE did not require phase 3 trials for approval for the treatment of uveitis. The effect is limited, lasting approximately 3 months [12].

No controlled trials have been performed, but retrospective studies have been published which show the benefit of intravitreal triamcinolone at a dose of 2–4 mg in 0.05–0.10 ml for the treatment of uveitis and uveitis-associated cystoid macular edema [47]. Studies have shown that the suppression of inflammation occurs rapidly and successfully with intravitreal triamcinolone acetonide [43].

The use of intravitreal triamcinolone for posterior and panuveitis secondary to Behcet's disease was studied by Un Chul Park et al. Forty-nine eyes of 49 patients with Behcet's were injected with intravitreal TRIESENCE. Besides improvement in vision, change in fluorescein angiographic evidence of activity was evaluated in 32 of the 49 eyes. Prior to injection, all eyes had vascular leakage and 71.9% of eyes had disc leakage. Angiography after injection showed resolution of all leakage in 25% of eyes, and 68.8% showed incomplete resolution of leakage. Cystoid macular edema on angiography was seen in 62.5% of the patients, and 85% of them had complete or partial resolution of that angiographic CME [48]. Intravitreal triamcinolone was an effective treatment for rapid improvement in inflammation and vision. Like other studies, however, vision gain was limited by cataract development [48].

As seen in the above study, other studies have shown intravitreal triamcinolone's ability to successfully treat cystoid macular edema. Kok et al. published a retrospective case series of 65 eyes in 54 patients with uveitis-associated cystoid macular edema. The presence of cystoid macular edema was confirmed by fluorescein angiography or OCT. The patients had been previously treated with oral steroids or periocular steroids without complete response. Patients received 4 mg in 0.1 ml intravitreal injection of triamcinolone. The patients had a mean follow-up period of 8 months. Visual acuity was best at a mean of 4 weeks post injection. Eighty-three percent of eyes had an improvement in visual acuity, with 51% gaining two lines on the Snellen visual acuity chart. Seventeen percent of eyes had no change in vision despite improvement in cystoid macular edema due to foveal damage from previous chronic cystoid macular edema. Those eyes with cystoid macular edema for less than 12 months had greatest improvement in visual acuity. In 7 of 17 patients on oral prednisone prior to enrollment, the dose was able to be reduced by greater than 5 mg after treatment. Sixteen patients were on both prednisone and another immunosuppressive agent at baseline. After intravitreal triamcinolone 51% of those patients reduced or stopped their second-line immunosuppressive agent [49].

Regarding duration of action, Steeples et al. published a retrospective cohort study of 66 injections of triamcinolone acetate to 44 eyes of 40 patients. Sixty-eight percent of patients underwent only a single injection, while 18% of patients received two injections, and 13% received three or more injections. Mean time to the second injection was 25.5 weeks and to the third injection was 52.7 weeks [50].

The side effects of intravitreal triamcinolone are similar to those of other steroids. The systemic side effects of intravitreal triamcinolone are minimal. The drug is limited to the eye and the serum level of the drug is not significant [51]. Patients experienced the expected side effects associated with local steroids including intraocular pressure rise and cataract formation. Previous studies have shown that the rate of cataract development is 15–30% after one injection of intravitreal steroid [47]. The rate of cataract progression has been shown to be increased fivefold, and rate of cataract formation increases with repeat injections of triamcinolone [52].

In the study published by Kok et al., after intravitreal injection of triamcinolone, 42 eyes (64%) had an IOP rise >5 mmHg, and 28 eyes (43%) had an IOP rise >10 mmHg. Severe IOP response was seen with 22 (34%) eyes having an IOP rise to greater than 30 and 7 eyes (11%) with an IOP greater than 40. Thirty-three eyes (51%) needed topical drops to lower intraocular pressure, while no patients needed incisional glaucoma surgery [49]. In the study by Steeples et al., 46% of patients had worsening of their cataract, and 45% had an IOP greater than 21 mmHg [50].

With intravitreal injections of triamcinolone, cases of infectious and noninfectious sterile inflammation can occur [53]. Moshfeghi et al. published a study where 0.87%, or 8 of 922 eyes, developed infectious endophthalmitis after intravitreal injection of triamcinolone. Three of the cases resulted in no light perception vision, and one patient underwent an enucleation [54]. Besides infectious endophthalmitis, pseudo-endophthalmitis can occur as a sterile inflammation. White triamcinolone crystals have been seen in the anterior chamber of patients and can create a pseudohypopyon [53]. Other patients can develop a significant anterior chamber inflammatory reaction with vitritis. This inflammatory debris is different than the pseudohypopyon of triamcinolone acetonide crystals. The inflammatory response that can develop may be in response to a component of the drug or to bacterial toxins that may be in sterile solutions [24]. Other complications associated with intravitreal injections, not unique to steroid, can occur including retinal detachment and vitreous hemorrhage [43].

Dexamethasone Implant

The dexamethasone implant (Ozurdex; Allergan, Inc., Irvine, California) is a bioerodible injectable steroid implant that releases 0.7 mg of dexamethasone. In September 2010, the FDA approved if for the treatment of noninfectious uveitis involving the posterior segment [9]. It is delivered with a prefilled auto-injector through a 22-gauge needle and can be injected in the office [55]. The drug is marketed to last up to 6 months [56].

In the HURON trial, eyes with noninfectious intermediate or posterior uveitis were randomized to a single treatment with a 0.7-mg dexamethasone implant, 0.35-mg dexamethasone implant, or sham procedure [57]. It was a 26-week, prospective, multicenter, masked, randomized, parallel-group, sham-controlled clinical trial. The primary outcome measure of the study was amount of vitreous haze that obscured visualization and the proportion of patients with a vitreous haze score of 0. A total of 229 patients were enrolled in the study, 77 received the 0.7 mg dexamethasone implant, 76 received the 0.35 mg implant, and 76 had sham injection [57]. At the initiation of the HURON study, the mean vitreous haze score was approximately 2 in all three randomization groups. At week 8, the percentage of eyes with a vitreous haze score of 0 was 47% in the 0.7 mg group, 36% in the 0.35 mg group, and only 12% in the sham group. Between weeks 6 and 26, the percentage of eyes with a vitreous haze score of 0 was statistically significantly higher in the 0.7 mg group vs. sham. There was not however a statistically significant difference between the two doses of dexamethasone [57]. The mean improvement from baseline BCVA was statistically significantly higher in the dexamethasone implant groups compared to sham. This difference was statistically significant for the 0.7-mg implant group at all time points and for the 0.35 mg at all time points except for week 26 [57]. Both the 0.35 mg and 0.7 mg groups had statistically significant improvement in OCT thickness compared to baseline. There was no statistically significant difference in OCT thickness from baseline in the sham group [57]. The beneficial effect on uveitis allowed for FDA approval of the dexamethasone implant for the treatment of noninfectious uveitis of the posterior segment.

For the treatment of uveitic macular edema Tomkins-Netzer et al. published a retrospective study of 38 eyes from 27 patients from Moorfields Eye Hospital of which 92.1% of patients received dexamethasone implants for the treatment of macular edema from uveitis. Three eyes in the study were treated for vitritis alone (7.89%). The average follow-up in the study was 17.3 months. Of the 38 eyes, 36.9% of eyes had a single implant, while 24 eyes (63.1%) had multiple implants. After the first injection, visual acuity improved significantly from 20/60 to 20/37 at 2-month follow-up. It decreased to 20/54 by 6 months. Central retinal thickness also decreased by 264 + − 33 micrometers at 1 month. Twenty-four of 38 eyes received repeat dexamethasone implants. In this study the median time to relapse was 6 months after the first injection, and overall 69% of eyes relapsed. Thirty-three eyes of 21 patients did not require a second injection. The study found that repeated dexamethasone implants led to a continuation of improvement in visual acuity and improvement and then stabilization of the retinal thickness [58].

Clinically, in patients not taking systemic immunosuppressive therapy, often the dexamethasone implant is not felt to last the 6 months marketed. Frequency of reinjection of the dexamethasone implant has been discussed in publications, but many patients are taking concurrent immunosuppression. There is not data on frequency of reinjection of the dexamethasone implant as monotherapy. Literature however does provided a sense of how immunosuppressive therapy can be adjusted when dexamethasone implants are used.

Eighty-two eyes in 63 patients received 142 implant injections over 35 months in a study by Zarranz-Ventura et al. At the time of enrollment in the study, 53.9% of the 63 patients were on a form of systemic immunosuppressive therapy. This included 14.3% of patients on prednisolone, 9.5% on one steroid-sparing immunosuppressive agent, 30.1% on a combination of prednisolone and another immunosuppressive agent, and 9.5% on triple therapy. The patients received a mean number of 1.7 injections over a mean follow-up period of 15.4 months. Over half, 52.4% of eyes received a single injection, 29.3% received two injections, and 18.2% underwent three or more injections. At 6 months 26% of patients had a second injection, at 9 months 51% had undergone their second injection, and at 12 months 51% had received their second implant [56]. At 1 month, 36% of patients were able to reduce the dose of steroid or immunosuppressive therapy, 42% were able to at 3 months, and 46% were able to at 6 months. At 12 months 62% of patients were able to reduce their dose of steroids or immunosuppression. The likelihood of stopping steroids was 8% at 1 and 3 months, 11% at 6 months, and 36% at 12 months [56].

As seen with other forms of steroids during the HURON trial, 5% of eyes had an intraocular pressure of >35 mmHg after injection with the dexamethasone implant. Less than 10% of patients had a pressure of 25 mmHg or higher, and in total, 23% of patients required topical drops to lower intraocular pressure. No patients required glaucoma surgery or laser. In the Tomkins-Netzer publication, patients who had previously been known as steroid responders did not have intraocular pressure response to the dexamethasone implant. No patients required incisional glaucoma surgery [58].

Regarding cataract development, 15% of patients in the 0.7 mg dexamethasone implant group of the HURON trial developed cataracts [57]. In the Tomkins-Netzer study, only one patient developed a cataract. The second eye developed a cataract after the third implant [58]. Other complications include endophthalmitis, which has been rarely reported for the dexamethasone implant [59]. Intravitreal injections carry the risk of retinal detachments as well. The HURON trial had two retinal detachments in the 0.7 mg group but also had two in the sham group [57].

Fluocinolone Implant/RETISERT

The fluocinolone acetonide 0.59 mg intravitreal implant (RETISERT; Bausch & Lomb, Rochester, NY) was approved by the FDA in 2005 for the treatment of non-infectious uveitis. It is a surgically placed implant that releases drug over a 3-year period. The Multicenter Uveitis Steroid Treatment (MUST) trial conducted a randomized, controlled comparative effectiveness trial to compare the outcomes of patients with fluocinolone implants versus systemic therapy. A total of 255 patients (479 eyes) were enrolled in the trial. While there was an advantage of visual acuity at 6 months for the implant group, at 2 years there was not a statistically significant difference between the two groups [60]. At each time point during the study, the fluocinolone implant group did have better control of inflammation however [60]. A subsequent publication evaluated 54-month follow-up of the MUST trial. At 54 months there was no statistically significant difference between the mean BCVA of the two groups, but the implant continued to control inflammation better over the 54-month period compared to systemic therapy. The implant also resolved macular edema faster than systemic therapy, but the percentage of patients who still had macular edema in the implant arm was similar to that of the systemic group after 36 months, and therefore at 54 months, there was no statistically significant difference between the two groups [61].

While acuity and macular edema were not statistically significantly different between the two groups, at 54 months it was likely the crossovers between treatment arms may have reduced the differences between the two groups. Most patients in the systemic therapy arm remained on systemic therapy; however approximately 20% of the systemic therapy arm had a fluocinolone implant placed. Only approximately 20% of the implant group was started on systemic therapy at the end of the study, and only 10% of the patients received two or more implants [61].

The fluocinolone implant had more associated ocular complications compared to systemic treatment. Those with an implant underwent more cataract and glaucoma surgeries than patients in the systemic therapy arm. In the first 2 years of the study, the incidence of glaucoma surgery was 31.1% vs. 4.5% (HR, 8.1) for the implant vs. systemic therapy. After 24 months, however, there was not a statistically significant difference in the incidence of glaucoma surgery between the two groups [62]. The 54-month incidence of initiation of IOP-lowering medications between the implant group and systemic therapy (77.9% vs. 34.0%; hazard ratio [HR], 3.9) was significantly higher in the implant group [62].

The risk of cataract development was high in both groups, but at 54-month follow-up, 98.9% of eyes in the implant group had a cataract, while 77.3% of the eyes in the systemic therapy group had a cataract [62]. Phakic eyes underwent cataract surgery at an approximate rate 4 times higher in the implant group. At the 54-month follow-up, 87.7% of eyes in the implant group had undergone cataract surgery, while only 43% of those in the systemic therapy arm underwent cataract surgery [62].

A Cochrane review was performed looking at corticosteroid implants compared to standard of care therapy. Only two randomized control trials were included which showed that the fluocinolone implant likely prevents recurrence of uveitis better than standard of care treatment with a relative risk of 0.29. It concluded that there was an increased rate of cataract surgery (RR 2.98) and glaucoma surgery (RR 7.48) in the patients receiving the implant compared to those who received standard of care therapy [44].

Both groups maintained good quality of life measures; however the fluocinolone group did tend to have a small advantage on vision-related quality of life and health-related quality of life measures at 12 months. At 24 months this became borderline significant [62]. There was a low rate of systemic complications from systemic therapy. The study concluded that if immunosuppression is given appropriately, then complications are not commonly seen [62]. The study made the conclusion that for bilateral cases systemic therapy is more cost-effective, but the implant is a reasonable option in patients who have unilateral disease or for those who do not tolerate systemic therapy [61].

In September 2014 the fluocinolone injectable implant (ILUVIEN; Alimera Sciences, Alpharetta, Georgia) became FDA approved for the treatment of diabetic macular edema. A similar unanchored nondegradable fluocinolone intravitreal implant (Medidur, pSivida Corp, Watertown, MA) is currently in phase 3 trials for the treatment of posterior uveitis. This implant is 0.19 mg compared to 0.59 mg in the RETISERT implant. If the results are favorable, it will seek FDA approval [55].

Jaffe et al. performed a small non-comparative prospective investigator-sponsored trial of the drug [63]. They evaluated implants with two different initial release rates. The lower release rate implant is thought to last 3 years, while the higher release rate implant lasts 1.5 years. Eleven eyes were treated in a 1:1 ratio. No patients had a flare of their uveitis during the follow-up period. At the start of the study, ten patients were on systemic prednisone, and at 24-month follow-up, six were still on prednisone, but the dose was decreased in four patients. Steroid-sparing immunosuppression was used in six patients and was reduced or stopped in four of the six patients. Visual acuity stabilized and improved in all patients at 12 and 24 months. At 12 months 50% of eyes had gained three lines, and at 24 months 73%

of eyes had gained three lines in vision. Visual acuity improved due to control of intraocular inflammation and improvement in cystoid macular edema [63]. Two eyes suffered hypotony during the follow-up period, and two eyes had glaucoma filtering surgery. Only one eye was phakic at time of implantation, and that patient did undergo cataract surgery during the study period [63]. The results of the phase 3 trials are still pending.

The fluocinolone implant is an important option for long-term control of intraocular inflammation. If the results from the fluocinolone injectable implant are promising, it remains to be seen whether or not this replaces the surgically placed fluocinolone implant despite significantly lower dose of the drug.

Compliance with Ethical Requirements Ashleigh Levison is a consultant for Santen Pharmaceutical and serves on the speaker's bureau for AbbVie. No human or animal studies were carried out by the author for this article.

References

1. Comstock TL, Decory HH. Advances in corticosteroid therapy for ocular inflammation: loteprednol etabonate. Int J Inflam. 2012;2012:789623. https://doi.org/10.1155/2012/789623 [published Online First: Epub Date].
2. Rhen T, Cidlowski JA. Antiinflammatory action of glucocorticoids—new mechanisms for old drugs. N Engl J Med. 2005;353(16):1711–23. https://doi.org/10.1056/NEJMra050541 [published Online First: Epub Date].
3. Stahn C, Buttgereit F. Genomic and nongenomic effects of glucocorticoids. Nat Clin Pract Rheumatol. 2008;4(10):525–33. https://doi.org/10.1038/ncprheum0898 [published Online First: Epub Date].
4. Karim R, Sykakis E, Lightman S, Fraser-Bell S. Interventions for the treatment of uveitic macular edema: a systematic review and meta-analysis. Clin Ophthalmol. 2013;7:1109–44. https://doi.org/10.2147/OPTH.S40268 [published Online First: Epub Date].
5. Lee K, Bajwa A, Freitas-Neto CA, Metzinger JL, Wentworth BA, Foster CS. A comprehensive review and update on the non-biologic treatment of adult noninfectious uveitis: part I. Expert Opin Pharmacother. 2014;15(15):2141–54. https://doi.org/10.1517/14656566.2014.948417 [published Online First: Epub Date].
6. Pavesio CE, Decory HH. Treatment of ocular inflammatory conditions with loteprednol etabonate. Br J Ophthalmol. 2008;92(4):455–9. https://doi.org/10.1136/bjo.2007.132621 [published Online First: Epub Date].
7. Kersey JP, Broadway DC. Corticosteroid-induced glaucoma: a review of the literature. Eye (Lond). 2006;20(4):407–16. https://doi.org/10.1038/sj.eye.6701895 [published Online First: Epub Date].
8. Jabs DA, Rosenbaum JT, Foster CS, et al. Guidelines for the use of immunosuppressive drugs in patients with ocular inflammatory disorders: recommendations of an expert panel. Am J Ophthalmol. 2000;130(4):492–513.
9. Saraiya NV, Goldstein DA. Dexamethasone for ocular inflammation. Expert Opin Pharmacother. 2011;12(7):1127–31. https://doi.org/10.1517/14656566.2011.571209 [published Online First: Epub Date].
10. Controlled evaluation of loteprednol etabonate and prednisolone acetate in the treatment of acute anterior uveitis. Loteprednol Etabonate US Uveitis Study Group. Am J Ophthalmol. 1999;127(5):537–44.
11. Samudre SS, Lattanzio FA, Williams PB, Sheppard JD. Comparison of topical steroids for acute anterior uveitis. J Ocul Pharmacol Ther. 2004;20(6):533–47. https://doi.org/10.1089/jop.2004.20.533 [published Online First: Epub Date].

12. Siddique SS, Shah R, Suelves AM, Foster CS. Road to remission: a comprehensive review of therapy in uveitis. Expert Opin Investig Drugs. 2011;20(11):1497–515. https://doi.org/10.1517/13543784.2011.617741 [published Online First: Epub Date].
13. Mulki L, Foster CS. Difluprednate for inflammatory eye disorders. Drugs Today (Barc). 2011;47(5):327–33. https://doi.org/10.1358/dot.2011.47.5.1590791 [published Online First: Epub Date].
14. Sheppard JD, Toyos MM, Kempen JH, Kaur P, Foster CS. Difluprednate 0.05% versus prednisolone acetate 1% for endogenous anterior uveitis: a phase III, multicenter, randomized study. Invest Ophthalmol Vis Sci. 2014;55(5):2993–3002. https://doi.org/10.1167/iovs.13-12660. [published Online First: Epub Date].
15. Tajika T, Isowaki A, Sakaki H. Ocular distribution of difluprednate ophthalmic emulsion 0.05% in rabbits. J Ocul Pharmacol Ther. 2011;27(1):43–9. https://doi.org/10.1089/jop.2010.0093 [published Online First: Epub Date].
16. Foster CS, Davanzo R, Flynn TE, McLeod K, Vogel R, Crockett RS. Durezol (Difluprednate Ophthalmic Emulsion 0.05%) compared with Pred Forte 1% ophthalmic suspension in the treatment of endogenous anterior uveitis. J Ocul Pharmacol Ther. 2010;26(5):475–83. https://doi.org/10.1089/jop.2010.0059 [published Online First: Epub Date].
17. Lu S, Taban M. Topical difluprednate for treatment of serous retinal detachment and panuveitis associated with Vogt-Koyanagi-Harada disease. Digit J Ophthalmol. 2016;22(2):54–7. https://doi.org/10.5693/djo.02.2015.05.004 [published Online First: Epub Date].
18. Onishi SM, Asahi MG, Chou C, Gallemore RP. Topical difluprednate for the treatment of Harada's disease. Clin Ophthalmol. 2015;9:157–67. https://doi.org/10.2147/OPTH.S72955 [published Online First: Epub Date].
19. Kurz PA, Chheda LV, Kurz DE. Effects of twice-daily topical difluprednate 0.05% emulsion in a child with pars planitis. Ocul Immunol Inflamm. 2011;19(1):84–5. https://doi.org/10.3109/09273948.2010.512993 [published Online First: Epub Date].
20. Bartlett JD, Horwitz B, Laibovitz R, Howes JF. Intraocular pressure response to loteprednol etabonate in known steroid responders. J Ocul Pharmacol. 1993;9(2):157–65.
21. Feiler DL, Srivastava SK, Pichi F, Bena J, Lowder CY. Resolution of noninfectious uveitic cystoid macular edema with topical difluprednate. Retina. 2016. https://doi.org/10.1097/IAE.0000000000001243 [published Online First: Epub Date].
22. Symes RJ, Forooghian F. Topical difluprednate monotherapy for uveitic macular edema. Can J Ophthalmol 2016;51(1):47–9. https://doi.org/10.1016/j.jcjo.2015.10.007 [published Online First: Epub Date].
23. Chalam K, Khetpal V, Patel CJ. Spectral domain optical coherence tomography documented rapid resolution of pseudophakic cystoid macular edema with topical difluprednate. Clin Ophthalmol. 2012;6:155–8. https://doi.org/10.2147/OPTH.S28151 [published Online First: Epub Date].
24. Jermak CM, Dellacroce JT, Heffez J, Peyman GA. Triamcinolone acetonide in ocular therapeutics. Surv Ophthalmol. 2007;52(5):503–22. https://doi.org/10.1016/j.survophthal.2007.06.004 [published Online First: Epub Date].
25. Kusne Y, Kang P, Fintelmann RE. A retrospective analysis of intraocular pressure changes after cataract surgery with the use of prednisolone acetate 1% versus difluprednate 0.05%. Clin Ophthalmol. 2016;10:2329–36. https://doi.org/10.2147/OPTH.S121849 [published Online First: Epub Date].
26. Slabaugh MA, Herlihy E, Ongchin S, van Gelder RN. Efficacy and potential complications of difluprednate use for pediatric uveitis. Am J Ophthalmol. 2012;153(5):932–8. https://doi.org/10.1016/j.ajo.2011.10.008 [published Online First: Epub Date].
27. Vedantham V. Periocular corticosteroid therapy: comments. Br J Ophthalmol. 2004;88(5):724–5.
28. Okada AA, Wakabayashi T, Morimura Y, et al. Trans-Tenon's retrobulbar triamcinolone infusion for the treatment of uveitis. Br J Ophthalmol. 2003;87(8):968–71.
29. Ferrante P, Ramsey A, Bunce C, Lightman S. Clinical trial to compare efficacy and side-effects of injection of posterior sub-Tenon triamcinolone versus orbital floor methylprednisolone in

the management of posterior uveitis. Clin Exp Ophthalmol. 2004;32(6):563–8. https://doi.org/10.1111/j.1442-9071.2004.00902.x [published Online First: Epub Date].
30. Thach AB, Dugel PU, Flindall RJ, Sipperley JO, Sneed SR. A comparison of retrobulbar versus sub-Tenon's corticosteroid therapy for cystoid macular edema refractory to topical medications. Ophthalmology. 1997;104(12):2003–8.
31. Freeman WR, Green RL, Smith RE. Echographic localization of corticosteroids after periocular injection. Am J Ophthalmol. 1987;103(3 Pt 1):281–8.
32. Sen HN, Vitale S, Gangaputra SS, et al. Periocular corticosteroid injections in uveitis: effects and complications. Ophthalmology. 2014;121(11):2275–86. https://doi.org/10.1016/j.ophtha.2014.05.021 [published Online First: Epub Date].
33. Helm CJ, Holland GN. The effects of posterior subtenon injection of triamcinolone acetonide in patients with intermediate uveitis. Am J Ophthalmol. 1995;120(1):55–64.
34. Salek SS, Leder HA, Butler NJ, Gan TJ, Dunn JP, Thorne JE. Periocular triamcinolone acetonide injections for control of intraocular inflammation associated with uveitis. Ocul Immunol Inflamm. 2013;21(4):257–63. https://doi.org/10.3109/09273948.2013.767353 [published Online First: Epub Date].
35. Leder HA, Jabs DA, Galor A, Dunn JP, Thorne JE. Periocular triamcinolone acetonide injections for cystoid macular edema complicating noninfectious uveitis. Am J Ophthalmol. 2011;152(3):441–48.e2. https://doi.org/10.1016/j.ajo.2011.02.009 [published Online First: Epub Date].
36. Iwao K, Inatani M, Kawaji T, Koga T, Mawatari Y, Tanihara H. Frequency and risk factors for intraocular pressure elevation after posterior sub-Tenon capsule triamcinolone acetonide injection. J Glaucoma. 2007;16(2):251–6. https://doi.org/10.1097/IJG.0b013e31802d696f [published Online First: Epub Date].
37. Nozik RA. Periocular injection of steroids. Trans Am Acad Ophthalmol Otolaryngol. 1972;76(3):695–705.
38. Bui Quoc E, Bodaghi B, Adam R, et al. Intraocular pressure elevation after subtenon injection of triamcinolone acetonide during uveitis. J Fr Ophtalmol. 2002;25(10):1048–56.
39. Giles CL. Bulbar perforation during periocular injection of corticosteroids. Am J Ophthalmol. 1974;77(4):438–41.
40. Ideta S, Noda M, Kawamura R, et al. Dehiscence of levator aponeurosis in ptosis after sub-Tenon injection of triamcinolone acetonide. Can J Ophthalmol. 2009;44(6):668–72. https://doi.org/10.3129/i09-188 [published Online First: Epub Date].
41. Nozik RA. Orbital rim fat atrophy after repository periocular corticosteroid injection. Am J Ophthalmol. 1976;82(6):928–30.
42. Byun YS, Park YH. Complications and safety profile of posterior subtenon injection of triamcinolone acetonide. J Ocul Pharmacol Ther. 2009;25(2):159–62. https://doi.org/10.1089/jop.2008.0087 [published Online First: Epub Date].
43. Ozkiris A. Intravitreal triamcinolone acetonide injection for the treatment of posterior uveitis. Ocul Immunol Inflamm. 2006;14(4):233–8. https://doi.org/10.1080/09273940600826604 [published Online First: Epub Date].
44. Habot-Wilner Z, Sallam A, Roufas A, et al. Periocular corticosteroid injection in the management of uveitis in children. Acta Ophthalmol. 2010;88(8):e299–304. https://doi.org/10.1111/j.1755-3768.2010.02025.x [published Online First: Epub Date].
45. Spitzer MS, Ziemssen F, Yörük E, Bartz-Schmidt KU, Schultheiss M, Szurman P. Preservative-free triamcinolone versus purified triamcinolone preparations. Klin Monatsbl Augenheilkd. 2011;228(7):626–30. https://doi.org/10.1055/s-0029-1245621 [published Online First: Epub Date].
46. Couch SM, Bakri SJ. Intravitreal triamcinolone for intraocular inflammation and associated macular edema. Clin Ophthalmol. 2009;3:41–7.
47. Sallam A, Taylor SR, Lightman S. Review and update of intraocular therapy in noninfectious uveitis. Curr Opin Ophthalmol. 2011;22(6):517–22. https://doi.org/10.1097/ICU.0b013e32834bbd68 [published Online First: Epub Date].

48. Park UC, Park JH, Yu HG. Long-term outcome of intravitreal triamcinolone acetonide injection for the treatment of uveitis attacks in Behçet disease. Ocul Immunol Inflamm. 2014;22(1):27–33. https://doi.org/10.3109/09273948.2013.829109 [published Online First: Epub Date].
49. Kok H, Lau C, Maycock N, McCluskey P, Lightman S. Outcome of intravitreal triamcinolone in uveitis. Ophthalmology. 2005;112(11):1916.e1–7. https://doi.org/10.1016/j.ophtha.2005.06.009 [published Online First: Epub Date].
50. Steeples LR, Anand N, Moraji J, Jones NP. Clinical Outcomes of Intravitreal Preservative-Free Triamcinolone Preparation (Triesence®) for Cystoid Macular Oedema and Inflammation in Patients with Uveitis. Ocul Immunol Inflamm. 2017:1–8. https://doi.org/10.1080/09273948.2017.1294185 [published Online First: Epub Date].
51. Kiernan DF, Mieler WF. The use of intraocular corticosteroids. Expert Opin Pharmacother. 2009;10(15):2511–25. https://doi.org/10.1517/14656560903160671 [published Online First: Epub Date].
52. Sallam A, Taylor SR, Habot-Wilner Z, et al. Repeat intravitreal triamcinolone acetonide injections in uveitic macular oedema. Acta Ophthalmol 2012;90(4):e323–5. https://doi.org/10.1111/j.1755-3768.2011.02247.x [published Online First: Epub Date].
53. Tay-Kearney ML. Intravitreal triamcinolone acetonide injection for the treatment of posterior uveitis. Ocul Immunol Inflamm. 2006;14(4):201–2. https://doi.org/10.1080/09273940600940926 [published Online First: Epub Date].
54. Moshfeghi DM, Kaiser PK, Scott IU, et al. Acute endophthalmitis following intravitreal triamcinolone acetonide injection. Am J Ophthalmol. 2003;136(5):791–6.
55. Cunningham ET, de Smet MD, Yeh S, Albini TA, Zierhut M. Sustained-release corticosteroids for uveitis. Ocul Immunol Inflamm. 2015;23(6):421–4. https://doi.org/10.3109/09273948.2015.1114778 [published Online First: Epub Date].
56. Zarranz-Ventura J, Carreño E, Johnston RL, et al. Multicenter study of intravitreal dexamethasone implant in noninfectious uveitis: indications, outcomes, and reinjection frequency. Am J Ophthalmol. 2014;158(6):1136–45.e5. https://doi.org/10.1016/j.ajo.2014.09.003 [published Online First: Epub Date].
57. Lowder C, Belfort R, Lightman S, et al. Dexamethasone intravitreal implant for noninfectious intermediate or posterior uveitis. Arch Ophthalmol. 2011;129(5):545–53. https://doi.org/10.1001/archophthalmol.2010.339 [published Online First: Epub Date].
58. Tomkins-Netzer O, Lightman S, Drye L, et al. Outcome of treatment of uveitic macular edema: the multicenter uveitis steroid treatment trial 2-year results. Ophthalmology. 2015;122(11):2351–9. https://doi.org/10.1016/j.ophtha.2015.07.036 [published Online First: Epub Date].
59. Goel N. Acute bacterial endophthalmitis following intravitreal dexamethasone implant: a case report and review of literature. Saudi J Ophthalmol. 2017;31(1):51–4. https://doi.org/10.1016/j.sjopt.2016.12.003 [published Online First: Epub Date].
60. Kempen JH, Altaweel MM, Holbrook JT, et al. Randomized comparison of systemic anti-inflammatory therapy versus fluocinolone acetonide implant for intermediate, posterior, and panuveitis: the multicenter uveitis steroid treatment trial. Ophthalmology. 2011;118(10):1916–26. https://doi.org/10.1016/j.ophtha.2011.07.027 [published Online First: Epub Date].
61. Kempen JH, Altaweel MM, Drye LT, et al. Benefits of systemic anti-inflammatory therapy versus fluocinolone acetonide intraocular implant for intermediate uveitis, posterior uveitis, and panuveitis: fifty-four-month results of the Multicenter Uveitis Steroid Treatment (MUST) trial and follow-up study. Ophthalmology. 2015;122(10):1967–75. https://doi.org/10.1016/j.ophtha.2015.06.042 [published Online First: Epub Date].
62. Group MUSTMTF-uSR. Quality of life and risks associated with systemic anti-inflammatory therapy versus fluocinolone acetonide intraocular implant for intermediate uveitis, posterior uveitis, or panuveitis: fifty-four-month results of the Multicenter Uveitis Steroid Treatment Trial and Follow-up Study. Ophthalmology. 2015;122(10):1976–86. https://doi.org/10.1016/j.ophtha.2015.06.043 [published Online First: Epub Date].
63. Jaffe GJ, Lin P, Keenan RT, Ashton P, Skalak C, Stinnett SS. Injectable fluocinolone acetonide long-acting implant for noninfectious intermediate uveitis, posterior uveitis, and panuveitis: two-year results. Ophthalmology. 2016;123(9):1940–8. https://doi.org/10.1016/j.ophtha.2016.05.025 [published Online First: Epub Date].

Noninfectious Uveitis: Immunomodulatory Agents and Biologicals

John A. Gonzales and Nisha Acharya

Antimetabolites

Corticosteroids remain the usual first-line agents in managing noninfectious uveitis. Whether administered in topical, oral, parenteral, periocular, or intraocular forms, they can be effective and, particularly when used for short periods of time, safe. However, corticosteroids have important side effects. While many of the side effects of steroids resolve after discontinuation, chronic uveitis requires chronic management, and the use of moderate to high doses of corticosteroids should be avoided. This is where corticosteroid-sparing immunomodulatory agents come into play. They provide a means to manage the uveitis while having a better side effect profile than high-dose or frequent administration of corticosteroids. Recently, there has been an impressive expansion in the therapeutics available to treat autoimmune diseases. Naturally, interest in using these medications that have indications in the realm of immunology and rheumatology for the management of uveitis has grown. Some of these medications, including the newer biologics, have very specific targets involved in inflammatory pathways. Antimetabolites, however, are still considered first-line therapy when corticosteroid-sparing management of uveitis is needed. Most uveitis specialists have extensive training and familiarity with the antimetabolites, and it makes sense from this perspective in utilizing them as one would an old friend.

J. A. Gonzales (✉) · N. Acharya
F.I. Proctor Foundation, University of California, San Francisco, San Francisco, CA, USA
e-mail: John.Gonzales@ucsf.edu; Nisha.Acharya@ucsf.edu

N. A. Rao et al. (eds.), *Posterior Uveitis*, Essentials in Ophthalmology,
https://doi.org/10.1007/978-3-030-03140-4_11

Interfering with metabolic pathways that are essential for cellular growth and involved in producing inflammatory mediators, the term "antimetabolites" are appropriately earned by this group of medications. In rheumatology, antimetabolites are commonly known as disease-modifying antirheumatic drugs (DMARDs). Antimetabolites have an even earlier history of being employed as chemotherapy for malignancies and organ transplant rejection prevention.

Much of our knowledge about the use of antimetabolites comes in the form of retrospective studies. Retrospective studies, however, have their limitations, including bias with respect to indications for using one particular antimetabolite over another (including bias of the treating center or physician), incomplete follow-up, and missing data (including reasons for discontinuing therapy). To date, there has been only one randomized clinical trial evaluating the efficacy of one particular antimetabolite compared to another for the management of uveitis [1]. Do uveitis specialists prefer one antimetabolite to another? Insight into the preferences and beliefs of uveitis specialists with respect to treatment can be seen in the responses provided by members of the American Uveitis Society. Members were surveyed about their practice patterns with 92% of respondents using methotrexate as their initial immunomodulatory agent for anterior uveitis. Only 5% used mycophenolate [2]. Other antimetabolites, such as azathioprine, were not as routinely used. For intermediate uveitis, 58% of the members responding commenced treatment with methotrexate, while 25% relied upon mycophenolate mofetil. Azathioprine was utilized by 3% of respondents in such a scenario. For posterior and panuveitis, 47% of respondents noted they would start with methotrexate, while an increasing number of specialists (27%) would use mycophenolate mofetil. However, the issue was not necessarily that members felt methotrexate was more effective than mycophenolate mofetil. Instead, when the AUS members were queried as to why they would not prescribe a particular medication, 47% noted lack of effectiveness was a reason not to prescribe methotrexate, while only 9% considered mycophenolate mofetil to ineffective. Mycophenolate mofetil was considered to be prohibitively expensive as first-line therapeutic.

Antimetabolites are a mainstay of corticosteroid-sparing therapy for uveitis. They are well tolerated by patients and represent, in general, the first line of medications that are utilized for chronic uveitis.

Azathioprine

6-Mercaptopurine was found to be effective in murine models of lymphoma [3]. 6-MP, however, is extensively metabolized, so efforts were made to synthesize derivatives with modified metabolism, thereby improving efficacy – azathioprine was the result of this labor [4].

Pharmacology and Pharmacokinetics

Azathioprine is a prodrug (an imidazolyl derivative of 6-mercaptopurine, 6-MP). Glutathione S-transferase activity in red blood cells converts azathioprine approximately 88% of azathioprine to 6-MP [5]. As a purine nucleoside analogue, 6-MP is then metabolized by hypoxanthine guanine phosphoribosyl transferase resulting in two active metabolites, thioinosinic and thioguanylic acid. The active metabolites then block purine metabolism and halt DNA synthesis. The enzyme thiopurine S-methyltransferase (TPMT) metabolizes 6-MP to the inactive metabolite, 6-methyl-mercaptopurine, as well as metabolizing the active metabolites (thioinosinic and thioguanylic acid). However, polymorphisms of the *TPMT* gene exist. In patients with homozygous mutations of *TPMT*, the enzyme is functionally inactive, which can lead to drug toxicity. In patients with heterozygous mutations of *TPMT*, the enzyme is partially functional, and a reduced dose of azathioprine should be used. An assay for homo- or heterozygosity of *TPMT* should be performed prior to instituting therapy with azathioprine. Those that are homozygous for TPMT deficiency should not be considered for azathioprine therapy as bone marrow toxicity with resultant cytopenias can occur early in the commencement of therapy. Heterozygous individuals may be dosed lower than in those homozygous for TPMT activity. In Han Chinese patients, TPMT mutations are not frequently encountered. However, side effects in this group of patients, particularly leukopenia, may be related to a genotype that leads to higher glutathione S-transferase activity [6].

Azathioprine is absorbed in the stomach and duodenum. Peak plasma levels (ranging from 27% to 83%) [5] are reached within 2 h of oral administration and taken up into cells with only 30% being protein bound. Up to 45% of azathioprine is excreted into the urine, while the remainder is converted to 6-MP in red blood cells.

Studies

A retrospective study of azathioprine's use in 34 patients with retinal vasculitis from a single center revealed that 56% of eyes exhibited a decrease in ocular inflammation and 64% of eyes either maintained or improved their visual acuities [7]. Relapse of ocular inflammation was also decreased in 10 patients who had data available prior to treatment with azathioprine. Patients who did not require an increase in their dose of prednisone were also considered treatment successes.

In the largest retrospective cohort studies evaluating azathioprine's use for treating noninfectious ocular inflammatory diseases involving 4 uveitis centers, 63% of patients (91 patients) had uveitis [8]. More patients with intermediate uveitis (90.3%) achieved inactive uveitis using the standardization of uveitis nomenclature (SUN) criteria [9] compared to anterior (51.4%) and posterior/panuveitis (74.4%). Additionally, corticosteroid-sparing control (less than 10 mg PO daily of prednisone) with azathioprine was most frequent in the setting of intermediate uveitis (adjusted hazard ratio 4.75 CI 1.23 to 13.58) compared to anterior uveitis. Posterior/panuveitis had less frequent corticosteroid-sparing control than intermediate uveitis when compared to anterior uveitis (adjusted HR 2.52, CI 0.64 to 9.86).

In the realm of pediatric, uveitis, a study of 40 children taking a variety of immunomodulatory agents over 5 years revealed that azathioprine was associated with a 61% improvement in visual acuity, which was lower than mycophenolate mofetil (91% improvement in visual acuity) [10]. Children were also on systemic corticosteroids in conjunction with their immunomodulatory medication. Similarly,

Arellanes-Garcia et al. performed a retrospective study of 160 Mexican children seen in her uveitis clinic. Her group found that azathioprine (in conjunction with systemic corticosteroids) was associated with a 61% improvement in visual activity in 34 patients with pars planitis [11].

The first study assessing azathioprine's efficacy in managing uveitis came in 1969 [12]. Mathews and colleagues enrolled a total of 16 patients with chronic anterior uveitis, and half were randomized by the pharmacist to receive azathioprine 100 mg PO daily or placebo daily, and the subjects were followed for 3 months. Interestingly, three patients from the placebo group (who had their data included with the other placebo group subjects) were crossed over to the azathioprine group, and their outcomes were included in the azathioprine group. Statistically speaking, these maneuvers are not typically performed today. The SUN criteria had not been developed during Mathews et al.'s assessment, and they used a scoring system in which a higher score was assigned to less cell and less flare. Additionally, they assessed patients' subjectively reported improvement or worsening of their vision. There was a trend toward improvement in both patient's reported vision and objective features (visual acuity, cell, and flare), but there was no statistically significant difference between the two groups.

More recently, azathioprine was used in a prospective clinical trial evaluating its efficacy in controlling Behçet's disease-related uveitis in 48 patients compared to placebo [13]. Mean visual acuity remained stable in the azathioprine group compared to a statistically significant decline in vision in the placebo group. Additionally, there were statistically significantly less occurrences of hypopyon uveitis in the azathioprine group compared to the placebo group. Moreover, in 25 patients without ocular disease at enrollment, 8 developed newly diagnosed uveitis in the placebo group compared to 1 in the azathioprine group, a statistically significant difference. In assessing long-term outcomes of the patients randomized to placebo or azathioprine [13], becoming blind and experiencing a two-line drop in visual acuity occurred more frequently in the placebo group compared to the azathioprine group [14].

Comparison with Other Antimetabolites and Immunomodulatory Therapies

A non-randomized trial was conducted utilizing azathioprine or chlorambucil in anterior uveitis [15]. In the 1970s, azathioprine was considered to be a cytotoxic agent by some [16], and the goal of this particular trial was to compare the relative efficacy of these two "cytotoxic" agents for chronic anterior endogenous (noninfectious) uveitis. Of the 25 patients enrolled, 22 received azathioprine, while 3 received chlorambucil. All patients were on doses of prednisone ranging from 10 to 15 mg daily. All but two patients were noted to manifest a response to azathioprine, but this included patients that would, by today's standards, still be considered to have active uveitis. For example, patients with 1+ anterior chamber cell were still considered to be responsive to azathioprine since such patients had exhibited more anterior chamber cell prior to enrollment. While this study did not fit the mold for an RCT, the authors recognized that long-term therapy with azathioprine was essential for preventing relapses of uveitis.

Side Effects

Side effects of azathioprine include gastrointestinal upset, cytopenias due to bone marrow suppression (leukopenia and thrombocytopenia in particular). Testing for TPMT activity is essential prior to utilizing azathioprine in a patient. Azathioprine is a pregnancy class D medication. As such, there is evidence of human fetal risk. Breastfeeding is considered reasonable in lactating mothers taking azathioprine with very low levels of the medication being found in breast milk [17].

Considerations

While azathioprine has been better at controlling inflammation than placebo [13], azathioprine may be the most effective for intermediate uveitis [8]. Compared to methotrexate and mycophenolate mofetil, azathioprine was associated with a longer time (6.5 months) for treatment success (control of uveitis with prednisone 10 mg PO daily or less) and a higher rate of side effects and discontinuation due to side effects [18]. Azathioprine has been combined with T-cell inhibitors and corticosteroids to achieve control of noninfectious uveitis, including serpiginous choroiditis [19] and sympathetic ophthalmia [20–23].

Leflunomide

The chemical name for leflunomide is 5-methyl-N-{4-(trifluoromethyl)phenyl]-1,2-oxazole-4-carboxamide. Its molecular formula is $C_{12}H_9F_3N2O_2$.

Leflunomide is a synthetic isoxazole derivative, which is converted to its active metabolite A77 1726 in the liver. Leflunomide was synthesized during the 1980s and ultimately approved by the FDA for the treatment of rheumatoid arthritis in the 1990s. Leflunomide has been shown to modulate inflammation via antagonizing lymphoproliferation by inhibiting dihydroorotate dehydrogenase, which leads to a reduction in the de novo synthesis of pyrimidines. A lack of pyrimidines results in halting of DNA synthesis and has particular effect on rapidly proliferating cells, including activated CD4+ T cells that are important in mediating inflammation. Specifically, proliferating cells are halted in G_1 phase. Moreover, leflunomide has been shown to have an effect on B-cell autoantibody synthesis [24]. A77 1726 modulates inflammation via other mechanisms as well. For example, it inhibits tyrosine kinase, which is important in mediating the progression of cells from G_0 phase to G_1 phase as well as activating the IL-2 receptor, which is involved in inflammation. Additionally, A77 1726 prevents degradation of IKB, which is the inhibitor of NF-KB [25]. Without activation, NF-KB is unable to translocate into the nucleus to result in transcription of genes that mediate inflammation.

The bioavailability of A77 1726 is not affected by the presence of food in the stomach or intestines. It is extensively bound to plasma proteins, and, as a result, its half-life is between 15 and 18 days [25]. Most of leflunomide is eliminated equally in urine and feces. Because of leflunomide's metabolism by the liver and its reliance upon enterohepatic recirculation for its clearance, those with hepatic dysfunction are not ideal candidates for leflunomide. The long half-life of leflunomide means that it can take up to 5 months for it to reach steady-state plasma concentration.

Efficacy

Leflunomide has been shown to be effective at decreasing ocular inflammation in murine models of uveitis [26, 27].

Comparison with Other Antimetabolites

While leflunomide has been used in the treatment of uveitis [28–30], it has been associated with more frequent rates of recurrences compared to methotrexate when used in the chronic anterior uveitis associated with juvenile idiopathic arthritis (JIA) [31]. Others have shown that leflunomide has been effective at managing the chronic anterior uveitis associated with JIA. Molina and colleagues performed a retrospective review of 13 patients with JIA-associated uveitis using leflunomide for at least 7 months [30]. They classified the uveitis response to leflunomide as having no response, improvement, complete remission, and persistent remission. They found that 50% of patients achieved and maintained complete remission, 25% showed improvement, 25% exhibited persistent remission, and 38.5% showed no response to leflunomide. Thus, overall, 61% of the cohort exhibited a favorable response to leflunomide.

Combination with Other Antimetabolites

Leflunomide has been used effectively in combination with methotrexate, particularly in rheumatoid arthritis [32]. While A77 1726 affects pyrimidine synthesis, methotrexate inhibits purine synthesis [33], thereby having a synergistic effect. While antimetabolites are typically used with the biologic infliximab, to prevent human anti-chimeric antibody (HACA) formation, using leflunomide with infliximab is associated with frequent adverse reactions [34]. Use of leflunomide with infliximab is, therefore, not recommended.

Side Effects

Side effects include nausea, diarrhea, rash, and reversible alopecia. Less frequent side effects include hypertension [35], upper respiratory tract infections, and hepatotoxicity. Additionally, there has been an association with increasing total cholesterol and LDL cholesterol with increasing length of time patients take leflunomide.

Other Considerations

Leflunomide has been used as a cheaper alternative to treatment cytomegalovirus (CMV). Additionally, leflunomide has been shown to be effective in the treatment of CMV that is resistant to its typical antiviral agents [36] (ganciclovir, foscarnet, and cidofovir) in organ transplant recipients [37–39]. Leflunomide affects the maturation of CMV's capsid [40], which is different than the inhibition of viral DNA polymerase that is employed by antivirals.

Methotrexate

The chemical name for methotrexate is N-{4-[[(2,4-diamino-6-pteridinyl)methyl] methylamino]benzoyl]-L-glutamic acid. Its empirical formula is $C_{20}H_{22}N_8O_5$.

Methotrexate is often employed as first-line corticosteroid-sparing therapy because it is relatively easy to take (once a week by mouth or subcutaneous injection) and relatively well tolerated. Methotrexate (previously known as amethopterin) is one of the newer antimetabolites, being synthesized in the 1940s. Initially, there was hope that folic acid (a water soluble B vitamin) and folate conjugates could be used in treating acute leukemia, but the use of these potential therapeutics actually potentiated the development of this hematologic malignancy. Deficiency in folate, however, was noted to effectively decrease peripheral leukemic cell count [41]. Thus began methotrexate's use a chemotherapeutic. Methotrexate proved to be effective in the 1950s for psoriasis (first-line therapies besides coal tar and ultraviolet light often included arsenic and mercury compounds). Cress and Deaver described a 27-year-old man with psoriatic arthritis [42]. He proved to be recalcitrant to numerous therapies, so methotrexate was commenced and not only did his psoriasis improve but his arthritis did as well. Methotrexate's use was then extended to rheumatoid arthritis in case reports during the 1960s [43–45]. A pilot study in the treatment of rheumatoid arthritis involving 32 patients demonstrated its efficacy in the majority of subjects [46, 47] and cemented its role not only in the treatment of rheumatoid arthritis but other rheumatologic conditions as well.

The enzyme dihydrofolate reductase (DHFR) has long been an attractive target for antibiotics, chemotherapeutics, and immunosuppressives given its importance in purine (adenine and guanine) and thymidylate synthesis. For example, trimethoprim is an antibiotic that targets bacterial DHFR. Methotrexate, on the other hand, targets mammalian DHFR. Cells that are rapidly growing and dividing, then, utilize DHFR more frequently than cells that are more senescent. In the case of methotrexate, there will be a more profound effect on cancer or inflammatory cells. However, side effects will manifest in other tissues that are not malignant or involved with immune function. For example, the stomach and small intestine epithelium have turnover rates ranging from 2 to 10 days. Neutrophils have turnover rates of 1–5 days, and cervical epithelium turns over every 5–6 days. Lymphomas have higher turnover rates [47, 48] so they can be particularly sensitive to folate antagonists.

Pharmacology and Pharmacokinetics

Methotrexate is polyglutamated after entering the cell, which has several functions. One is that it allows for the accumulation of intracellular methotrexate (as the concentration of monoglutamate methotrexate outside of the cell is much lower than inside) [49]. Additionally, the polyglutamation of methotrexate increases its intracellular life. Finally, polyglutamation enhances methotrexate's enzyme inhibitory potency. Methotrexate inhibits DHFR, an enzyme that reduces dihydrofolic acid to tetrahydrofolic acid, which can be converted to cofactors utilized in one-carbon transfer chemistry (one carbon units include methyl, methylene, and formate).

Tetrahydrofolate is required for the de novo synthesis of purines (important for nucleic acid synthesis) [33], thymidylic acid, and certain amino acids. These molecules are, in turn, required for cell growth and proliferation. Moreover, methotrexate inhibits thymidylate synthase, which is involved in the de novo synthesis of pyrimidines. Since methotrexate primarily enters the cells that make up various tissues, it is minimally bound to plasma proteins. In addition to disrupting purine synthesis, methotrexate exhibits other actions that can be therapeutic. Methotrexate inhibits transmethylation reactions [50, 51], important in metabolism, and inhibits the formation of polyamines [52]. Polyamines play a role in inflammation as seen in the synovial fluid and tissues in patients with rheumatoid arthritis [53]. Additionally, methotrexate promotes adenosine release [54], which can have anti-inflammatory effects [55, 56].

After oral consumption, methotrexate is absorbed from the proximal jejunum, and peak serum levels are attained in 1 to 2 h. The bioavailability of methotrexate is approximately 60–80%. Food does not affect the absorption of methotrexate [57], but it can delay absorption and reduce peak concentration. When administered parenterally (e.g., intramuscularly and subcutaneously), complete absorption occurs, and peak serum concentrations are attained in under an hour. The half-life of methotrexate varies from 3 to 10 h. Methotrexate is eliminated by the renal glomerular filtration and active tubular secretion so use in those with renal dysfunction should be adjusted according to the creatinine clearance. Delayed drug clearance is a major factor influencing methotrexate toxicity.

Studies

In a retrospective cohort study of 384 patients commenced on methotrexate for corticosteroid-sparing monotherapy of ocular inflammation (including uveitis, scleritis, and ocular cicatricial pemphigoid), 66% of patients were able to achieve inactivity of ocular inflammation that was sustained for at least 4 weeks within 1 year of therapy [58]. Approximately 58% of patients were able to achieve corticosteroid-sparing control of inflammation (being on 10 mg or less of daily oral prednisone).

Methotrexate is extensively used in the setting of JIA-associated uveitis. In the past, children with juvenile idiopathic arthritis (JIA)-associated uveitis were noted to achieve control of their ocular inflammation with systemic corticosteroids but also exhibited significant steroid-related side effects. Foster's group performed a retrospective review of children with JIA-associated uveitis from the late 1970s to late 1980s [59]. Of twenty-six JIA patients, 8 had used systemic immunomodulatory therapy, including 3 taking methotrexate with doses ranging from 5 to 15 mg PO weekly and 1 patient taking both methotrexate and azathioprine. Two of three patients taking methotrexate achieved control of inflammation, while the patient taking both methotrexate and azathioprine did not achieve control. This was a small study but important in demonstrating the use and good tolerance of methotrexate in the pediatric uveitis population. In a later retrospective study, Weiss et al. reported that six of seven children requiring advancement to methotrexate due to active uveitis despite topical corticosteroids or occurrence of corticosteroid-related side effect were associated with improvement of uveitis [60]. Later, Foeldvari and Wierk showed that methotrexate was effective in treating JIA-associated uveitis in 84% of their cohort after an average of 4.5 months [61]. The mean dose of methotrexate used in this cohort was 15.6 mg/m^2. Malik and Pavesio also demonstrated that methotrexate was effective in the management of JIA-associated uveitis in 10 children [62]. More recently, Heiligenhaus and colleagues assessed 31 patients with JIA-associated uveitis with 21 (67.7%) achieving control of inflammation (with or without the use of concomitant topical corticosteroids) [63].

If ocular inflammation is not responding to oral methotrexate, consideration should be made, if indicated, for subcutaneous administration. Extrapolating from the rheumatoid arthritis literature [64], switching from oral administration to subcutaneous administration of methotrexate may result in more satisfactory control of uveitis.

Methotrexate Resistance

Resistance to methotrexate has been noted in conditions ranging from the rheumatologic (as in rheumatoid arthritis) [65–67] to the ophthalmologic (in the case of primary vitreoretinal lymphoma) [68]. Such resistance mediates lack of control of inflammation or tumor proliferation. Additionally, in methotrexate resistance has been suggested to be responsible for the side effects experienced by some patients [69]. In the future, it may become practice to assess each patient's potential response to different immunomodulatory agents based upon their gene expression of proteins involved in therapeutic responses.

Side Effects

Methotrexate can be hepatotoxic, causing fibrosis and cirrhosis. For this reason, liver transaminases (including aspartate aminotransferase and alanine aminotransferase) should be routinely monitored. In psoriasis, liver fibrosis and cirrhosis can occur without overt abnormalities in serologically assessed liver transaminases. For this reason, some recommend performing liver biopsies periodically to evaluate for histologic evidence of hepatitis. In the rheumatoid arthritis literature, age when methotrexate was commenced, duration of use, and cumulative dose have been risk factors identified for liver damage [70, 71]. Methotrexate can rarely cause a direct toxic effect to lung parenchymal tissue, characterized by a nonproductive cough and wheezing. Patients should be assessed for pulmonary symptoms while on methotrexate and, should complaints arise, be examined with auscultation of the lungs and consideration for pulmonary radiographic imaging, which can reveal a diffuse interstitial pattern [72]. An ulcerative stomatitis/mucositis can occur [73].

Folic acid or folinic acid (leucovorin) is typically administered to abrogate or abolish the side effects of methotrexate without affecting methotrexate's efficacy [74–76]. Folic acid is typically dosed at 1 mg orally each day. Some specialists will hold folic acid on the day that methotrexate is administered, but there is no data that suggests that taking folic acid on the day of methotrexate administration decreases the efficacy of methotrexate. If side effects continue to persist, then the dose of folic acid may be increased to 3–5 mg daily. Folinic acid may be administered for especially recalcitrant side effects (10 mg orally taken 12 h after methotrexate administration). Methotrexate is absolutely contraindicated in pregnancy (pregnancy class X) and can induce teratogenic effects and induce fetal death when taken by a pregnant woman. In fact, methotrexate is used in high doses as an abortive medication. Typically women wishing to conceive are recommended to wait 3 months after cessation of methotrexate. Methotrexate can be detected in human breast milk, and breastfeeding should cease if a mother is utilizing methotrexate. Occasionally, fatal opportunistic infections (*Pneumocystis jirovecii* pneumonia) have occurred with methotrexate. Caution should be practiced when using methotrexate in patients experiencing an active infection. Additionally, methotrexate can be contraindicated in some patients with immunodeficiencies (whether acquired or primary).

Mycophenolate Mofetil

Mycophenolate mofetil, synthesized in the late 1980s [77], was shown to be effective in preventing organ allograft rejection in animal models [78–80], and this discovery ultimately leads to trials involving reversal of human allograft rejection [81].

Pharmacology and Pharmacokinetics

After oral administration, mycophenolate mofetil is absorbed in the small intestine and metabolized to mycophenolic acid, which then undergoes glucuronidation via glucuronyl transferase to yield the phenolic glucuronide of mycophenolic acid (MPAG). MPAG is converted to mycophenolic acid during enterohepatic recirculation. As the morpholinoethyl ester of mycophenolic acid, mycophenolate mofetil exhibits more bioavailability than mycophenolic acid [77], which ranges up to 94% [82]. Carboxylesterases in the small intestine then convert mycophenolate mofetil to mycophenolic acid [82]. As a noncompetitive and reversible inhibitor of inosine monophosphate dehydrogenase, mycophenolate acid blocks de novo purine synthesis, thereby hindering DNA synthesis, affecting proliferation of lymphocytes.

Mycophenolic acid is metabolized by glucuronyl transferase to yield mycophenolic acid glucuronide (which has no pharmacologic activity) and is then eliminated in the urine.

Food consumption with mycophenolate mofetil can result in a lower peak concentration. Thus, it is recommended that mycophenolate be taken on an empty stomach. Mycophenolic acid is 97% bound to serum albumin, and the mean half-life is approximately 18 h. Most of the medication is excreted in the urine as MPAG. Renal insufficiency can result in a higher bioavailability, which has the potential to lead to more untoward side effects.

Studies

The largest retrospective study involving the use of mycophenolate mofetil in uveitis comes from Siepmann and colleagues in Germany [83]. Of 106 patients studied, 92 (nearly 87%) experienced less than or equal to one recurrence of uveitis.

Follow-up in this cohort ranged from 6 months to 41 months. Visual acuity was particularly well preserved in patients with anterior and intermediate uveitis (vision was either stable or improved). Only four patients exhibited a lack of control of their uveitis with mycophenolate mofetil. Another study from Germany, involving 60 noninfectious uveitis patients, revealed that corticosteroid-sparing control (defined as ≤10 mg PO daily of prednisolone) of uveitis was achieved in 72% of patients after 1 year of treatment [84]. Relapses, while occurring in 50% of the cohort, exhibited a rate of only 0.23 relapses/year during the treatment period, and most were managed with either increasing the dose of prednisone, mycophenolate, or both. This particular cohort had a large component made up of intermediate uveitis patients (70%), and 32% of these patients failed mycophenolate mofetil due to efficacy, in particular most often due to uveitic macular edema.

Another large retrospective study involved a cohort of patients from North America at the Wilmer Eye Institute [85]. Fifty-one patients with noninfectious uveitis were included in the study. Most patients achieved control of uveitis with a total daily dose of 2 g. Most patients who did not achieve control with 2 g daily did so with 3 g daily. The median time to treatment success with mycophenolate mofetil 2 g daily was 3.5 months. In those patients requiring 3 g daily, the median time to treatment success was 4.7 months, though this was not statistically different from the lower dosage.

A more recent study involving exclusively Hispanic patients (including 21 with uveitis) revealed that most patients achieved control of ocular inflammation at 6 months after previously failing other immunomodulatory medications [86]. Five patients (23.8%) had active uveitis at 6 months' follow-up. Control of ocular inflammation in general (patients with uveitis only were not independently assessed though they made up the majority of cases) was achieved with doses of 10 mg daily or less.

Mycophenolate mofetil is not used as frequently as methotrexate for uveitis in children. However, mycophenolate demonstrates effective control of pediatric systemic autoimmune diseases including systemic lupus erythematosus [87]. Mycophenolate is typically dosed in children similar to that used in renal transplantation: 600 mg/m^2 PO BID. In one of the largest retrospective studies evaluating the use of mycophenolate mofetil in the setting of pediatric uveitis [88], 17 children that were commenced on mycophenolate mofetil, 88% were able to achieve ≤5 mg PO daily of prednisolone. While only 24% of patients during a mean follow-up of 3 years exhibited no relapses, all patients exhibited a reduction in relapses compared to the number experienced prior to starting mycophenolate mofetil.

Mycophenolate mofetil has also been effective in controlling uveitis in patients failing methotrexate. Sobrin and colleagues performed a retrospective review of their patients with noninfectious ocular inflammation failing methotrexate (either due to efficacy or due to intolerance) [89]. Approximately half of their patients were able to achieve control of inflammation with mycophenolate. However, the odds of control of uveitis in patients with JIA-associated uveitis were lower than for those patients without this type of ocular inflammation.

Side Effects

The most common side effects of mycophenolate mofetil are gastrointestinal in nature and include gastric pain, diarrhea, and nausea [83]. Fatigue and pruritus are other common side effects. Gastrointestinal bleeding and perforations are rarely encountered. These cases have typically occurred in the organ transplantation literature. Additionally, infections involving opportunistic organisms as well as herpetic viral infections are more frequent than in azathioprine, but again, these have been encountered in organ transplant patients. There is an increased risk of malignancy, particularly skin cancers, in transplant patients taking mycophenolate mofetil.

Fetal loss and congenital malformations are noted with mycophenolate. Consequently, contraception must be practiced while taking mycophenolate mofetil. Additionally, patients taking oral contraceptives should be made aware that mycophenolate mofetil can decrease the serum levels of contraceptive hormones with a theoretically reduced efficacy of the contraceptive.

Other Considerations

The use of proton-pump inhibitors (PPI) for peptic ulcer disease and gastroesophageal reflux disease decreases both the serum concentration and bioavailability of mycophenolate mofetil. Patients who are on a PPI who are to commence mycophenolate mofetil for their uveitis management should be considered to switch to a histamine-2 receptor antagonist (e.g., famotidine).

Mycophenolic Acid

Mycophenolic acid was originally recognized to have antibiotic properties. *Penicillium brevicompactum*, a mold (recall that the Greek root word "myco" means fungus), was noted to secrete a substance (mycophenolic acid) that inhibited the growth of *Staphylococcus aureus*. Bartolomeo Gosio, an Italian physician, is credited with this discovery [90]. Gosio was looking to implicate different molds as a cause of niacin deficiency (pellagra).

Pharmacology and Pharmacokinetics

After oral consumption, mycophenolic acid is absorbed into the small intestine. Because mycophenolic acid is enteric-coated, it often exhibits better gastrointestinal tolerability than mycophenolate mofetil [91]. Mycophenolic acid inhibits inosine 5'-monophosphate dehydrogenase. After oral consumption, the bioavailability of mycophenolic acid is 72%. As noted for mycophenolate mofetil (which is converted to mycophenolic acid), 97% of mycophenolic acid is bound to albumin. Mycophenolic acid's mechanism of action, metabolism, and excretion is the same as that for mycophenolate mofetil.

Use in Uveitis

Mycophenolic acid has been suggested as a possible therapy for intraocular use, but this continues to be entirely experimental and is not being utilized in humans.

However, toxicity of human retinal pigment epithelium and Müller cells was not seen for doses of mycophenolic acid lower than 50 μg/mL or less [92].

There is a Phase 3 clinical trial aimed at determining the efficacy, safety, and tolerability of mycophenolic acid in patients with intermediate uveitis (ClinicalTrials.gov Identifier NCT01092533).

Sulfasalazine

While sulfasalazine is not an antimetabolite, it bears mentioning since it has certainly been used as a DMARD in rheumatology and has been used occasionally in the treatment of uveitis. The IUPAC name for sulfasalazine is 2-Hydroxy-5-[[4-(2-pyridinylsulfamoyl)phenyl]diazenyl]benzoic acid. Its molecular formula is $C_{18}H_{14}N_4O_5S$.

Pharmacology and Pharmacokinetics

Sulfasalazine is either absorbed in the upper gastrointestinal system (up to 30% of the intact drug) or is cleaved into sulfapyridine and 5-amino salicylate by colonic bacteria. The cleavage products are thought to be involved in inhibiting folate absorption and metabolism [93–95]. Additionally, sulfasalazine and 5-amino salicylate inhibit in vitro leukocyte motility [96].

Placebo-Controlled Trials

In a small placebo-controlled trial, 22 patients with ankylosing spondylitis-associated recurrent anterior uveitis were randomized either to sulfasalazine (10 patients) or placebo (12 patients) and followed for 3 years. Uveitis activity was assessed by fluorophotometry. The number of recurrences was less than one for each year in the patients taking sulfasalazine (with the highest number of mean recurrences during year two with 0.6 +/−0.84 recurrences). In the placebo group, the number of recurrences was statistically significantly higher (with the highest recurrences occurring during the first year of follow up at 1.33 +/−1.23 recurrences). Additionally, the formation of posterior synechiae was less frequently encountered in the sulfasalazine group.

Studies

Ten patients with recurrent anterior uveitis were commenced on sulfasalazine and followed for 1 year [97]. In the year prior to the institution of sulfasalazine, there was a mean of 3.4 flares, which was statistically significantly less during the year the patients were on the DMARD (less than 1 flare).

In a study involving chronic uveitis, four Taiwanese children with JIA- or ankylosing spondylitis-related were committed to sulfasalazine due to failing to taper off of steroid drops as well as exhibiting a lack of uveitis control with oral nonsteroidal anti-inflammatory drugs. Two children with JIA-associated uveitis and the child with ankylosing spondylitis-associated uveitis showed improvement in their anterior chamber cell and visual acuity. The medication was tolerated well by all four children.

Side Effects

Common side effects include gastrointestinal discomfort and rash. Stevens-Johnson and neutropenia are less frequent but serious side effects.

General Considerations with the Antimetabolites

In a large retrospective study in which patients with noninfectious ocular inflammatory diseases were assessed, three of the most commonly used antimetabolites to control ocular inflammation (including uveitis) were assessed [18]. The median time to treatment success (on ≤10 mg prednisone PO daily) with methotrexate was 6.5 months compared to that of mycophenolate mofetil (4 months) and azathioprine (4.8 months). It was noted that methotrexate was frequently started at a low dose and increased over time, whereas mycophenolate mofetil and azathioprine were typically started at more therapeutic doses. After 6 months of therapy, the proportion of all ocular inflammation patients achieving treatment success with mycophenolate was 70% compared to 42% of those on methotrexate and 48% of those taking azathioprine. While these results are intriguing, there still remains the issue of determining the best antimetabolite to use as first-line therapy for corticosteroid-sparing control of uveitis. To address this important issue, Acharya and colleagues compared methotrexate and mycophenolate mofetil (two of the most commonly used antimetabolites) for initial corticosteroid-sparing control of noninfectious intermediate, posterior, and panuveitis. While past retrospective studies have suggested that mycophenolate mofetil may be more effective in the management of uveitis, Acharya's RCT found that a higher proportion of those randomized to methotrexate achieved control of their uveitis compared to those randomized to mycophenolate mofetil [1]. Control of uveitis was defined as less than 1+ anterior chamber cell or vitreous haze or inactive retinal or choroidal lesions. However, while the maximum dose of methotrexate was used (25 mg PO weekly), the maximum dose for mycophenolate mofetil in the trial was 1 g PO BID rather than the typical maximum dose of 1.5 g PO BID. To address this issue, Acharya is currently conducting a National Eye Institute-sponsored randomized controlled trial, which is powered to detect a smaller difference (20%) between the two randomization groups and utilizing the typical maximum doses of these medications. The data gathered from this pivotal study will provide uveitis specialists with much needed evidence to support the initial use of either methotrexate or mycophenolate mofetil as initial corticosteroid-sparing therapy.

In general, as with all other immunomodulatory agents, live vaccines should not be administered to those taking antimetabolites. Additionally, patients considering vaccinations with killed agents may proceed but should be informed that they may mount a truncated immune response due to the iatrogenic immunosuppression.

Contraception should be practiced while on antimetabolites. Developing fetuses with their rapid cell turnover are especially vulnerable to the effects of antimetabolites that affect nucleic acid synthesis. In fact, high-dose methotrexate is utilized as an abortive agent. It is recommended that in those wishing to become pregnant, discontinue use and wait at least 3 months prior to conceiving.

Antimetabolites can be used in conjunction with other immunomodulatory agents, particularly from other classes such as the T-cell inhibitors (e.g., cyclosporine [98, 99]) or with biologics. In the case of biologics, antimetabolites may help decrease the frequency of developing antibodies (e.g., human anti-chimeric antibodies, HACAs) against monoclonal antibodies (e.g., rituximab, infliximab, adalimumab).

Much of the information regarding cancer and systemic immunomodulatory therapy with antimetabolites comes from the transplant literature. For example, renal transplant patients on azathioprine have 50- to 100-fold increase in the relative risk of malignancy. However, it has been noted that rheumatoid arthritis carries a background risk of cancer development compared to patients without rheumatoid arthritis. Rheumatoid arthritis patients have been noted to have a fivefold increase in cancer compared to the general population. Azathioprine-treated RA patients have a tenfold increase in cancer compared to the general population [100]. The most common neoplasias include squamous cell carcinoma of the skin, non-Hodgkin's lymphoma, and Kaposi's sarcoma [101].

In a retrospective cohort study evaluating nearly 8000 patients with ocular inflammatory diseases (1155 patients with uveitis), the antimetabolites were not associated with an increased risk in overall mortality and were not associated with an increased risk in cancer-related mortality [102]. Conveying this information to patients or the parents of patients can do much to mollify their concerns about starting antimetabolite therapy. Oftentimes in uveitis, advancement to systemic immunomodulatory therapy must be made, and the knowledge that these medications are not only effective, but also safe, can do much to treat the mind *and* body of the person in the uveitis specialist's examination chair.

Calcineurin Inhibitors

Calcineurin is a phosphatase, an enzyme that is involved in the phosphorylation of the nuclear factor of activated T cells (NFAT), allowing this transcription factor to translocate from the cytosol into the nucleus of T cells. In the nucleus, NFAT can then transcribe mRNA to be utilized in the production of lymphokines including interleukin 2 and *others*.

Cyclosporine

While cyclosporine proved its efficacy in the world of organ transplantation, it made its debut in the realm of uveitis when Nussenblatt and colleagues used it in the management of experimental autoimmune uveitis utilizing retinal S antigen in a murine model [103].

Pharmacology and Pharmacokinetics

Cyclosporine binds to cyclophilin, which is an intracellular cytoplasmic protein in T cells. It is metabolized by the CYP3A4 hepatic enzymatic system. Thus, it is important not to consume grapefruit juice when taking oral cyclosporine as grapefruit juice inhibits CYP3A4, which would increase bioavailability. The metabolites of cyclosporine (none of which have immunosuppressive effects) are excreted mainly in the bile. Cyclosporine is not very soluble in water. The micro-emulsion form of the original cyclosporine (Sandimmune, Novartis) known as Neoral (from Novartis) has more consistent absorption rates and, thus, bioavailability.

Studies

Nussenblatt and colleagues' results in the murine model were so encouraging that his group used cyclosporine for the first time to treat uveitis in eight humans [104]. They noted that most patients had a relatively abrupt response (less than 2 weeks) in terms of improvement in inflammation and visual acuity.

The Systemic Immunosuppressive Therapy for Eye Diseases (SITE) cohort evaluated cyclosporine's efficacy in noninfectious ocular inflammation (including uveitis and scleritis). One definition of control of inflammation used by the SITE study was no inflammation (as defined by the SUN criteria) on ≤10 mg PO daily of prednisone. Using this definition, SITE found that inflammation was controlled in 22.1% of cohort participants (95% CI: 17.7 to 27.3) at 6 months and 36.1% of cohort participants (95% CI: 30.5 to 42.2) at 12 months [105].

Side Effects

Common side effects with cyclosporine include fatigue, paresthesias, tremors, headaches, gum hyperplasia, and nausea [105, 106]. Nephrotoxicity can be an issue, though in the SITE study, only 10.7% discontinued cyclosporine in the first year of starting the medication due to nephrotoxicity [105]. Additionally, the SITE study evaluating cyclosporine showed that patients older than 55 years of age were severalfold more likely to develop side effects limiting the use of cyclosporine compared to those aged 18–39 years.

Tacrolimus

Tacrolimus was born from a desire for an immunosuppressive and naturally occurring compound that could be used for transplant medicine. The Fujisawa Pharmaceutical Company Ltd. in Japan isolated a macrolide antibiotic from the fermentation broth of *Streptomyces tsukubaensis* "strain no. 9993, in a 2-ton tank" [107]. Tacrolimus was initially designated FK506 because it (as well as rapamycin) binds to the immunophilin family member, FK-binding protein (FKBP), which functions as a protein folding chaperone. Tacrolimus suppressed human and murine cytotoxic T-cell generation in cell cultures at concentrations lower than cyclosporine. Thus, tacrolimus was noted to be more potent than cyclosporine, to suppress immune responses and suppress the expression of IL-2, IL-3, and IFN-gamma [108]. Like cyclosporine, tacrolimus suppresses T-cell activity.

Pharmacology and Pharmacokinetics

Tacrolimus is incompletely and erratically absorbed from the gut reaching peak plasma concentrations in 1–4 h. The mean half-life is around 9 h (though this is calculated from intravenous administration in humans), though it is prolonged when there is liver dysfunction (as it is extensively metabolized by the CYP450 enzymatic system). Its mean bioavailability is 27%, and most of tacrolimus is excreted in the feces [109]. For uveitis, the oral dosing ranges from 0.15 to 0.3 mg/kg daily.

Studies

Shortly after tacrolimus found its utility in transplant medicine, Mochizuki and colleagues studied tacrolimus and found it to be effective in the management posterior uveitis in 53 patients [110].

Hogan et al. evaluated tacrolimus in their retrospective study of 62 patients with uveitis [111]. All required steroid-sparing therapy, over half had failed alternative systemic immunomodulatory therapy, and nearly a third of patients had failed a second systemic immunomodulatory medication. Control of uveitis was achieved in over half of patients (such that tacrolimus was continued or allowed for discontinuation of medication). Others noted that tacrolimus was an effective and reliable medication, particularly when uveitis patients had failed with cyclosporine [112, 113].

Side Effects

Hypercholesterolemia, hypertension, and nephrotoxicity are the most common side effects of tacrolimus.

Tacrolimus Versus Cyclosporine

In an unmasked randomized trial comparing tacrolimus (19 patients) to cyclosporine (18 patients) in noninfectious posterior uveitis, Murphy and colleagues found that the efficacy of cyclosporine and tacrolimus was comparable [106]. Control of uveitis and improvement in visual acuity was found in 67% of the cyclosporine patients and 68% of the tacrolimus patients. Additionally failure with the randomized T-cell inhibitor mediation was similar between the two groups, though tacrolimus would have been slightly lower than cyclosporine when one considers that one of the patients randomized to tacrolimus was ultimately diagnosed with intraocular lymphoma. Cyclosporine was associated with more side effects than tacrolimus. Hypercholesterolemia and hypertension were less frequent with tacrolimus compared to cyclosporine. This group also assessed quality of life by using questionnaires for vision and health. Interestingly, there was no significant change in quality of life measures in either treatment group suggesting that while therapies in uveitis can be effective, there are still factors, possibly associated with side effects or the fact of having a chronic disease that need to be addressed. These issues are not unique to tacrolimus or cyclosporine, however, and are germane to any immunosuppressive agent used to treat uveitis.

Alkylating Agents

Intense research on the mustard gases (most of which were actually liquids) during World War II. It was found that the nitrogen mustards were as mutagenic in the fruit fly (*Drosophila melanogaster*) as were X-rays [114]. The alkylation of DNA leading to its cross-linking results in inhibition of DNA synthesis. This feature proved useful in the treatment of cancers, but it was readily recognized that they were useful in rheumatologic diseases [115, 116].

Cyclophosphamide

Brock described his time as head of the Pharmacological Department at ASTA Werke AG in the late 1940s. ASTA Werke's original claim to fame in pharmacology was the pain medication Quadronal. The Brock group's goal, however, was to further the development of cancer chemotherapeutic drugs. Cyclophosphamide was originally known as B 518-ASTA.

Cyclophosphamide is an oxazaphosphorine and represents a prodrug of nitrogen mustard that is activated by the liver enzyme cytochrome P450 [117]. Interestingly, the idea of a "prodrug" or "latent drug," a form of a drug that is not chemically active, but can later be activated once administered, was coined by H. Druckrey, a member of the Brock group.

Pharmacology and Pharmacokinetics

When administered orally, cyclophosphamide is absorbed in the gut. It is metabolized by the liver's cytochrome P450 system yielding compounds with alkylating properties.

Monthly intravenous administration of cyclophosphamide can also be utilized at 0.75–1 g/m^2 of body surface area with the dose titrated to a white blood cell count between 1500 to 3000/μL. Mesna, which conjugates to toxic metabolites of cyclophosphamide, can help decrease hemorrhagic cystitis. Hydration is also important when taking cyclophosphamide.

Studies

In the retrospective SITE study of cyclophosphamide used to treat ocular inflammation (including uveitis), 76% of patients achieved control of inflammatory activity [118]. Most patients were also able to achieve a corticosteroid-sparing dose of prednisone (less than 10 mg daily of oral prednisone). Ocular inflammatory disease remission can be a benefit of cyclophosphamide treatment (at a rate of 0.32/person-year in the SITE study), but cyclophosphamide is typically reserved for especially sight-threatening inflammation given its significant side effect profile (discontinued by 33.5% of patients within 1 year).

Side Effects

Side effects include gastrointestinal upset, myelosuppression with resultant cytopenias, gonadal failure, susceptibility for infections, hemorrhagic cystitis, and bladder cancer [119].

Chlorambucil

Similar to cyclophosphamide, chlorambucil works by replacing a hydrogen ion for an alkyl group. The resultant alkylated DNA is unable to be replicated.

Pharmacology and Pharmacokinetics

Chlorambucil is metabolized by the livers CYP450 enzyme system to phenylacetic acid mustard [120]. Food consumption with chlorambucil slightly increases the time to reach maximum plasma concentration compared to the fasting state, but does not decrease its bioavailability [121].

Studies

Chlorambucil's use has been typically reserved for uveitis in which blindness is imminent, particularly in the setting of Behçet's disease and sympathetic ophthalmia. Because of its side effect profile, a preference has been to use it for a relatively short period of time [122, 123]. Nonetheless, chlorambucil has proven effective especially when uveitis patients have failed numerous other therapies (particularly prior to the availability of biologic agents for the treatment of uveitis) [124].

Side Effects

Gonadal dysfunction, secondary amenorrhea, and myelosuppression are important side effects.

Biologics

Immune responses are initiated, propagated, and terminated by a variety of cell signaling proteins. Biologics are themselves proteins that are engineered to modulate the immune system in ways that tend to have more specific targets than antimetabolites, alkylating agents, and even calcineurin inhibitors. The biologics are made up of a variety of medications including monoclonal antibodies and fusion proteins.

Tumor Necrosis Factor Inhibitors

The cytokine tumor necrosis factor is produced by macrophages and lymphocytes and is important mediator of inflammation, septic shock, and cytotoxicity. When TNF is aberrantly expresses, as in autoimmune disease, it can mediate the production of more proinflammatory cytokines such as leukotrienes and prostaglandins [125, 126]. TNF inhibition, then, have been a source of intense investigation for pharmaceutical companies developing clinical indications for autoimmune diseases. Most of the TNF inhibitors are aimed at treating rheumatic diseases, but there has been significant interest in their use in uveitis. Indeed, TNF inhibitors have been shown to not only effective for adults with uveitis but children as well [127].

Adalimumab

Adalimumab is the only nonsteroid medication that is approved by the US Food and Drug Administration for noninfectious intermediate, posterior, and panuveitis. With a half-life of 15–19 days, adalimumab is effective when administered every 14 days. The half-life of adalimumab is longer than chimeric or artificially fused human peptides because its structure and function are the same as naturally occurring human immunoglobulin G1. Naturally occurring immunoglobulin has a life span of approximately 2 weeks [128, 129].

Studies

Adalimumab (Humira, AbbVie Inc.) is a fully humanized monoclonal antibody targeting TNF-alpha. A prospective multicenter open label examining the benefits of adalimumab in refractory (unable to taper off steroids and one other immunomodulatory agent or intolerant to such therapy) noninfectious uveitis in adults found that 68% of participants achieved control at 10 weeks and 39% maintained durable control at 1 year [130]. This study, however, did not include a loading dose (of 80 mg); to address the utility of such a loading dose, a multicenter clinical trial recently concluded with the results pending.

Uveitis associated with JIA has been shown to respond to adalimumab as well as 65.3–88% in some studies [131, 132]. However, such successes are not experienced by all JIA cases, and consideration for other agents should be made should there be a lack of adequate response to adalimumab [133].

While one study examined the use of intravitreal adalimumab in eight patients with uveitic macular edema without demonstration of efficacy [134], other studies using intravitreal TNF inhibitors have been far more sobering [135, 136]. Intravitreal injections of TNF inhibitors are not recommended.

Side Effects

Upper respiratory tract infection, rash, injection site reaction, transaminitis, and headache are more common reactions. Less common but serious reactions include lymphoproliferative disorders (lymphoma and leukemia), reactivation of hepatitis B or latent tuberculosis, and opportunistic or non-opportunistic infections.

Infliximab

Infliximab (Remicade, Janssen Biotech, Inc.) is a chimeric monoclonal antibody that targets TNF-alpha. Fusion of the TNF-alpha binding site on the murine antibody A2 to the constant region of human IgG1 kappa immunoglobulin leads to the formation of the chimeric monoclonal antibody, infliximab. Chimeric monoclonal antibodies can be distinguished by the nomenclature utilized for the biologics. For monoclonal antibodies, the generic name will end in "mab" (as in infliximab). The "x" in the generic name of a monoclonal antibody identifies it as a chimeric antibody (from the Greek letter χ (chi), which looks similar to the Latin letter X). Infliximab's serum concentrations are proportional to the dose of medication administered. The half-life of infliximab is 8–9 days.

Studies

In a prospective study examining the use of infliximab in noninfectious uveitis refractory to systemic corticosteroids and at least one other immunomodulatory agent (or intolerance to such therapy), control of uveitis was achieved in 78% effect at 10 weeks and 48% at 1 year [137, 138]. In sarcoid uveitis failing conventional therapy with antimetabolites, TNF inhibitors (infliximab, adalimumab, or golimumab) showed efficacy in achieving improvements in features of inflammation and macular edema [139]. Infliximab has been useful in JIA-associated uveitis as well [140, 141].

Final Words on Adalimumab and Infliximab

An expert panel has suggested using either adalimumab or infliximab as first-line therapy for the uveitis associated with Behçet's disease and as second-line therapy for the uveitis associated with juvenile inflammatory arthritis [142]. The French Uveitis Network has reported that adalimumab and infliximab exhibit similar efficacy in the management of uveitis. The multicenter network performed an observational study in which uveitis patients who had failed conventional therapies were treated with either adalimumab or infliximab. The complete response rate (anterior chamber and vitreous haze scores of 0, regression of retinal vasculitis, resolution of macular edema, and ≤10 mg/day of corticosteroids) was 26% at 6 months and 28% at 12 months (though overall response rates at 6 and 12 months were 87% and 93%, respectively, when considering improvement in inflammation or macular edema by at least 50%, and reduction of initial corticosteroid dose) [143]. Randomized prospective trials comparing these two important players are needed.

Golimumab

There are small case reports that golimumab (Simponi, Janssen Biotech, Inc.) suggesting efficacy in uveitis. Golimumab has shown to be effective in patients with refractory recurrent anterior uveitis in the setting of ankylosing spondyloarthropathies with most patients achieving improvement or remission of uveitis [144, 145]. While in some cases patients had not previously tried infliximab, in other cases many patients had actually failed infliximab but showed improvement in inflammation with golimumab [146].

Etanercept

The fusion protein etanercept (Enbrel, Amgen, Inc., and Pfizer Inc.) targets both TNF-alpha and TNF-beta. Etanercept, however, exhibits minimal efficacy in ocular inflammation [147]. Historically, there was the thought that, unlike adalimumab and infliximab, etanercept did not bind membrane-bound (cell surface) TNF nor did it activate complement. In vitro studies have shown that while etanercept has superior binding of soluble TNF compared to adalimumab and infliximab, all three agents exhibit similar affinity for membrane TNF [148]. Additionally, none of these agents were able to induce complement-dependent cytotoxicity in vitro [148]. Instead, the ability of one monoclonal antibody (either infliximab or adalimumab) to bind *numerous* membrane-bound TNF results in pro-apoptotic signaling that is not achieved when a single etanercept molecule binds to only one membrane TNF [149].

Side Effects

The TNF inhibitors have a 4–5% risk of serious infection (including reactivation of tuberculosis, fulminant hepatitis B, or fungal infections) as well as approximately a 1/1000 risk of lymphoma. There is at least a 15% risk of skin reaction, which is usually manageable with topical therapy. As these are antibodies, there is a risk of developing anti-drug antibodies (particularly with the chimeric antibodies) and increased clearance of the drug, which can lead to reduced effectiveness of the medication and possible side effects. In such cases, combining these medications with an antimetabolite can help decrease such reactions.

Interferon

Interferons are cytokines originally found in the late 1950s that are produced by host cells in the setting of viral infections. Their name comes from the fact that they exhibit the ability to interfere with viral replication (originally studied with influenza virus A) [150].

Pegylated interferon alpha is produced by recombinant DNA vector technology; it is produced gene expression in bacterial cells. There are two types of interferons, type I and type II. Interferon alpha-2a and -2b belong to the type 1 family. Dendritic cells are major producers of interferon alpha in the setting of certain viral infections and tumor genesis inhibiting these destructive processes from progressing [151, 152]. However, when interferon is aberrantly expressed, autoimmune diseases, such as systemic lupus erythematosus to rheumatoid arthritis, may result [153, 154].

Studies

Interferon alpha was shown to be effective in animal models of experimental autoimmune uveitis, which lead to its consideration for use in uveitis in humans [155–157].

In a Parisian study, interferon alpha-2a was used for uveitis patients experiencing a relapse on their prednisone/immunomodulatory combination. Behçet's disease-related uveitis made up just over half of the patients studied with 82.6% of cases exhibiting control after administration of interferon alpha-2a. Those with uveitis other than Behçet's in the study group exhibited control of their uveitis to the tune of 59% [158]. This same group has noted that interferon alpha-2a is especially effective for Behçet's disease uveitis [159], and in Turkey and Korea, interferon alpha-2a is useful in decreasing flare-ups of Behçet's disease uveitis when first-line immunomodulatory therapy has failed [160, 161]. Interferon alpha-2b has also been utilized for Behçet's disease, ocular sarcoidosis, and has demonstrated efficacy for refractory uveitic macular edema [162–164].

Side Effects

Side effects of interferon therapy can commonly include flu-like symptoms, abdominal pain and diarrhea, headache, and rash. Less common, but more severe reactions include cardiomyopathy, myelosuppression, depression, psychosis, lupus-like reactions, and a severe skin reaction that resembles pemphigus [165, 166].

Anti-CD20

Uveitis has traditionally been thought of as a primarily T-cell-mediated process. This knowledge comes from the study of other autoimmune diseases as well as knowledge from studies of uveitis including experimental autoimmune uveitis [167–169]. However, B cells are important players in many types of inflammatory conditions. Insight into the potential for B-cell-directed therapy is reflected in the case of a boy with refractory JIA-associated uveitis who was tried and failed on numerous medications from antimetabolites to TNF inhibitors. Unfortunately, one of his eyes became phthisical and required enucleation. Histopathology performed by Narsing Rao showed that there was a predominance of a B-cell infiltrate (characterized by such activity that Russell bodies were clearly identified) [170].

Rituximab (Rituxan, Genentech) is a chimeric (human and murine) monoclonal antibody that was developed at the National Institutes of Health (NIH) National Cancer Institute (NCI) to treat B-cell non-Hodgkin's lymphoma (NHL). Given that B cells express CD20, this was a prime target for developing therapy that specifically targeted B-cell lymphoproliferative processes. Rituximab (originally developed by Biogen Idec) has been a major playing in improving outcomes in NHL [171].

Studies

Rituximab demonstrated it effectiveness in the setting of scleritis and orbital inflammation in granulomatosis with polyangiitis [172], but rituximab has also been effective in a group of patients with especially refractory posterior uveitis [173, 174]. Harkening back to the infiltration of B cells in the enucleated eye of the boy with JIA, rituximab has found utility in treating severe and refractory uveitis in JIA [175, 176].

Anti-IL-2

Daclizumab (Zinbryta, Biogen, Inc.), introduced in 1997 under the work of Thomas Waldman, MD at the NIH NCI (and at that time known under the trade name Zenapax), is a humanized monoclonal antibody that targets the "Tac" portion of the IL-2 receptor. It was originally developed to prevent allograft transplant rejection. Shortly after its introduction, daclizumab's potential utility in uveitis was recognized. Collaborating with Laboratory of Immunology at the National Eye Institute, daclizumab was found to be effective in managing experimental autoimmune uveoretinitis in a primate model [177]. Shortly thereafter, Dr. Waldmann collaborated with Robert Nussenblatt, MD at National Eye Institute to use it in uveitis patients demonstrating its safety and efficacy [178, 179]. Daclizumab has been effective in preventing the onward march of visual decline that has dogged the treatment of birdshot chorioretinopathy in a small study [180]. Interestingly, when daclizumab or placebo added to pre-existing standard immunosuppression in a small study of Behçet's disease-related uveitis, daclizumab was not any more effective than the placebo. However, both groups (and, in particular, the placebo group) had very infrequent uveitis flare-ups during the study [181].

Daclizumab was pulled off the market in 2009 because it was not performing well commercially as other biologics began to populate the market. However, daclizumab has reemerged, and studies will assess its efficacy in uveitis once again.

Anti-IL-6

Tocilizumab (Actemra, Genentech) is an interleukin (IL)-6 inhibitor. Inflammatory cells that mediate uveitis express IL-6 in high concentrations [182, 183].

Studies

Tocilizumab (Actemra, Genentech, Inc.) has been prospectively studied in the setting of JIA-associated uveitis refractory to biologic therapy including TNF inhibitors, T-cell costimulatory blockers, and anti-CD20 therapy [184]. After 6 months, most patients showed improvement in anterior chamber cell with even more patients showing improvement at 1 year. Seventy-six percent of patients attained remission in this study. Tocilizumab has also been effective in managing uveitic CME refractory to other therapies. In one retrospective study, eight eyes in five patients who had failed other biologic therapy achieved improvement of CME as well as remission of their uveitis [185].

T-cell Costimulatory Blockade

Abatacept (Orencia, Bristol-Myers Squibb Co.) is a fusion protein that inhibits the CD28 co-stimulatory molecule, which results in T-cell inactivation [186, 187]. Abatacept has been shown to be effective when used as either first-line or second-line (after failing TNF inhibitors) therapy in refractory JIA-associated uveitis [188].

A Word on the Biosimilars

A biosimilar or follow-on biologic is similar to an original biologic medication and can be colloquially thought of as a "generic" version of the original biologic. In 2015, it was reported that there were over 700 biosimilars in various stages of development [189]. The creation of biosimilars to adalimumab, infliximab, and rituximab is especially popular [190]. There is great potential for biosimilars to possibly take the place of some biologics for managing chronic inflammatory disorders. However, developing clinical, US FDA-approved indications for biologics (let alone biosimilars) in uveitis remains an important obstacle. Insurance companies will typically look to FDA-approved indications prior to approving a medicine for a patient, particularly when the medication is as expensive as a biologic. Despite the potential for biosimilars to be alternative, cheaper therapies, it will be important to demonstrate that they are at least just as effective as the original biologic and have a similar side effect profile. Randomized controlled trials will be needed to make these comparisons.

Compliance with Ethical Requirements John Gonzales and Nisha Acharya declare that they have no conflict of interest. No human or animal studies were carried out by the authors for this chapter.

References

1. Rathinam SR, Babu M, Thundikandy R, et al. A randomized clinical trial comparing methotrexate and mycophenolate mofetil for noninfectious uveitis. Ophthalmology. 2014;121(10):1863–70.
2. Esterberg E, Acharya NR. Corticosteroid-sparing therapy: practice patterns among uveitis specialists. J Ophthalmic Inflamm Infect. 2012;2(1):21–8.
3. Elion GB, Hitchings GH, Vanderwerff H. Antagonists of nucleic acid derivatives. VI. Purines. J Biol Chem. 1951;192(2):505–18.
4. Elion GB. Nobel Lecture. The purine path to chemotherapy. Biosci Rep. 1989;9(5):509–29.
5. Hoffmann M, Rychlewski J, Chrzanowska M, Hermann T. Mechanism of activation of an immunosuppressive drug: azathioprine. Quantum chemical study on the reaction of azathioprine with cysteine. J Am Chem Soc. 2001;123(26):6404–9.
6. Liu H, Ding L, Zhang F, et al. The impact of glutathione S-transferase genotype and phenotype on the adverse drug reactions to azathioprine in patients with inflammatory bowel diseases. J Pharmacol Sci. 2015;129(2):95–100.
7. Greenwood AJ, Stanford MR, Graham EM. The role of azathioprine in the management of retinal vasculitis. Eye (London, England). 1998;12(Pt 5):783–8.
8. Pasadhika S, Kempen JH, Newcomb CW, et al. Azathioprine for ocular inflammatory diseases. Am J Ophthalmol. 2009;148(4):500–509.e502.
9. Jabs DA, Nussenblatt RB, Rosenbaum JT. Standardization of uveitis nomenclature for reporting clinical data. Results of the First International Workshop. Am J Ophthalmol. 2005;140(3):509–16.
10. Schatz CS, Uzel JL, Leininger L, Danner S, Terzic J, Fischbach M. Immunosuppressants used in a steroid-sparing strategy for childhood uveitis. J Pediatr Ophthalmol Strabismus. 2007;44(1):28–34.
11. Arellanes-Garcia L, Navarro-Lopez L, Recillas-Gispert C. Pars planitis in the Mexican Mestizo population: ocular findings, treatment, and visual outcome. Ocul Immunol Inflamm. 2003;11(1):53–60.
12. Mathews JD, Crawford BA, Bignell JL, Mackay IR. Azathioprine in active chronic iridocyclitis. A double-blind controlled trial. Br J Ophthalmol. 1969;53(5):327–30.
13. Yazici H, Pazarli H, Barnes CG, et al. A controlled trial of azathioprine in Behcet's syndrome. N Engl J Med. 1990;322(5):281–5.
14. Hamuryudan V, Ozyazgan Y, Hizli N, et al. Azathioprine in Behcet's syndrome: effects on long-term prognosis. Arthritis Rheum. 1997;40(4):769–74.
15. Andrasch RH, Pirofsky B, Burns RP. Immunosuppressive therapy for severe chronic uveitis. Arch Ophthalmol (Chicago, Ill.: 1960). 1978;96(2):247–51.
16. Cytotoxic drugs in treatment of nonmalignant diseases. Ann Intern Med. 1972;76(4):619–42.
17. Nielsen OH, Maxwell C, Hendel J. IBD medications during pregnancy and lactation. Nat Rev Gastroenterol Hepatol. 2014;11(2):116–27.
18. Galor A, Jabs DA, Leder HA, et al. Comparison of antimetabolite drugs as corticosteroid-sparing therapy for noninfectious ocular inflammation. Ophthalmology. 2008;115(10):1826–32.

19. Hooper PL, Kaplan HJ. Triple agent immunosuppression in serpiginous choroiditis. Ophthalmology. 1991;98(6):944–51; discussion 951-942.
20. Moore CE. Sympathetic ophthalmitis treated with azathioprine. Br J Ophthalmol. 1968;52(9):688–90.
21. Hakin KN, Pearson RV, Lightman SL. Sympathetic ophthalmia: visual results with modern immunosuppressive therapy. Eye (London, England). 1992;6(Pt 5):453–5.
22. Hellmund K, Fruhauf A, Seiler T, Naumann GO. Sympathetic ophthalmia 50 years after penetrating injury. A case report. Klin Monbl Augenheilkd. 1998;213(3):182–5.
23. Sisk RA, Davis JL, Dubovy SR, Smiddy WE. Sympathetic ophthalmia following vitrectomy for endophthalmitis after intravitreal bevacizumab. Ocul Immunol Inflamm. 2008;16(5): 236–8.
24. Siemasko KF, Chong AS, Williams JW, Bremer EG, Finnegan A. Regulation of B cell function by the immunosuppressive agent leflunomide. Transplantation. 1996;61(4):635–42.
25. Manna SK, Aggarwal BB. Immunosuppressive leflunomide metabolite (A77 1726) blocks TNF-dependent nuclear factor-kappa B activation and gene expression. J Immunol (Baltimore, Md.: 1950). 1999;162(4):2095–102.
26. Robertson SM, Lang LS. Leflunomide: inhibition of S-antigen induced autoimmune uveitis in Lewis rats. Agents Actions. 1994;42(3–4):167–72.
27. Fang CB, Zhou DX, Zhan SX, et al. Amelioration of experimental autoimmune uveitis by leflunomide in Lewis rats. PLoS One. 2013;8(4):e62071.
28. Wang J, Xie QB, Zhao Y, Liu Y. Flare up of rheumatoid arthritis associated with Vogt-Koyanagi-Harada syndrome treated with leflunomide. Int J Ophthalmol. 2014;7(5):909–11.
29. Steigerwalt RD Jr, Bacci S, Valesini G. Severe uveitis successfully treated with leflunomide. Retin Cases Brief Rep. 2007;1(1):54–5.
30. Molina C, Modesto C, Martin-Begue N, Arnal C. Leflunomide, a valid and safe drug for the treatment of chronic anterior uveitis associated with juvenile idiopathic arthritis. Clin Rheumatol. 2013;32(11):1673–5.
31. Bichler J, Benseler SM, Krumrey-Langkammerer M, Haas JP, Hugle B. Leflunomide is associated with a higher flare rate compared to methotrexate in the treatment of chronic uveitis in juvenile idiopathic arthritis. Scand J Rheumatol. 2015;44(4):280–3.
32. Kremer JM, Genovese MC, Cannon GW, et al. Concomitant leflunomide therapy in patients with active rheumatoid arthritis despite stable doses of methotrexate. A randomized, double-blind, placebo-controlled trial. Ann Intern Med. 2002;137(9):726–33.
33. Fairbanks LD, Ruckemann K, Qiu Y, et al. Methotrexate inhibits the first committed step of purine biosynthesis in mitogen-stimulated human T-lymphocytes: a metabolic basis for efficacy in rheumatoid arthritis? Biochem J. 1999;342(Pt 1):143–52.
34. Kiely PD, Johnson DM. Infliximab and leflunomide combination therapy in rheumatoid arthritis: an open-label study. Rheumatology (Oxford, England). 2002;41(6):631–7.
35. Nurmohamed MT, van Halm VP, Dijkmans BA. Cardiovascular risk profile of antirheumatic agents in patients with osteoarthritis and rheumatoid arthritis. Drugs. 2002;62(11):1599–609.
36. Erice A. Resistance of human cytomegalovirus to antiviral drugs. Clin Microbiol Rev. 1999;12(2):286–97.
37. Andrassy J, Illner WD, Rentsch M, Jaeger G, Jauch KW, Fischereder M. Leflunomide: a treatment option for ganciclovir-resistant cytomegalovirus infection after renal transplantation. NDT Plus. 2009;2(2):149–51.
38. Chon WJ, Kadambi PV, Xu C, et al. Use of leflunomide in renal transplant recipients with ganciclovir-resistant/refractory cytomegalovirus infection: a case series from the University of Chicago. Case Rep Nephrol Dial. 2015;5(1):96–105.
39. Verkaik NJ, Hoek RA, van Bergeijk H, et al. Leflunomide as part of the treatment for multidrug-resistant cytomegalovirus disease after lung transplantation: case report and review of the literature. Transpl Infect Dis. 2013;15(6):E243–9.
40. Waldman WJ, Knight DA, Blinder L, et al. Inhibition of cytomegalovirus in vitro and in vivo by the experimental immunosuppressive agent leflunomide. Intervirology. 1999;42(5–6):412–8.

41. Heinle RW, Welch AD. Experiments with pteroylglutamic acid and pteroylglutamic acid deficiency in human leukemia. J Clin Invest. 1948;27(4):539.
42. Cress RH, Deaver NL. Methotrexate in the Management of Severe Psoriasis and Arthritis: report of a case. South Med J. 1964;57:1088–90.
43. Enderlin M. Experiences with antimetabolite therapy of malignant forms of progressive chronic polyarthritis. Helv Med Acta Suppl. 1966;46:171.
44. Gross D, Enderlin M, Fehr K. Immunosuppressive therapy of progredient chronic polyarthritis using antimetabolites and cytostatics. Schweiz Med Wochenschr. 1967;97(40):1301–10.
45. Fosdick WM. Cytotoxic therapy in rheumatoid arthritis. Med Clin North Am. 1968;52(3):747–57.
46. Wilke WS, Calabrese LH, Scherbel AL. Methotrexate in the treatment of rheumatoid arthritis; pilot study. Cleve Clin Q. 1980;47(4):305–9.
47. Hall PA, Levison DA. Review: assessment of cell proliferation in histological material. J Clin Pathol. 1990;43(3):184–92.
48. Spina D, Leoncini L, Del Vecchio MT, et al. Low versus high cell turnover in diffusely growing non-Hodgkin's lymphomas. J Pathol. 1995;177(4):335–41.
49. Day RO, Furst DE, Riel PLCM, van Bresnihan B, editors. Antirheumatic therapy: actions and outcomes: Birhäuser Verlag. ISBN 978-3-7643-7726-7.
50. Jurgensen CH, Huber BE, Zimmerman TP, Wolberg G. 3-deazaadenosine inhibits leukocyte adhesion and ICAM-1 biosynthesis in tumor necrosis factor-stimulated human endothelial cells. J Immunol (Baltimore, Md.: 1950). 1990;144(2):653–61.
51. Jurgensen CH, Wolberg G, Zimmerman TP. Inhibition of neutrophil adherence to endothelial cells by 3-deazaadenosine. Agents Actions. 1989;27(3–4):398–400.
52. Nesher G, Moore TL. The in vitro effects of methotrexate on peripheral blood mononuclear cells. Modulation by methyl donors and spermidine. Arthritis Rheum. 1990;33(7):954–9.
53. Yukioka K, Wakitani S, Yukioka M, et al. Polyamine levels in synovial tissues and synovial fluids of patients with rheumatoid arthritis. J Rheumatol. 1992;19(5):689–92.
54. Morabito L, Montesinos MC, Schreibman DM, et al. Methotrexate and sulfasalazine promote adenosine release by a mechanism that requires ecto-5′-nucleotidase-mediated conversion of adenine nucleotides. J Clin Invest. 1998;101(2):295–300.
55. Cronstein BN, Rosenstein ED, Kramer SB, Weissmann G, Hirschhorn R. Adenosine; a physiologic modulator of superoxide anion generation by human neutrophils. Adenosine acts via an A2 receptor on human neutrophils. J Immunol (Baltimore, Md.: 1950). 1985;135(2):1366–71.
56. Cronstein BN, Daguma L, Nichols D, Hutchison AJ, Williams M. The adenosine/neutrophil paradox resolved: human neutrophils possess both A1 and A2 receptors that promote chemotaxis and inhibit O2 generation, respectively. J Clin Invest. 1990;85(4):1150–7.
57. Jundt JW, Browne BA, Fiocco GP, Steele AD, Mock D. A comparison of low dose methotrexate bioavailability: oral solution, oral tablet, subcutaneous and intramuscular dosing. J Rheumatol. 1993;20(11):1845–9.
58. Gangaputra S, Newcomb CW, Liesegang TL, et al. Methotrexate for ocular inflammatory diseases. Ophthalmology. 2009;116(11):2188–2198.e2181.
59. Hemady RK, Baer JC, Foster CS. Immunosuppressive drugs in the management of progressive, corticosteroid-resistant uveitis associated with juvenile rheumatoid arthritis. Int Ophthalmol Clin. 1992;32(1):241–52.
60. Weiss AH, Wallace CA, Sherry DD. Methotrexate for resistant chronic uveitis in children with juvenile rheumatoid arthritis. J Pediatr. 1998;133(2):266–8.
61. Foeldvari I, Wierk A. Methotrexate is an effective treatment for chronic uveitis associated with juvenile idiopathic arthritis. J Rheumatol. 2005;32(2):362–5.
62. Malik AR, Pavesio C. The use of low dose methotrexate in children with chronic anterior and intermediate uveitis. Br J Ophthalmol. 2005;89(7):806–8.
63. Heiligenhaus A, Mingels A, Heinz C, Ganser G. Methotrexate for uveitis associated with juvenile idiopathic arthritis: value and requirement for additional anti-inflammatory medication. Eur J Ophthalmol. 2007;17(5):743–8.

64. Herman RA, Veng-Pedersen P, Hoffman J, Koehnke R, Furst DE. Pharmacokinetics of low-dose methotrexate in rheumatoid arthritis patients. J Pharm Sci. 1989;78(2):165–71.
65. Prasad S, Tripathi D, Rai MK, Aggarwal S, Mittal B, Agarwal V. Multidrug resistance protein-1 expression, function and polymorphisms in patients with rheumatoid arthritis not responding to methotrexate. Int J Rheum Dis. 2014;17(8):878–86.
66. Wessels JA, van der Kooij SM, le Cessie S, et al. A clinical pharmacogenetic model to predict the efficacy of methotrexate monotherapy in recent-onset rheumatoid arthritis. Arthritis Rheum. 2007;56(6):1765–75.
67. Wessels JA, Kooloos WM, De Jonge R, et al. Relationship between genetic variants in the adenosine pathway and outcome of methotrexate treatment in patients with recent-onset rheumatoid arthritis. Arthritis Rheum. 2006;54(9):2830–9.
68. Sen HN, Chan CC, Byrnes G, Fariss RN, Nussenblatt RB, Buggage RR. Intravitreal methotrexate resistance in a patient with primary intraocular lymphoma. Ocul Immunol Inflamm. 2008;16(1):29–33.
69. Micsik T, Lorincz A, Gal J, Schwab R, Petak I. MDR-1 and MRP-1 activity in peripheral blood leukocytes of rheumatoid arthritis patients. Diagn Pathol. 2015;10(1):216.
70. Sotoudehmanesh R, Anvari B, Akhlaghi M, Shahraeeni S, Kolahdoozan S. Methotrexate hepatotoxicity in patients with rheumatoid arthritis. Middle East J Dig Dis. 2010;2(2):104–9.
71. Sakthiswary R, Chan GY, Koh ET, Leong KP, Thong BY. Methotrexate-associated nonalcoholic fatty liver disease with transaminitis in rheumatoid arthritis. TheScientificWorldJournal. 2014;2014:823763.
72. Jakubovic BD, Donovan A, Webster PM, Shear NH. Methotrexate-induced pulmonary toxicity. Can Respir J. 2013;20(3):153–5.
73. Troeltzsch M, von Blohn G, Kriegelstein S, et al. Oral mucositis in patients receiving low-dose methotrexate therapy for rheumatoid arthritis: report of 2 cases and literature review. Oral Surg Oral Med Oral Pathol Oral Radiol. 2013;115(5):e28–33.
74. Morgan SL, Baggott JE, Vaughn WH, et al. Supplementation with folic acid during methotrexate therapy for rheumatoid arthritis. A double-blind, placebo-controlled trial. Ann Intern Med. 1994;121(11):833–41.
75. Morgan SL, Baggott JE, Vaughn WH, et al. The effect of folic acid supplementation on the toxicity of low-dose methotrexate in patients with rheumatoid arthritis. Arthritis Rheum. 1990;33(1):9–18.
76. Shea B, Swinden MV, Ghogomu ET, et al. Folic acid and folinic acid for reducing side effects in patients receiving methotrexate for rheumatoid arthritis. J Rheumatol. 2014;41(6):1049–60.
77. Lee WA, Gu L, Miksztal AR, Chu N, Leung K, Nelson PH. Bioavailability improvement of mycophenolic acid through amino ester derivatization. Pharm Res. 1990;7(2):161–6.
78. Morris RE, Hoyt EG, Murphy MP, Eugui EM, Allison AC. Mycophenolic acid morpholinoethylester (RS-61443) is a new immunosuppressant that prevents and halts heart allograft rejection by selective inhibition of T- and B-cell purine synthesis. Transplant Proc. 1990;22(4):1659–62.
79. Platz KP, Sollinger HW, Hullett DA, Eckhoff DE, Eugui EM, Allison AC. RS-61443—a new, potent immunosuppressive agent. Transplantation. 1991;51(1):27–31.
80. Platz KP, Bechstein WO, Eckhoff DE, Suzuki Y, Sollinger HW. RS-61443 reverses acute allograft rejection in dogs. Surgery. 1991;110(4):736–40; discussion 740-731.
81. Sollinger HW, Deierhoi MH, Belzer FO, Diethelm AG, Kauffman RS. RS-61443—a phase I clinical trial and pilot rescue study. Transplantation. 1992;53(2):428–32.
82. Staatz CE, Tett SE. Clinical pharmacokinetics and pharmacodynamics of mycophenolate in solid organ transplant recipients. Clin Pharmacokinet. 2007;46(1):13–58.
83. Siepmann K, Huber M, Stubiger N, Deuter C, Zierhut M. Mycophenolate mofetil is a highly effective and safe immunosuppressive agent for the treatment of uveitis : a retrospective analysis of 106 patients. Graefe's Arch Clin Exp Ophthalmol. 2006;244(7):788–94.
84. Doycheva D, Zierhut M, Blumenstock G, Stuebiger N, Deuter C. Long-term results of therapy with mycophenolate mofetil in chronic non-infectious uveitis. Graefe's Arch Clin Exp Ophthalmol. 2011;249(8):1235–43.

85. Thorne JE, Jabs DA, Qazi FA, Nguyen QD, Kempen JH, Dunn JP. Mycophenolate mofetil therapy for inflammatory eye disease. Ophthalmology. 2005;112(8):1472–7.
86. Cuchacovich M, Solanes F, Perez C, et al. Mycophenolate mofetil therapy in refractory inflammatory eye disease. J Ocul Pharmacol Ther. 2016;32(1):55–61.
87. Filler G, Hansen M, LeBlanc C, et al. Pharmacokinetics of mycophenolate mofetil for autoimmune disease in children. Pediatr Nephrol (Berlin, Germany). 2003;18(5):445–9.
88. Doycheva D, Deuter C, Stuebiger N, Biester S, Zierhut M. Mycophenolate mofetil in the treatment of uveitis in children. Br J Ophthalmol. 2007;91(2):180–4.
89. Sobrin L, Christen W, Foster CS. Mycophenolate mofetil after methotrexate failure or intolerance in the treatment of scleritis and uveitis. Ophthalmology. 2008;115(8):1416–21, 1421.e1411.
90. Bentley R. Mycophenolic Acid: a one hundred year odyssey from antibiotic to immunosuppressant. Chem Rev. 2000;100(10):3801–26.
91. Doycheva D, Jagle H, Zierhut M, et al. Mycophenolic acid in the treatment of birdshot chorioretinopathy: long-term follow-up. Br J Ophthalmol. 2015;99(1):87–91.
92. Zacharias LC, Damico FM, Kenney MC, et al. In vitro evidence for mycophenolic acid dose-related cytotoxicity in human retinal cells. Retina (Philadelphia, Pa.). 2013;33(10):2155–61.
93. Franklin JL, Rosenberg HH. Impaired folic acid absorption in inflammatory bowel disease: effects of salicylazosulfapyridine (Azulfidine). Gastroenterology. 1973;64(4):517–25.
94. Selhub J, Dhar GJ, Rosenberg IH. Inhibition of folate enzymes by sulfasalazine. J Clin Invest. 1978;61(1):221–4.
95. Baum CL, Selhub J, Rosenberg IH. Antifolate actions of sulfasalazine on intact lymphocytes. J Lab Clin Med. 1981;97(6):779–84.
96. Rhodes JM, Jewell DP. Motility of neutrophils and monocytes in Crohn's disease and ulcerative colitis. Gut. 1983;24(1):73–7.
97. Munoz-Fernandez S, Hidalgo V, Fernandez-Melon J, et al. Sulfasalazine reduces the number of flares of acute anterior uveitis over a one-year period. J Rheumatol. 2003;30(6):1277–9.
98. Kaklamani VG, Kaklamanis PG. Treatment of Behcet's disease—an update. Semin Arthritis Rheum. 2001;30(5):299–312.
99. Arcinue CA, Radwan A, Lebanan MO, Foster CS. Comparison of two different combination immunosuppressive therapies in the treatment of Vogt-Koyonagi-Harada syndrome. Ocul Immunol Inflamm. 2013;21(1):47–52.
100. Silman AJ, Petrie J, Hazleman B, Evans SJ. Lymphoproliferative cancer and other malignancy in patients with rheumatoid arthritis treated with azathioprine: a 20 year follow up study. Ann Rheum Dis. 1988;47(12):988–92.
101. Penn I. Cancers complicating organ transplantation. N Engl J Med. 1990;323(25):1767–9.
102. Kempen JH, Daniel E, Dunn JP, et al. Overall and cancer related mortality among patients with ocular inflammation treated with immunosuppressive drugs: retrospective cohort study. BMJ (Clinical research ed.). 2009;339:b2480.
103. Nussenblatt RB, Rodrigues MM, Wacker WB, Cevario SJ, Salinas-Carmona MC, Gery I. Cyclosporin a. Inhibition of experimental autoimmune uveitis in Lewis rats. J Clin Invest. 1981;67(4):1228–31.
104. Nussenblatt RB, Palestine AG, Rook AH, Scher I, Wacker WB, Gery I. Treatment of intraocular inflammatory disease with cyclosporin a. Lancet (London, England). 1983;2(8344):235–8.
105. Kacmaz RO, Kempen JH, Newcomb C, et al. Cyclosporine for ocular inflammatory diseases. Ophthalmology. 2010;117(3):576–84.
106. Murphy CC, Greiner K, Plskova J, et al. Cyclosporine vs tacrolimus therapy for posterior and intermediate uveitis. Arch Ophthalmol (Chicago, Ill.: 1960). 2005;123(5):634–41.
107. Tanaka H, Kuroda A, Marusawa H, et al. Physicochemical properties of FK-506, a novel immunosuppressant isolated from Streptomyces tsukubaensis. Transplant Proc. 1987;19(5 Suppl 6):11–6.
108. Kino T, Hatanaka H, Hashimoto M, et al. FK-506, a novel immunosuppressant isolated from a Streptomyces. I. Fermentation, isolation, and physico-chemical and biological characteristics. J Antibiot. 1987;40(9):1249–55.

109. Venkataramanan R, Jain A, Cadoff E, et al. Pharmacokinetics of FK 506: preclinical and clinical studies. Transplant Proc. 1990;22(1):52–6.
110. Mochizuki M, Masuda K, Sakane T, et al. A multicenter clinical open trial of FK 506 in refractory uveitis, including Behcet's disease. Japanese FK 506 Study Group on Refractory Uveitis. Transplant Proc. 1991;23(6):3343–6.
111. Hogan AC, McAvoy CE, Dick AD, Lee RW. Long-term efficacy and tolerance of tacrolimus for the treatment of uveitis. Ophthalmology. 2007;114(5):1000–6.
112. Sloper CM, Powell RJ, Dua HS. Tacrolimus (FK506) in the treatment of posterior uveitis refractory to cyclosporine. Ophthalmology. 1999;106(4):723–8.
113. Kilmartin DJ, Forrester JV, Dick AD. Tacrolimus (FK506) in failed cyclosporin a therapy in endogenous posterior uveitis. Ocul Immunol Inflamm. 1998;6(2):101–9.
114. Auerbach C, Robson JM. Chemical production of mutations. Nature. 1946;157:302.
115. Osborne ED, Jordon JW, et al. Nitrogen mustard therapy in cutaneous blastomatous disease. J Am Med Assoc. 1947;135(17):1123–8.
116. Gubner R, August S, Ginsberg V. Therapeutic suppression of tissue reactivity. II. Effect of aminopterin in rheumatoid arthritis and psoriasis. Am J Med Sci. 1951;221(2):176–82.
117. Arnold H, Bourseaux F, Brock N. Chemotherapeutic action of a cyclic nitrogen mustard phosphamide ester (B 518-ASTA) in experimental tumours of the rat. Nature. 1958;181(4613):931.
118. Pujari SS, Kempen JH, Newcomb CW, et al. Cyclophosphamide for ocular inflammatory diseases. Ophthalmology. 2010;117(2):356–65.
119. Houssiau FA. Cyclophosphamide in lupus nephritis. Lupus. 2005;14(1):53–8.
120. Alberts DS, Chang SY, Chen HS, Larcom BJ, Evans TL. Comparative pharmacokinetics of chlorambucil and melphalan in man. Recent Results Cancer Res. 1980;74:124–31.
121. Ehrsson H, Wallin I, Simonsson B, Hartvig P, Oberg G. Effect of food on pharmacokinetics of chlorambucil and its main metabolite, phenylacetic acid mustard. Eur J Clin Pharmacol. 1984;27(1):111–4.
122. Tessler HH, Jennings T. High-dose short-term chlorambucil for intractable sympathetic ophthalmia and Behcet's disease. Br J Ophthalmol. 1990;74(6):353–7.
123. Goldstein DA, Fontanilla FA, Kaul S, Sahin O, Tessler HH. Long-term follow-up of patients treated with short-term high-dose chlorambucil for sight-threatening ocular inflammation. Ophthalmology. 2002;109(2):370–7.
124. Miserocchi E, Baltatzis S, Ekong A, Roque M, Foster CS. Efficacy and safety of chlorambucil in intractable noninfectious uveitis: the Massachusetts Eye and Ear Infirmary experience. Ophthalmology. 2002;109(1):137–42.
125. Fiers W. Tumor necrosis factor. Characterization at the molecular, cellular and in vivo level. FEBS Lett. 1991;285(2):199–212.
126. Heller RA, Kronke M. Tumor necrosis factor receptor-mediated signaling pathways. J Cell Biol. 1994;126(1):5–9.
127. Lerman MA, Burnham JM, Chang PY, et al. Response of pediatric uveitis to tumor necrosis factor-alpha inhibitors. J Rheumatol. 2013;40(8):1394–403.
128. Rau R. Adalimumab (a fully human anti-tumour necrosis factor alpha monoclonal antibody) in the treatment of active rheumatoid arthritis: the initial results of five trials. Ann Rheum Dis. 2002;61(Suppl 2):ii70–3.
129. Weisman MH, Moreland LW, Furst DE, et al. Efficacy, pharmacokinetic, and safety assessment of adalimumab, a fully human anti-tumor necrosis factor-alpha monoclonal antibody, in adults with rheumatoid arthritis receiving concomitant methotrexate: a pilot study. Clin Ther. 2003;25(6):1700–21.
130. Suhler EB, Lowder CY, Goldstein DA, et al. Adalimumab therapy for refractory uveitis: results of a multicentre, open-label, prospective trial. Br J Ophthalmol. 2013;97(4):481–6.
131. Biester S, Deuter C, Michels H, et al. Adalimumab in the therapy of uveitis in childhood. Br J Ophthalmol. 2007;91(3):319–24.
132. Diaz-Llopis M, Garcia-Delpech S, Salom D, et al. Adalimumab therapy for refractory uveitis: a pilot study. J Ocul Pharmacol Ther. 2008;24(3):351–61.

133. Tynjala P, Kotaniemi K, Lindahl P, et al. Adalimumab in juvenile idiopathic arthritis-associated chronic anterior uveitis. Rheumatology (Oxford, England). 2008;47(3):339–44.
134. Androudi S, Tsironi E, Kalogeropoulos C, Theodoridou A, Brazitikos P. Intravitreal adalimumab for refractory uveitis-related macular edema. Ophthalmology. 2010;117(8):1612–6.
135. Giganti M, Beer PM, Lemanski N, Hartman C, Schartman J, Falk N. Adverse events after intravitreal infliximab (Remicade). Retina (Philadelphia, Pa.). 2010;30(1):71–80.
136. Pulido JS, Pulido JE, Michet CJ, Vile RG. More questions than answers: a call for a moratorium on the use of intravitreal infliximab outside of a well-designed trial. Retina (Philadelphia, Pa.). 2010;30(1):1–5.
137. Suhler EB, Smith JR, Wertheim MS, et al. A prospective trial of infliximab therapy for refractory uveitis: preliminary safety and efficacy outcomes. Arch Ophthalmol (Chicago, Ill.: 1960). 2005;123(7):903–12.
138. Suhler EB, Smith JR, Giles TR, et al. Infliximab therapy for refractory uveitis: 2-year results of a prospective trial. Arch Ophthalmol (Chicago, Ill.: 1960). 2009;127(6):819–22.
139. Riancho-Zarrabeitia L, Calvo-Rio V, Blanco R, et al. Anti-TNF-alpha therapy in refractory uveitis associated with sarcoidosis: multicenter study of 17 patients. Semin Arthritis Rheum. 2015;45(3):361–8.
140. Ardoin SP, Kredich D, Rabinovich E, Schanberg LE, Jaffe GJ. Infliximab to treat chronic noninfectious uveitis in children: retrospective case series with long-term follow-up. Am J Ophthalmol. 2007;144(6):844–9.
141. Rajaraman RT, Kimura Y, Li S, Haines K, Chu DS. Retrospective case review of pediatric patients with uveitis treated with infliximab. Ophthalmology. 2006;113(2):308–14.
142. Levy-Clarke G, Jabs DA, Read RW, Rosenbaum JT, Vitale A, Van Gelder RN. Expert panel recommendations for the use of anti-tumor necrosis factor biologic agents in patients with ocular inflammatory disorders. Ophthalmology. 2014;121(3):785–796.e783.
143. Vallet H, Seve P, Biard L, et al. Infliximab versus adalimumab in the treatment of refractory inflammatory uveitis: a multicenter study from the French Uveitis Network. Arthritis Rheumatol (Hoboken, N.J.). 2016;68(6):1522–30.
144. Yazgan S, Celik U, Isik M, et al. Efficacy of golimumab on recurrent uveitis in HLA-B27-positive ankylosing spondylitis. Int Ophthalmol. 2017;37(1):139–45.
145. Calvo-Rio V, Blanco R, Santos-Gomez M, et al. Golimumab in refractory uveitis related to spondyloarthritis. Multicenter study of 15 patients. Semin Arthritis Rheum. 2016;46(1):95–101.
146. Miserocchi E, Modorati G, Pontikaki I, Meroni PL, Gerloni V. Long-term treatment with golimumab for severe uveitis. Ocul Immunol Inflamm. 2014;22(2):90–5.
147. Galor A, Perez VL, Hammel JP, Lowder CY. Differential effectiveness of etanercept and infliximab in the treatment of ocular inflammation. Ophthalmology. 2006;113(12):2317–23.
148. Kaymakcalan Z, Sakorafas P, Bose S, et al. Comparisons of affinities, avidities, and complement activation of adalimumab, infliximab, and etanercept in binding to soluble and membrane tumor necrosis factor. Clin Immunol (Orlando, Fla.). 2009;131(2):308–16.
149. Van den Brande JM, Braat H, van den Brink GR, et al. Infliximab but not etanercept induces apoptosis in lamina propria T-lymphocytes from patients with Crohn's disease. Gastroenterology. 2003;124(7):1774–85.
150. Isaacs A, Lindenmann J. Virus interference. I. The interferon. By A. Isaacs and J. Lindenmann, 1957. J Interf Res. 1987;7(5):429–38.
151. Zou W, Machelon V, Coulomb-L'Hermin A, et al. Stromal-derived factor-1 in human tumors recruits and alters the function of plasmacytoid precursor dendritic cells. Nat Med. 2001;7(12):1339–46.
152. Colonna M, Krug A, Cella M. Interferon-producing cells: on the front line in immune responses against pathogens. Curr Opin Immunol. 2002;14(3):373–9.
153. Vallin H, Perers A, Alm GV, Ronnblom L. Anti-double-stranded DNA antibodies and immunostimulatory plasmid DNA in combination mimic the endogenous IFN-alpha inducer in systemic lupus erythematosus. J Immunol (Baltimore, Md.: 1950). 1999;163(11):6306–13.

154. Wampler Muskardin T, Vashisht P, Dorschner JM, et al. Increased pretreatment serum IFN-beta/alpha ratio predicts non-response to tumour necrosis factor alpha inhibition in rheumatoid arthritis. Ann Rheum Dis. 2016;75(10):1757–62.
155. Okada AA, Keino H, Suzuki J, Sakai J, Usui M, Mizuguchi J. Kinetics of intraocular cytokines in the suppression of experimental autoimmune uveoretinitis by type I IFN. Int Immunol. 1998;10(12):1917–22.
156. Okada AA, Keino H, Fukai T, Sakai J, Usui M, Mizuguchi J. Effect of type I interferon on experimental autoimmune uveoretinitis in rats. Ocul Immunol Inflamm. 1998;6(4):215–26.
157. Stubiger N, Crane IJ, Kotter I, et al. Interferon alpha 2a in IRPB-derived peptide-induced EAU—part I. Adv Exp Med Biol. 2003;528:537–40.
158. Bodaghi B, Gendron G, Wechsler B, et al. Efficacy of interferon alpha in the treatment of refractory and sight threatening uveitis: a retrospective monocentric study of 45 patients. Br J Ophthalmol. 2007;91(3):335–9.
159. Gueudry J, Wechsler B, Terrada C, et al. Long-term efficacy and safety of low-dose interferon alpha2a therapy in severe uveitis associated with Behcet disease. Am J Ophthalmol. 2008;146(6):837–844.e831.
160. Hasanreisoglu M, Cubuk MO, Ozdek S, Gurelik G, Aktas Z, Hasanreisoglu B. Interferon alpha-2a therapy in patients with refractory Behcet uveitis. Ocul Immunol Inflamm. 2017;25(1):71–5.
161. Park JY, Chung YR, Lee K, Song JH, Lee ES. Clinical experience of interferon alfa-2a treatment for refractory uveitis in Behcet's disease. Yonsei Med J. 2015;56(4):1158–62.
162. Butler NJ, Suhler EB, Rosenbaum JT. Interferon alpha 2b in the treatment of uveitic cystoid macular edema. Ocul Immunol Inflamm. 2012;20(2):86–90.
163. Doycheva D, Deuter C, Stuebiger N, Zierhut M. Interferon-alpha-associated presumed ocular sarcoidosis. Graefes Arch Clin Exp Ophthalmol. 2009;247(5):675–80.
164. Durand JM, Soubeyrand J. Interferon-alpha 2b for refractory ocular Behcet's disease. Lancet (London, England). 1994;344(8918):333.
165. Fleischmann M, Celerier P, Bernard P, Litoux P, Dreno B. Long-term interferon-alpha therapy induces autoantibodies against epidermis. Dermatology (Basel, Switzerland). 1996;192(1):50–5.
166. Schilling PJ, Kurzrock R, Kantarjian H, Gutterman JU, Talpaz M. Development of systemic lupus erythematosus after interferon therapy for chronic myelogenous leukemia. Cancer. 1991;68(7):1536–7.
167. Becker MD, Adamus G, Davey MP, Rosenbaum JT. The role of T cells in autoimmune uveitis. Ocul Immunol Inflamm. 2000;8(2):93–100.
168. Caspi RR, Sun B, Agarwal RK, et al. T cell mechanisms in experimental autoimmune uveoretinitis: susceptibility is a function of the cytokine response profile. Eye (London, England). 1997;11(Pt 2):209–12.
169. Whitcup SM, Pleyer U, Lai JC, Lutz S, Mochizuki M, Chan CC. Topical liposome-encapsulated FK506 for the treatment of endotoxin-induced uveitis. Ocul Immunol Inflamm. 1998;6(1):51–6.
170. Parikh JG, Tawansy KA, Rao NA. Immunohistochemical study of chronic nongranulomatous anterior uveitis in juvenile idiopathic arthritis. Ophthalmology. 2008;115(10):1833–6.
171. Maloney DG, Grillo-Lopez AJ, White CA, et al. IDEC-C2B8 (Rituximab) anti-CD20 monoclonal antibody therapy in patients with relapsed low-grade non-Hodgkin's lymphoma. Blood. 1997;90(6):2188–95.
172. Keogh KA, Wylam ME, Stone JH, Specks U. Induction of remission by B lymphocyte depletion in eleven patients with refractory antineutrophil cytoplasmic antibody-associated vasculitis. Arthritis Rheum. 2005;52(1):262–8.
173. Lasave AF, You C, Ma L, et al. Long-term outcomes of rituximab therapy in patients with noninfectious posterior uveitis refractory to conventional immunosuppressive therapy. Retina. 2018;38(2):395–402.
174. Lopez-Gonzalez R, Loza E, Jover JA, et al. Treatment of refractory posterior uveitis with infliximab: a 7-year follow-up study. Scand J Rheumatol. 2009;38(1):58–62.

175. Miserocchi E, Modorati G, Berchicci L, Pontikaki I, Meroni P, Gerloni V. Long-term treatment with rituximab in severe juvenile idiopathic arthritis-associated uveitis. Br J Ophthalmol. 2016;100(6):782–6.
176. Heiligenhaus A, Miserocchi E, Heinz C, Gerloni V, Kotaniemi K. Treatment of severe uveitis associated with juvenile idiopathic arthritis with anti-CD20 monoclonal antibody (rituximab). Rheumatology (Oxford, England). 2011;50(8):1390–4.
177. Guex-Crosier Y, Raber J, Chan CC, et al. Humanized antibodies against the alpha-chain of the IL-2 receptor and against the beta-chain shared by the IL-2 and IL-15 receptors in a monkey uveitis model of autoimmune diseases. J Immunol (Baltimore, Md.: 1950). 1997;158(1):452–8.
178. Nussenblatt RB, Thompson DJ, Li Z, et al. Humanized anti-interleukin-2 (IL-2) receptor alpha therapy: long-term results in uveitis patients and preliminary safety and activity data for establishing parameters for subcutaneous administration. J Autoimmun. 2003;21(3):283–93.
179. Nussenblatt RB, Peterson JS, Foster CS, et al. Initial evaluation of subcutaneous daclizumab treatments for noninfectious uveitis: a multicenter noncomparative interventional case series. Ophthalmology. 2005;112(5):764–70.
180. Sobrin L, Huang JJ, Christen W, Kafkala C, Choopong P, Foster CS. Daclizumab for treatment of birdshot chorioretinopathy. Arch Ophthalmol (Chicago, Ill.: 1960). 2008;126(2):186–91.
181. Buggage RR, Levy-Clarke G, Sen HN, et al. A double-masked, randomized study to investigate the safety and efficacy of daclizumab to treat the ocular complications related to Behcet's disease. Ocul Immunol Inflamm. 2007;15(2):63–70.
182. Murray PI, Hoekzema R, van Haren MA, de Hon FD, Kijlstra A. Aqueous humor interleukin-6 levels in uveitis. Invest Ophthalmol Vis Sci. 1990;31(5):917–20.
183. Kramer M, Monselise Y, Bahar I, Cohen Y, Weinberger D, Goldenberg-Cohen N. Serum cytokine levels in active uveitis and remission. Curr Eye Res. 2007;32(7–8):669–75.
184. Calvo-Rio V, Santos-Gomez M, Calvo I, et al. Anti-Interleukin-6 receptor tocilizumab for severe juvenile idiopathic arthritis-associated uveitis refractory to anti-tumor necrosis factor therapy: a multicenter study of twenty-five patients. Arthritis Rheumatol (Hoboken, NJ). 2017;69(3):668–75.
185. Adan A, Mesquida M, Llorenc V, et al. Tocilizumab treatment for refractory uveitis-related cystoid macular edema. Graefes Arch Clin Exp Ophthalmol. 2013;251(11):2627–32.
186. Yamada A, Salama AD, Sayegh MH. The role of novel T cell costimulatory pathways in autoimmunity and transplantation. J Am Soc Nephrol. 2002;13(2):559–75.
187. Sayegh MH, Turka LA. The role of T-cell costimulatory activation pathways in transplant rejection. N Engl J Med. 1998;338(25):1813–21.
188. Birolo C, Zannin ME, Arsenyeva S, et al. Comparable efficacy of Abatacept used as first-line or second-line biological agent for severe juvenile idiopathic arthritis-related uveitis. J Rheumatol. 2016;43(11):2068–73.
189. Megget K. FEATURE: Follow the leader. 2015; http://www.pharmatimes.com/news/feature_follow_the_leader_971332. Accessed 12 Mar 2017.
190. Jacobs I, Petersel D, Isakov L, Lula S, Lea Sewell K. Biosimilars for the treatment of chronic inflammatory diseases: a systematic review of published evidence. BioDrugs. 2016;30(6):525–70.

Noninfectious Uveitis: Emerging Therapies

Julie Schallhorn

Introduction

Few would argue that our current tools for managing uveitis are perfect. Although the current armamentarium of antimetabolite, biologic, and steroid therapies is able to treat the vast majority of noninfectious uveitis cases, the incidence of serious and occasionally vision- or life-threatening side effects remains stubbornly high. The perfect treatment – one able to simply flip the pro-inflammatory switch in uveitis to "off" – remains in the future. However, the new generation of therapies promises better, more targeted inflammatory control while minimizing ocular and systemic side effects.

The next generation of uveitic therapies clusters into two areas. The first is novel biologic and small-molecule drugs that are specifically targeted to the dysregulated immune system, and the second is bioengineered drug delivery systems that promise targeted delivery to the eye while sparing systemic side effects.

Novel Drug Approaches

The road to uveitis therapy is littered with phase III clinical trials that have yielded disappointing results with novel biologics after having promising phase I/II trials. Gevokizumab [1], targeting IL-1β, and secukinumab [2] (trade name Cosentyx®), targeted at IL-17, have failed to meet their primary endpoints in large, well-constructed trials, and daclizumab [3] (trade name Zinbryta®), targeting the IL-2 receptor, likewise had disappointing results in a trial for Behcet's disease with

J. Schallhorn (✉)
Department of Ophthalmology and Francis I. Proctor Foundation, University of California, San Francisco, San Francisco, CA, USA
e-mail: Julie.schallhorn@ucsf.edu

N. A. Rao et al. (eds.), *Posterior Uveitis*, Essentials in Ophthalmology,
https://doi.org/10.1007/978-3-030-03140-4_12

uveitis. Fortunately, there are many more therapies in the pipeline. As our knowledge of the inflammatory mediators involved in the complex inflammatory cascade improves, more targets are becoming available for potential therapeutic development. These have already yielded multiple medications that are approved for non-uveitic disease but have potential activity in uveitis.

Biologics

Biologic drugs remain an active area of investigation for systemic immune-mediated inflammatory diseases. Multiple trials are currently in process, and approvals of new drugs are occurring at a record rate.

As IL-17 has been implicated as a major cytokine in multiple inflammatory diseases, there are several anti-IL-17 antibodies and IL-17 receptor blockers that are currently under investigation [4]. In addition to secukinumab, ixekizumab and bimekizumab are both anti-1L-17 antibodies that have been under investigation and have proven efficacy in treating psoriasis and psoriatic arthritis [5, 6]. Secukinumab, however, has shown only moderate efficacy in rheumatoid arthritis and actually caused worsening of Crohn's disease in a well-constructed clinical trial [7]. An IL-17 receptor blocker, brodalumab, has likewise shown good efficacy in psoriasis but was not effective for rheumatoid arthritis [8, 9]. With the exception of secukinumab, which did not meet its primary endpoint in phase III trials for uveitis [2], none of these have been tested in uveitis. Unfortunately, the IL-17-blocking antibodies have yielded somewhat disappointing results except in treating psoriasis, demonstrating the challenges as we try to understand complexities of the immune system.

The differentiation of CD4 + T cells to Th17 cells is a major step in the genesis of the inflammatory response. Ustekinumab, trade name Stelara®, is active against IL-12 and IL-23, both of which are central to Th17 differentiation. It is approved for the treatment of psoriasis, psoriatic arthritis, and Crohn's disease, and although it has theoretic benefit in uveitis, current evidence is scant [10]. Unexpectedly, it has been shown to be inferior to secukinumab in the treatment of psoriasis [11].

The interferon (IFN) signaling pathway is a pro-inflammatory pathway active during viral infections and has been shown to be upregulated in multiple autoimmune diseases including lupus and rheumatoid arthritis [12]. As such, it has become a target for immunomodulatory therapies. Of the three subtypes of IFN, type I (which includes IFN-α and IFN-β, as well as IFN-ε, IFN-κ, IFN-ω) seems to be the biggest player in autoimmunity, and efforts to modulate the IFN receptor system have been targeted toward this. An anti-IFN-α antibody, sifalimumab, has shown promise for the treatment of systemic lupus erythematosus (SLE) and dermatomyositis but was ineffective for psoriasis [4, 13]. A different anti-IFN-α antibody, rontalizumab, did not achieve its primary endpoint in trials for SLE [14]. A receptor blocker for IFN-α, anifrolumab, is also under investigation and was recently shown to be effective in treating SLE [15]. A major side effect of this class of biologics is viral infections, in particular herpes zoster, which occurred in all studies. Earlier preclinical and phase I studies are being conducted to look at other modes of IFN blockage, including blocking type II IFN and downregulating dendritic cells which are involved in IFN trafficking [4].

Although not a true biologic, a vaccine-type approach to inducing autoimmunity against IFN-α is also undergoing. In this, inactivated IFN-α is coupled to an activator, keyhole limpet hemocyanin, in order to induce autoantibodies against IFN-α. In a phase I/II dose escalation trial, the vaccine was successful in inducing the autoantibodies [16]. Further studies are needed to establish the role of this approach.

Given the success of rituximab in treating autoimmune disorders, multiple biologics are in development directed against B cells. Currently approved for SLE, belimumab (Benlysta®) is targeted against soluble B-cell activating factor (BAFF) [17]. However, two other anti-BAFFs, tabalumab and blisibimod, did not meet their endpoints in phase III trials, and BAFFs have been ineffective in rheumatoid arthritis [4, 18]. Ocrelizumab (trade name Ocrevus®), like rituximab, is an anti-CD20 antibody and has demonstrated efficacy in multiple sclerosis [19]. Trials in psoriasis and SLE were terminated due to a high rate of adverse events [4].

Although no therapeutics are currently in clinical use, an intriguing area of research is directed toward encouraging the development of regulatory T cells (Treg), which downregulate inflammatory responses and help to restore homeostasis. Any approach which is able to re-induce homeostasis carries the possibility of inducing long-term remission of inflammatory disease, which is a very worthy goal. Low-dose IL-2 infusions selectively promote Treg cell differentiation and have shown efficacy in small studies in graft-versus-host disease, SLE, and type I diabetes mellitus [20–22]. Pursuing this pathway is not without risk, however. A phase I trial of TGN-1412, a CD-28 agonist, precipitated a life-threatening cytokine storm in volunteers, which was not anticipated based on the preclinical animal trials, and raised numerous questions on the safe conduct of clinical trials [23]. However, this approach is currently undergoing renewed interest, as it can induce Treg differentiation under much lower dosing conditions [24, 25]. Also under investigation are highly conserved protein sequences on IgG antibodies that induce a Treg response, so-called Tregitopes [26]. Although not currently in human studies, they have shown promise in preclinical animal models.

Small Molecules

Multiple small molecules and peptides are under investigation as potential therapeutics, either in preclinical studies or early clinical studies (Table 1). Some, such as tofacitinib (trade name Xeljanz®), are well-known treatments for rheumatologic disease [27]; others are novel molecules designed to target important parts of the inflammatory cascade. The common thread that runs among them is the increasing understanding of the complex interplay of the regulatory mechanisms of the immune system and the progressively eloquent methods being devised to redirect the inflammatory pathway.

The molecule furthest along in development in this category is sirolimus. On the back of favorable phase II results, a large phase III trial of intravitreal sirolimus was

Table 1 Small molecules and peptides currently under investigation for the treatment of uveitis

Class	Drug	Mechanism	Status
α-4 integrin inhibitors [33]	α-4api	Inhibit T-cell adhesion	Preclinical studies
Aldolase reductase inhibitors [58–60]	Zopolrestat Fidarestat Epalrestat BF-5M	Block oxidative stress molecular signaling, NF-κB	Fidarestat – phase III trials for diabetic neuropathy BF-5M – preclinical
JAK (Janus kinase) inhibitors [41]	Tofacitinib Baricitinib	Prevent activation of JAK and subsequent intracellular signaling pathway via STAT	Tofacitinib – Approved for use in rheumatoid arthritis Baricitinib – under review for FDA approval for rheumatoid arthritis
STAT3 inhibitors [42–44]	ORLL-NIH001	Suppress CD4+ T cell into TH17 differentiation	Preclinical studies
AMPK (adenosine monophosphate-activated protein kinase) analogs [61]	AICAR	Inhibition of JAK-STAT signaling, inhibition of NF-κB, inhibition of leukocyte infiltration	Preclinical studies
PDE4 (phosphodiesterase 4) inhibitors [50, 51]	Dipyridamole Rolipram Apremilast	Intracellular accumulation of CAMP in leukocytes resulting in downregulation of inflammatory response	Dipyridamole – approved for use in combination with warfarin in prevention of thromboembolism from cardiac valve replacement Apremilast – approved for use in psoriasis Rolipram – preclinical uveitis studies, initially developed as an antidepressant but discontinued
S1P (sphingosine-1) antagonists [35, 36]	Fingolimod	Block T-cell migration	Approved for use in multiple sclerosis [37], preclinical uveitis studies
DHODH (dihydroorotate dehydrogenase inhibitor) [49]	Leflunomide Teriflunomide PP-001	Pyrimidine synthesis inhibitor	Leflunomide and teriflunomide approved for use in rheumatoid arthritis and psoriasis, PP-001 in phase I intravitreal injection trial
mTOR inhibitor [62]	Sirolimus	T-cell activation inhibitor	Phase III clinical trials

conducted. The SAKURA trial demonstrated statistically increase in number of patients reaching the primary endpoint (vitreous haze grade of 0) at 6 months in the 440 μg injection group as compared to the active control and the higher-dose 880 μg group. Despite this, the Food and Drug Administration (FDA) recently requested further proof of effectiveness prior to approval, and further studies are ongoing [28].

Ultimately, the role of sirolimus in the treatment of uveitis has yet to be determined.

The inhibition of T-cell migration is a potential target for therapeutics that is under investigation. The process of T-cell migration involves complex signaling through multiple cellular adhesion molecules, the integrins. Recently, a topical anti-T-cell adhesion molecule that blocks LFA-1, lifitegrast, trade name Xiidra®, was approved for the treatment of dry eye disease, but its use has not been investigated in uveitis [29–31]. A different intracellular adhesion blocker, the α-4 integrin inhibitors disrupt binding of α-4 integrin to VCAM-1 and thus impair T-cell migration [32]. In a mouse model of EAU, α-4api, a small peptide α-4 integrin blocker, demonstrated a significant reduction in inflammation as compared to control [33]. The integrin-blocking monoclonal antibody natalizumab (trade name Tysabri®) has been found to carry the risk of increased incidence of progressive multifocal leukoencephalopathy, which makes local administration of this class of drugs much more attractive [34].

The sphingosine-1 (SP-1) antagonist, fingolimod, causes retention of T cells within lymphoid organs, preventing them from migrating out to affect the end actions of the disease. It is currently approved for use in multiple sclerosis and is marketed under the trade name Gilenya® by Novartis. In models of EAU, it suppresses intraocular inflammation but does not induce remission [35, 36]. When used systemically as a treatment for multiple sclerosis, it carries the notable side effect of drug-induced cystoid macular edema, which is estimated to occur in up to 1% of cases and appears to be dose-dependent [37].

Another active area of inquiry is the JAK-STAT pathway. This pathway regulates the external reception of inflammatory signals via JAK (Janus kinase) and transmits them to the nucleus for transcription via STAT (signal transducers and activation of transcription) [38]. Two JAK inhibitors are currently in clinical use for the treatment of rheumatoid arthritis. Tofacitinib (trade name Xeljanz®) [39] is currently approved for use in the United States, and baricitinib [40] (trade name Incyte®) is currently under review by the FDA. Ample evidence supports these drugs as being effective for the treatment of rheumatoid arthritis. Data in the treatment of uveitis, however, is scanty and limited to demonstration of effectiveness in EAU that was presented in an ARVO poster [41]. Further investigation, particularly in rheumatoid arthritis-related ocular inflammation, would be much welcome.

A STAT-3 inhibitor is also currently under investigation. STAT-3 is responsible for enabling differentiation of CD4+ T cells into Th-17 cells, and blocking this pathway has been shown to inhibit the development of EAU in experimental models [42, 43]. A novel STAT-3 blocker, ORLL-NIH001, has had promising results in preclinical studies [44].

Dihydroorotate dehydrogenase (DHODH) is responsible for a necessary step in pyrimidine synthesis pathway. Two currently available DHODH inhibitors, leflunomide (Arava®) and teriflunomide (Aubagio®), are in use for treatment of rheumatoid arthritis and psoriasis [45]. There is data to support the use of leflunomide as an effective treatment in juvenile idiopathic arthritis [46]; however there is some concern that it may be less effective than methotrexate [47]. Modes of EAU have demonstrated improvement with leflunomide administration [48]. A novel DHODH, PP-001, has been shown to decrease relapse rate in EAU [49] and is under development by a pharmaceutical company for use in humans.

Phosphodiesterase inhibitors may have some role in uveitis treatment. Phosphodiesterase-4 (PDE-4) is expressed mainly in inflammatory cells and is responsible for the degradation of cyclic AMP and cyclic GMP [50]. Inhibitors of this enzyme, including rolipram and apremilast, have been shown to be effective in treating models of EAU [50, 51]. Apremilast (trade name Otezla®) is currently in use for the treatment of psoriasis and psoriatic arthritis [52].

Oxidative stress has been implicated in potentiating autoimmunity and worsening inflammatory conditions [53]. Oxidative mitochondrial stress is one of the first events to occur in models of EAU [54, 55]. Cellular destruction and death lead to the release of oxidized lipids, which act as pro-inflammatory signals through activation of the nuclear factor κB pathway [56, 57]. Based upon this, aldolase reductase inhibitors have been studied for utility in uveitis. Aldolase reductase generates lipid aldehydes in cells that are subjected to oxidative stress, which then activate the nuclear factor κB pathway that leads to an inflammatory signaling cascade. Multiple aldolase reductase inhibitors have been studied in models of EAU (Table 1), as well as in other entities [58–60].

Adjuvant Therapies

A number of drugs have been investigated as adjuvants to immunosuppressive therapies for uveitis (Table 2). These drugs are either approved for other uses (statins and diltiazem) or, in the case of curcumin and plant flavonoids, come from traditional medicine approaches. The statins and diltiazem have been subjected to rigorous studies when undergoing evaluation for their approved indications; however, plant extracts and curcumin have not been subjected to the same degree of rigor. Thus, it is important to advise patients who may be interested in these "alternative medicine" therapies that, although there is some evidence to suggest that they may have a benefit, the full side effect profile and dosing are unknown.

Novel Drug Delivery Systems

Noninfectious uveitis without systemic involvement is an ideal target for sustained, localized drug delivery systems that can provide local immunosuppression while sparing systemic toxicity and side effects. An ideal delivery system would be easy to implant or place, deliver stable dissolution kinetics over its lifetime, have minimal ocular side effects, and leave no residue inside the eye. Some of the most promising advances in therapeutics for noninfectious uveitis are likely to come from this arena.

Table 2 Adjuvant therapies for uveitis treatment

Drug	Mechanism	Dose	Evidence	Design
Curcumin [63]	Inhibition of NF-κB	1200 mg of curcumin-phosphatidylcholine complex twice a day	Statistically significant reduction in anterior uveitis flares	Prospective, open label
Statins [64]	3-Hydroxy-3-methylglutaryl coenzyme A reductase inhibitor with unknown anti-inflammatory effect	Simvastatin, 40 mg/day	Patients treated with simvastatin had significantly higher rates of steroid-sparing uveitis control than control group	Randomized, non-masked clinical trial
Diltiazem [65]	Calcium channel blocker, inhibition of metabolism of cyclosporine	30–60 mg/day, weight-dependent	Patients treated with diltiazem required lower dose of oral cyclosporine to achieve uveitis control	Randomized, open-label trial
Plant flavonoids [53]	Prevention of oxidative stress	Varies	Multiple models of experimental autoimmune uveitis	

Reservoir Systems

The first generation of sustained release drug delivery systems was based on a pellet or reservoir of drug in a nondissolvable container and was developed for corticosteroid delivery. The first available device, the Retisert, a sustained fluocinolone acetonide intravitreal implant, delivers a stable dose of 0.59 μg/day over the course of 30 months [66]. After elution of the steroid, the plastic plinth and cup remain in the eye, and a new device must be placed for further treatment. Ample evidence, reviewed in detail in the chapter on corticosteroids, supports the Retisert as effective for noninfectious uveitis. There have been reports of dislocations of the empty steroid cup from the plinth, which is estimated to occur in up to 5% of eyes after an average of 5 years of follow-up [67].

The sustained release intravitreal fluocinolone acetonide pellet, the Iluvien, provides 0.2 μg per day of fluocinolone acetonide [68]. The implant is a cylindrical non-biodegradable shell filled with 0.19 mg of fluocinolone acetonide. One end is capped with a permeable polyvinyl alcohol membrane that allows for steady release of the steroid into the vitreous for a duration of 3 years. It is implanted through an in-office injection through the pars plana on a 25 g needle [68]. Much like other corticosteroid preparations, the risk for cataract and intraocular pressure elevation is increased with the implant [68]. Although approved for the treatment of diabetic macular edema, it is currently not approved for the treatment of noninfectious uveitis. Early evidence in uveitis suggests that the implant may be effective for uveitic macular edema [69]. A larger, 11-person trial comparing a low-dose (0.2 μg per day release) implant to a high-dose (0.5 μg per day release) implant demonstrated that both were effective uveitis control [70]. In this study, patients had improvement in best-corrected visual acuity and a decrease in the need for topical corticosteroids and systemic immunosuppressive therapy at 2 years after implantation. Altogether, results of the injectable fluocinolone implant are promising but need further study to ultimately verify its effectiveness.

A refillable subconjunctival micro pump reservoir device connected to a pars plana infusion cannula (the Posterior MicroPump, Replenish Inc., Pasadena, CA) has been developed and implanted in human eyes to deliver ranibizumab for the treatment of diabetic macular edema [71]. The device utilizes a controlled electrolysis reaction to convert water to hydrogen and oxygen gas and increase pressure in the reservoir to expel the expected dose of the medication. It is controlled through a telemetry system that can modulate the dose and timing of drug delivery, providing a potentially widely adaptable and customizable interface. It is currently in early clinical trials and holds great promise for conditions requiring repeated intravitreal injections. Another refillable port delivery system held by Genentech for ranibizumab is currently in clinical trials for the treatment of age-related macular edema [72].

Dissolvible Polymers

Biodegradable polymers with embedded medications are particularly attractive as a method of drug delivery. The polymers are composed of repeats of nontoxic components of the poly-α-hydroxy acid family and include polylactic acid (PLA), a poly[D,L- lactic-co-glycolide] (PLGA), or poly[d,l-lactide-co-ε-caprolactone] (PLC) [73, 74]. The therapeutic drug of choice is embedded in to the polymer, which can then be shaped as desired, including into a pellet shape or a sheet, for implantation and delivery. The polymers undergo hydrolysis, which releases the encapsulated drugs, and themselves are broken down into their monomer components, which are then broken down via the Krebs cycle. There is some indication, at least in the case of PLGA polymers, that the size and shape of the implant can have an effect on the toxicity of the device, with microspheres ranging from 3 to 100 μm inducing an inflammatory response in rabbit eyes but rods of the same mass inducing no inflammatory response [75].

The intravitreal dexamethasone sustained release pellet (Ozurdex) is the most widely known example of the biodegradable polymer delivery system. It consists of a PLGA polymer embedded with 0.7 mg of dexamethasone, which provides stable release of dexamethasone over a period of 60 days, and can have continued release up to 6 months [76, 77]. Dissolution of the carrier enables release of the dexamethasone, and the carrier is entirely broken down and absorbed, with no residual material left inside the eye. The pellet is delivered via a 22-gauge needle through the pars plana and can be placed with topical anesthesia in clinic. It is approved for the treatment of noninfectious intermediate and posterior uveitis, as well as cystoid macular edema, and the clinical impression has been very favorable. Clinical results with this device are covered in the chapter on Steroids.

Multiple studies have been conducted looking at incorporating T-cell inhibitors, such as cyclosporine and tacrolimus, into biodegradable polymers for sustained delivery. Intravitreal or intrascleral PLGA or PLC implants embedded with tacrolimus [78, 79] and cyclosporine [80, 81] have been developed and tested in animal models with good tolerability; however human studies are lacking at this time. A subconjunctival pellet PLC cyclosporine delivery system has been developed and tested in corneal graft rejection in humans [82]. It is able to deliver inhibitory levels of cyclosporine over a 1-year time frame. Although promising in animal models and in early studies looking at corneal transplant graft rejection [82, 83], it ultimately failed to prevent neovascularization of high-risk corneal grafts [84], and its future remains uncertain.

Polymers of PLC have been formulated into microfilms for subconjunctival placement [74]. These microfilms have been embedded with prednisolone acetate as well as tacrolimus and have been shown to deliver therapeutic levels of drug over a 6-week time period. The biofilms were effective at preventing corneal allograft rejection (prednisolone) [85] and for the treatment of allergic conjunctivitis (tacrolimus) [86] but have not been evaluated in the setting of uveitis.

A novel delivery system for methotrexate involving chitosan-methotrexate fibrils coated in PLA has been developed and evaluated in a rabbit model [87]. In this system, PLA acts as a barrier for the rapid dissolution of methotrexate, which is extremely hydrophilic and rapidly dissolves and is cleared from the vitreous. The chitosan is lysosomally degraded into its component sugars. In the animal model, the implant was able to sustain therapeutic release of methotrexate over a 1-month time period [88]. Studies in animal models of uveitis and humans are yet to be conducted.

A proprietary dissolvable non-polymer-based drug delivery system, Verisome® from Icon Bioscience, Newark, NJ, is currently in clinical or preclinical trials with multiple drugs, including nonsteroidals and anti-inflammatories. There is little available information as to how the platform functions, and no published outcomes data, so its utility and future applicability remains unknown at the time of this printing [89].

Nanoparticles

Nanoparticles are a novel approach to drug delivery designed to overcome the absorption barriers of the ocular surface to allow improved intraocular delivery. The target drug is linked to or packaged within the particle, which then navigates entry into the eye through the ocular surface and is able to deliver its contents. Currently, all nanoparticle delivery systems are preclinical [90]. For a comprehensive overview of the current state of ocular nanoparticle development, consult Janagam et al., "Nanoparticles for drug delivery to the anterior segment of the eye" in Advanced Drug Delivery Reviews, 2017, Volume 122.

Self-assembling cubosomes of monoolein, water, and dexamethasone have been formulated which resulted in an eightfold increase in intraocular delivery of the dexamethasone as compared to a standard solution [91]. A similar cubosome-containing flurbiprofen has also been formulated, which likewise resulted in enhanced intraocular penetration [92].

A different cationic nanoparticle platform consisting of poly[ethylacrylate, methyl-methacrylate, and chlorotrimethyl-ammonioethyl methacrylate], known commercially as Eudragit® [93], has been studied as a carrier for nonsteroidals [94] including piroxicam [95] and naproxen [93] as well as methylprednisolone [96]. In models of rabbit experimental autoimmune uveitis (EAU), the methylprednisolone and piroxicam preparations demonstrated superiority in calming inflammation over the standard suspensions of each. This platform is used in multiple targeted drug delivery systems beyond the eye.

Non-PLA-encapsulated chitosan has been successfully used to formulate nanoparticle carriers for cyclosporine [97] and indomethacin [98] that result in increased intraocular permeability of the topical solutions as well as increased dwell time on the ocular surface [99]. Besides being cationic, chitosan has the advantage of being able to transiently open tight junctions between epithelial cells, increasing permeability [100]. Chitosan is also being investigated as a carrier for multiple other ophthalmic medications [100].

Curcumin, a spice, has been demonstrated to have anti-inflammatory activity and to have potential as an adjuvant for the suppression of inflammation in uveitis, as discussed previously. However, it has poor bioavailability and a rapid half-life when administered orally or topically. Recently, a calix[4]arene–curcumin nano aggregate has been described that has good intraocular penetration and was able to avert lipopolysaccharide-induced EAU in a rat model [101]. Human studies have not been undertaken, to date.

Liposomes

Liposomes function differently than nanoparticles in that their main purpose is to increase drug dwell time inside the eye rather than to enhance permeability. Many drugs are rapidly cleared from the intraocular space, requiring frequent repeat dosing to maintain therapeutic levels. Liposomes are an approach to overcome this problem. Liposomal drug preparations result in a central, aqueous phase containing the therapeutic agent surrounded by an amphiphilic shell of lipid molecules. The exterior lipophilic portion of the shell prevents rapid clearance of the therapeutic agent and results in longer-term release. There are multiple currently available medications for systemic administration that come in liposomal preparations, including one notable ocular drug. Verteporfin, used in photodynamic therapy, is a liposomal preparation of a photoactive benzoporphyrin derivative that is given systemically and activated with 689 nm wavelength light shined upon the area of treatment [102].

Prior to the development of highly active antiretroviral therapy (HAART) for the human immunodeficiency virus (HIV), cytomegalovirus (CMV) retinitis was an insidious and all-too-frequent cause of loss of vision. Given the rapid clearance of foscarnet and ganciclovir from the intravitreal space and the frequent need for repeat injection, a significant amount of work was done on developing liposomal formulations of anti-CMV drugs for intravitreal delivery. These yielded stable liposomal preparations of cidofovir [103] and ganciclovir [104, 105], the latter of which was tested in early phase clinical trials. Interestingly, this era also yielded the novel antisense antiviral drug fomivirsen, which was the first in its class to win FDA approval [106]. The advent of HAART and the dramatic reduction in CMV retinitis burden resulted in the discontinuation of this line of inquiry for the anti-CMV treatments; however, the building blocks established have the potential to be applied to the current challenges in uveitis.

Preclinical experiments with EAU in a rat model demonstrated a significant reduction in inflammatory activity with intravitreal injection of liposomal-encapsulated infliximab as compared to bare infliximab [107]. Likewise, liposomal tacrolimus demonstrated a more rapid resolution of EAU in a mouse model as compared to bare tacrolimus, with no intraocular toxicity [107].

In addition to potentially improved delivery of anti-inflammatory medications that are currently used in uveitis, liposomal encapsulation provides the possibility of the introduction of novel anti-inflammatory mediators. Vasoactive intestinal peptide encapsulated in liposomes and injected intravitreally has been shown to downregulate EAU in a rat model [108, 109]. Transduction of liposomally delivered plasmid DNA has been demonstrated with β-galactosidase gene transfer via intravitreal injection in rats [110]. Although this work was a proof of concept without specific uveitic applications, it opens the door to a potential transient gene therapy approach to inflammation.

Iontophoresis

Iontophoresis utilizes an ionic charge gradient generated by an annular electrode applied to the ocular surface to drive charged particles through the ocular surface and into the eye [111]. This can, in theory, work with multiple different charged molecules, but its utility has been demonstrated only with dexamethasone phosphate. The advantage of this treatment is that it can achieve very high concentrations of steroid within the eye with a single treatment, eliminating or reducing the need for topical steroid drop application. A phase I/II trial demonstrated resolution of all anterior chamber cell in 60% of patients after a single treatment [111]; phase III trials are currently pending. There is only a single iontophoresis device available on the market, the Eyegate II from Eyegate Pharma, Waltham, MA.

Suprachoroidal Delivery

The suprachoroidal space has recently demonstrated promise as an effective route for corticosteroid delivery. First proposed as a surgical procedure in 2006 [112], the technique has been refined and a disposable injector developed to enable repeatable, nonsurgical delivery of triamcinolone to the suprachoroidal space [113]. This technique caries the advantage of targeted posterior segment steroid delivery. Animal studies in rabbits have demonstrated that, after a suprachoroidal injection, triamcinolone levels in the retina are over 500,000 times greater than in the aqueous and 25,000 times greater than systemically [114].

A series of phase I through III trials have investigated the safety and efficacy of a suprachoroidal injection of 4 mg of triamcinolone for the treatment of uveitic macular edema associated with noninfectious uveitis and have yielded promising results [113, 115]. The phase III PEACHTREE trial demonstrated a significantly greater proportion of patients gaining three or more lines of vision in the treatment arm than the sham arm (47% vs 16%, respectively), meeting the primary endpoint of the study [115]. The trial also met its secondary endpoint, with a significant reduction in central retinal thickness from baseline to the 24-week endpoint in the treatment group versus the sham (157 vs 19 microns, respectively) [115].

Compliance with Ethical Requirements Julie Schallhorn declares she does not have any conflict of interest. No human studies were carried out by the authors of this book. No animal studies were carried out by the authors of this book.

References

1. Tugal-Tutkun I, Pavesio C, De Cordoue A, Bernard-Poenaru O, Gul A. Use of Gevokizumab in patients with Behcet's disease uveitis: an international, randomized, double-masked, placebo-controlled study and open-label extension study. Ocul Immunol Inflamm. 2018;26(7):1023–33.
2. Dick AD, Tugal-Tutkun I, Foster S, et al. Secukinumab in the treatment of noninfectious uveitis: results of three randomized, controlled clinical trials. Ophthalmology. 2013;120(4):777–87.
3. Buggage RR, Levy-Clarke G, Sen HN, et al. A double-masked, randomized study to investigate the safety and efficacy of daclizumab to treat the ocular complications related to Behcet's disease. Ocul Immunol Inflamm. 2007;15(2):63–70.
4. Baker KF, Isaacs JD. Novel therapies for immune-mediated inflammatory diseases: what can we learn from their use in rheumatoid arthritis, spondyloarthritis, systemic lupus erythematosus, psoriasis, Crohn's disease and ulcerative colitis? Ann Rheum Dis. 2018;77(2):175–87.
5. Glatt S, Helmer E, Haier B, et al. First-in-human randomized study of bimekizumab, a humanized monoclonal antibody and selective dual inhibitor of IL-17A and IL-17F, in mild psoriasis. Br J Clin Pharmacol. 2017;83(5):991–1001.
6. Griffiths CE, Reich K, Lebwohl M, et al. Comparison of ixekizumab with etanercept or placebo in moderate-to-severe psoriasis (UNCOVER-2 and UNCOVER-3): results from two phase 3 randomised trials. Lancet. 2015;386(9993):541–51.
7. Hueber W, Sands BE, Lewitzky S, et al. Secukinumab, a human anti-IL-17A monoclonal antibody, for moderate to severe Crohn's disease: unexpected results of a randomised, double-blind placebo-controlled trial. Gut. 2012;61(12):1693–700.
8. Nirula A, Nilsen J, Klekotka P, et al. Effect of IL-17 receptor a blockade with brodalumab in inflammatory diseases. Rheumatology (Oxford). 2016;55(suppl 2):ii43–55.
9. Pavelka K, Chon Y, Newmark R, Lin SL, Baumgartner S, Erondu N. A study to evaluate the safety, tolerability, and efficacy of brodalumab in subjects with rheumatoid arthritis and an inadequate response to methotrexate. J Rheumatol. 2015;42(6):912–9.
10. Mugheddu C, Atzori L, Del Piano M, et al. Successful ustekinumab treatment of noninfectious uveitis and concomitant severe psoriatic arthritis and plaque psoriasis. Dermatol Ther. 2017;30(5):e12527.

11. Blauvelt A, Reich K, Tsai TF, et al. Secukinumab is superior to ustekinumab in clearing skin of subjects with moderate-to-severe plaque psoriasis up to 1 year: results from the CLEAR study. J Am Acad Dermatol. 2017;76(1):60–9. e69
12. Schneider WM, Chevillotte MD, Rice CM. Interferon-stimulated genes: a complex web of host defenses. Annu Rev Immunol. 2014;32:513–45.
13. Khamashta M, Merrill JT, Werth VP, et al. Sifalimumab, an anti-interferon-alpha monoclonal antibody, in moderate to severe systemic lupus erythematosus: a randomised, double-blind, placebo-controlled study. Ann Rheum Dis. 2016;75(11):1909–16.
14. Kalunian KC, Merrill JT, Maciuca R, et al. A phase II study of the efficacy and safety of rontalizumab (rhuMAb interferon-alpha) in patients with systemic lupus erythematosus (ROSE). Ann Rheum Dis. 2016;75(1):196–202.
15. Furie R, Khamashta M, Merrill JT, et al. Anifrolumab, an anti-interferon-alpha receptor monoclonal antibody, in moderate-to-severe systemic lupus erythematosus. Arthritis Rheum (Hoboken, NJ). 2017;69(2):376–86.
16. Bernard R. Lauwerys, Eric Hachulla, François Spertini, Estibaliz Lazaro, Christian Jorgensen, Xavier Mariette, Edwige Haelterman, Géraldine Grouard-Vogel, Bernard Fanget, Olivier Dhellin, Pierre Vandepapelière, Frédéric A. Houssiau, (2013) Down-regulation of interferon signature in systemic lupus erythematosus patients by active immunization with interferon Î±-kinoid. Arthritis & Rheumatism 65 (2):447–56
17. Guerreiro Castro S, Isenberg DA. Belimumab in systemic lupus erythematosus (SLE): evidence-to-date and clinical usefulness. Ther Adv Musculoskelet Dis. 2017;9(3):75–85.
18. Merrill JT, van Vollenhoven RF, Buyon JP, et al. Efficacy and safety of subcutaneous tabalumab, a monoclonal antibody to B-cell activating factor, in patients with systemic lupus erythematosus: results from ILLUMINATE-2, a 52-week, phase III, multicentre, randomised, double-blind, placebo-controlled study. Ann Rheum Dis. 2016;75(2):332–40.
19. Hauser SL, Bar-Or A, Comi G, et al. Ocrelizumab versus interferon Beta-1a in relapsing multiple sclerosis. N Engl J Med. 2017;376(3):221–34.
20. Hartemann A, Bensimon G, Payan CA, et al. Low-dose interleukin 2 in patients with type 1 diabetes: a phase 1/2 randomised, double-blind, placebo-controlled trial. Lancet Diabetes Endocrinol. 2013;1(4):295–305.
21. Koreth J, Matsuoka K, Kim HT, et al. Interleukin-2 and regulatory T cells in graft-versus-host disease. N Engl J Med. 2011;365(22):2055–66.
22. von Spee-Mayer C, Siegert E, Abdirama D, et al. Low-dose interleukin-2 selectively corrects regulatory T cell defects in patients with systemic lupus erythematosus. Ann Rheum Dis. 2016;75(7):1407–15.
23. Goodyear M. Learning from the TGN1412 trial. BMJ (Clinical research ed). 2006;332(7543):677–8.
24. Tyrsin D, Chuvpilo S, Matskevich A, et al. From TGN1412 to TAB08: the return of CD28 superagonist therapy to clinical development for the treatment of rheumatoid arthritis. Clin Exp Rheumatol. 2016;34(4 Suppl 98):45–8.
25. Konig M, Rharbaoui F, Aigner S, Dalken B, Schuttrumpf J. Tregalizumab – a monoclonal antibody to target regulatory T cells. Front Immunol. 2016;7:11.
26. De Groot AS, Moise L, McMurry JA, et al. Activation of natural regulatory T cells by IgG fc-derived peptide "Tregitopes". Blood. 2008;112(8):3303–11.
27. Dhillon S. Tofacitinib: a review in rheumatoid arthritis. Drugs. 2017;77(18):1987–2001.
28. Healio. https://www.healio.com/ophthalmology/retina-vitreous/news/online/%7B7acf5955-5299-42c0-bcde-56687839e439%7D/santens-intravitreal-sirolimus-for-noninfectious-posterior-segment-uveitis-not-approved. Accessed 10 Jan 2018.
29. Holland EJ, Luchs J, Karpecki PM, et al. Lifitegrast for the treatment of dry eye disease: results of a phase III, randomized, double-masked, placebo-controlled trial (OPUS-3). Ophthalmology. 2017;124(1):53–60.
30. Sheppard JD, Torkildsen GL, Lonsdale JD, et al. Lifitegrast ophthalmic solution 5.0% for treatment of dry eye disease: results of the OPUS-1 phase 3 study. Ophthalmology. 2014;121(2):475–83.

31. Tauber J, Karpecki P, Latkany R, et al. Lifitegrast ophthalmic solution 5.0% versus placebo for treatment of dry eye disease: results of the randomized phase III OPUS-2 study. Ophthalmology. 2015;122(12):2423–31.
32. Madri JA, Graesser D, Haas T. The roles of adhesion molecules and proteinases in lymphocyte transendothelial migration. Biochem Cell Biol. 1996;74(6):749–57.
33. Martin AP, de Moraes LV, Tadokoro CE, et al. Administration of a peptide inhibitor of alpha4-integrin inhibits the development of experimental autoimmune uveitis. Invest Ophthalmol Vis Sci. 2005;46(6):2056–63.
34. Bloomgren G, Richman S, Hotermans C, et al. Risk of natalizumab-associated progressive multifocal leukoencephalopathy. N Engl J Med. 2012;366(20):1870–80.
35. Kurose S, Ikeda E, Tokiwa M, Hikita N, Mochizuki M. Effects of FTY720, a novel immunosuppressant, on experimental autoimmune uveoretinitis in rats. Exp Eye Res. 2000;70(1):7–15.
36. Commodaro AG, Peron JP, Lopes CT, et al. Evaluation of experimental autoimmune uveitis in mice treated with FTY720. Invest Ophthalmol Vis Sci. 2010;51(5):2568–74.
37. Zarbin MA, Jampol LM, Jager RD, et al. Ophthalmic evaluations in clinical studies of fingolimod (FTY720) in multiple sclerosis. Ophthalmology. 2013;120(7):1432–9.
38. Egwuagu CE, Larkin IJ. Therapeutic targeting of STAT pathways in CNS autoimmune diseases. JAK-STAT. 2013;2(1):e24134.
39. Lee EB, Fleischmann R, Hall S, et al. Tofacitinib versus methotrexate in rheumatoid arthritis. N Engl J Med. 2014;370(25):2377–86.
40. Taylor PC, Keystone EC, van der Heijde D, et al. Baricitinib versus placebo or adalimumab in rheumatoid arthritis. N Engl J Med. 2017;376(7):652–62.
41. Huang J-F, Zhang Y, Hirakawa B. Evaluation of JAK inhibition with topical tofacitinib in an experimental autoimmune uveitis model (EAU). Association for Research in Vision and Ophthalmology Annual Meeting; 2013; Ft. Lauderdale.
42. Harris TJ, Grosso JF, Yen HR, et al. Cutting edge: an in vivo requirement for STAT3 signaling in TH17 development and TH17-dependent autoimmunity. J Immunol. 2007;179(7):4313–7.
43. Liu X, Lee YS, Yu CR, Egwuagu CE. Loss of STAT3 in CD4+ T cells prevents development of experimental autoimmune diseases. J Immunol. 2008;180(9):6070–6.
44. Yu CR, Lee YS, Mahdi RM, Surendran N, Egwuagu CE. Therapeutic targeting of STAT3 (signal transducers and activators of transcription 3) pathway inhibits experimental autoimmune uveitis. PLoS One. 2012;7(1):e29742.
45. Bae SC, Lee YH. Comparative efficacy and tolerability of monotherapy with leflunomide or tacrolimus for the treatment of rheumatoid arthritis: a Bayesian network meta-analysis of randomized controlled trials. Clin Rheumatol. 2018;37(2):323–30.
46. Molina C, Modesto C, Martin-Begue N, Arnal C. Leflunomide, a valid and safe drug for the treatment of chronic anterior uveitis associated with juvenile idiopathic arthritis. Clin Rheumatol. 2013;32(11):1673–5.
47. Bichler J, Benseler SM, Krumrey-Langkammerer M, Haas JP, Hugle B. Leflunomide is associated with a higher flare rate compared to methotrexate in the treatment of chronic uveitis in juvenile idiopathic arthritis. Scand J Rheumatol. 2015;44(4):280–3.
48. Fang CB, Zhou DX, Zhan SX, et al. Amelioration of experimental autoimmune uveitis by leflunomide in Lewis rats. PLoS One. 2013;8(4):e62071.
49. Diedrichs-Mohring M, Leban J, Strobl S, Obermayr F, Wildner G. A new small molecule for treating inflammation and chorioretinal neovascularization in relapsing-remitting and chronic experimental autoimmune uveitis. Invest Ophthalmol Vis Sci. 2014;56(2):1147–57.
50. Kumar N, Goldminz AM, Kim N, Gottlieb AB. Phosphodiesterase 4-targeted treatments for autoimmune diseases. BMC Med. 2013;11:96.
51. Xu H, Strassmann G, Chan CC, et al. Protective effect of the type IV phosphodiesterase inhibitor rolipram in EAU: protection is independent of IL-10-inducing activity. Invest Ophthalmol Vis Sci. 1999;40(5):942–50.
52. Gooderham M, Papp K. Apremilast in the treatment of psoriasis and psoriatic arthritis. Skin Therapy Lett. 2015;20(5):1–6.

53. Yadav UC, Kalariya NM, Ramana KV. Emerging role of antioxidants in the protection of uveitis complications. Curr Med Chem. 2011;18(6):931–42.
54. Nguyen AM, Rao NA. Oxidative photoreceptor cell damage in autoimmune uveitis. J Ophthalmic Inflamm Infect. 2010;1(1):7–13.
55. Saraswathy S, Rao NA. Photoreceptor mitochondrial oxidative stress in experimental autoimmune uveitis. Ophthalmic Res. 2008;40(3–4):160–4.
56. Lawrence T. The nuclear factor NF-kappaB pathway in inflammation. Cold Spring Harb Perspect Biol. 2009;1(6):a001651.
57. Wright JG, Christman JW. The role of nuclear factor kappa B in the pathogenesis of pulmonary diseases: implications for therapy. Am J Respir Med. 2003;2(3):211–9.
58. Yadav UC, Shoeb M, Srivastava SK, Ramana KV. Amelioration of experimental autoimmune uveoretinitis by aldose reductase inhibition in Lewis rats. Invest Ophthalmol Vis Sci. 2011;52(11):8033–41.
59. Yadav UC, Srivastava SK, Ramana KV. Aldose reductase inhibition prevents endotoxin-induced uveitis in rats. Invest Ophthalmol Vis Sci. 2007;48(10):4634–42.
60. Di Filippo C, Zippo MV, Maisto R, et al. Inhibition of ocular aldose reductase by a new benzofuroxane derivative ameliorates rat endotoxic uveitis. Mediat Inflamm. 2014;2014:857958.
61. Suzuki J, Yoshimura T, Simeonova M, et al. Aminoimidazole carboxamide ribonucleotide ameliorates experimental autoimmune uveitis. Invest Ophthalmol Vis Sci. 2012;53(7):4158–69.
62. Nguyen QD, Merrill PT, Clark WL, et al. Intravitreal sirolimus for noninfectious uveitis: a phase III sirolimus study assessing double-masKed Uveitis TReAtment (SAKURA). Ophthalmology. 2016;123(11):2413–23.
63. Allegri P, Mastromarino A, Neri P. Management of chronic anterior uveitis relapses: efficacy of oral phospholipidic curcumin treatment. Long-term follow-up. Clin Ophthalmol. 2010;4:1201–6.
64. Shirinsky IV, Biryukova AA, Shirinsky VS. Simvastatin as an adjunct to conventional therapy of non-infectious uveitis: a randomized, open-label pilot study. Curr Eye Res. 2017;42(12):1713–8.
65. Shalaby U. Diltiazem co treatment with cyclosporine for induction of disease remission in sight-threatening non-infectious intraocular inflammation. Jpn J Ophthalmol. 2017;61(2):169–78.
66. Driot JY, Novack GD, Rittenhouse KD, Milazzo C, Pearson PA. Ocular pharmacokinetics of fluocinolone acetonide after Retisert intravitreal implantation in rabbits over a 1-year period. J Ocul Pharmacol Ther. 2004;20(3):269–75.
67. Holbrook JT, Sugar EA, Burke AE, et al. Dissociations of the fluocinolone acetonide implant: the multicenter uveitis steroid treatment (MUST) trial and follow-up study. Am J Ophthalmol. 2016;164:29–36.
68. Campochiaro PA, Hafiz G, Shah SM, et al. Sustained ocular delivery of fluocinolone acetonide by an intravitreal insert. Ophthalmology. 2010;117(7):1393–9. e1393
69. Reddy AK, Burkholder BM, Khan IR, Thorne JE. Iluvien implantation for uveitis and uveitic macular Edema. Ocul Immunol Inflamm. 2018;26(2):315–16.
70. Jaffe GJ, Lin P, Keenan RT, Ashton P, Skalak C, Stinnett SS. Injectable fluocinolone acetonide long-acting implant for noninfectious intermediate uveitis, posterior uveitis, and panuveitis: two-year results. Ophthalmology. 2016;123(9):1940–8.
71. Humayun M, Santos A, Altamirano JC, et al. Implantable MicroPump for drug delivery in patients with diabetic macular Edema. Transl Vis Sci Technol. 2014;3(6):5.
72. clinicaltrials.gov. https://clinicaltrials.gov/ct2/show/NCT02510794. Accessed 5 Nov 2017.
73. Rawas-Qalaji M, Williams CA. Advances in ocular drug delivery. Curr Eye Res. 2012;37(5):345–56.
74. Liu YC, Peng Y, Lwin NC, Wong TT, Venkatraman SS, Mehta JS. Optimization of subconjunctival biodegradable microfilms for sustained drug delivery to the anterior segment in a small animal model. Invest Ophthalmol Vis Sci. 2013;54(4):2607–15.
75. Thackaberry EA, Farman C, Zhong F, et al. Evaluation of the toxicity of intravitreally injected PLGA microspheres and rods in monkeys and rabbits: effects of depot size on inflammatory response. Invest Ophthalmol Vis Sci. 2017;58(10):4274–85.

76. Chang-Lin JE, Attar M, Acheampong AA, et al. Pharmacokinetics and pharmacodynamics of a sustained-release dexamethasone intravitreal implant. Invest Ophthalmol Vis Sci. 2011;52(1):80–6.
77. Whitcup SM, Robinson MR. Development of a dexamethasone intravitreal implant for the treatment of noninfectious posterior segment uveitis. Ann N Y Acad Sci. 2015;1358:1–12.
78. Souza MC, Fialho SL, Souza PA, Fulgencio GO, Da Silva GR, Silva-Cunha A. Tacrolimus-loaded PLGA implants: in vivo release and ocular toxicity. Curr Eye Res. 2014;39(1):99–102.
79. Sakurai E, Nozaki M, Okabe K, Kunou N, Kimura H, Ogura Y. Scleral plug of biodegradable polymers containing tacrolimus (FK506) for experimental uveitis. Invest Ophthalmol Vis Sci. 2003;44(11):4845–52.
80. Jaffe GJ, Yang CS, Wang XC, Cousins SW, Gallemore RP, Ashton P. Intravitreal sustained-release cyclosporine in the treatment of experimental uveitis. Ophthalmology. 1998;105(1):46–56.
81. Dong X, Shi W, Yuan G, Xie L, Wang S, Lin P. Intravitreal implantation of the biodegradable cyclosporin a drug delivery system for experimental chronic uveitis. Graefes Arch Clin Exp Ophthalmol. 2006;244(4):492–7.
82. Shi W, Chen M, Xie L, et al. A novel cyclosporine a drug-delivery system for prevention of human corneal rejection after high-risk keratoplasty: a clinical study. Ophthalmology. 2013;120(4):695–702.
83. Lee SS, Kim H, Wang NS, et al. A pharmacokinetic and safety evaluation of an episcleral cyclosporine implant for potential use in high-risk keratoplasty rejection. Invest Ophthalmol Vis Sci. 2007;48(5):2023–9.
84. Bock F, Matthaei M, Reinhard T, et al. High-dose subconjunctival cyclosporine a implants do not affect corneal neovascularization after high-risk keratoplasty. Ophthalmology. 2014;121(9):1677–82.
85. Liu YC, Peng Y, Lwin NC, Venkatraman SS, Wong TT, Mehta JS. A biodegradable, sustained-released, prednisolone acetate microfilm drug delivery system effectively prolongs corneal allograft survival in the rat keratoplasty model. PLoS One. 2013;8(8):e70419.
86. Liu YC, Ng XW, Teo EPW, et al. A biodegradable, sustained-released, tacrolimus microfilm drug delivery system for the management of allergic conjunctivitis in a mouse model. Invest Ophthalmol Vis Sci. 2018;59(2):675–84.
87. Manna S, Augsburger JJ, Correa ZM, Landero JA, Banerjee RK. Development of chitosan and polylactic acid based methotrexate intravitreal micro-implants to treat primary intraocular lymphoma: an in vitro study. J Biomech Eng. 2014;136(2):021018.
88. Manna S, Banerjee RK, Augsburger JJ, Al-Rjoub MF, Donnell A, Correa ZM. Biodegradable chitosan and polylactic acid-based intraocular micro-implant for sustained release of methotrexate into vitreous: analysis of pharmacokinetics and toxicity in rabbit eyes. Graefes Arch Clin Exp Ophthalmol. 2015;253(8):1297–305.
89. Bioscience I. http://iconbioscience.com/verisome-drug-delivery-technology/. Accessed 13 Nov 2017.
90. Janagam DR, Wu L, Lowe TL. Nanoparticles for drug delivery to the anterior segment of the eye. Adv Drug Deliv Rev. 2017;122:31–64.
91. Gan L, Han S, Shen J, et al. Self-assembled liquid crystalline nanoparticles as a novel ophthalmic delivery system for dexamethasone: improving preocular retention and ocular bioavailability. Int J Pharm. 2010;396(1–2):179–87.
92. Han S, Shen JQ, Gan Y, et al. Novel vehicle based on cubosomes for ophthalmic delivery of flurbiprofen with low irritancy and high bioavailability. Acta Pharmacol Sin. 2010;31(8):990–8.
93. Adibkia K, Javadzadeh Y, Dastmalchi S, Mohammadi G, Niri FK, Alaei-Beirami M. Naproxen-eudragit RS100 nanoparticles: preparation and physicochemical characterization. Colloids Surf B Biointerfaces. 2011;83(1):155–9.
94. Katara R, Majumdar DK. Eudragit RL 100-based nanoparticulate system of aceclofenac for ocular delivery. Colloids Surf B Biointerfaces. 2013;103:455–62.
95. Adibkia K, Siahi Shadbad MR, Nokhodchi A, et al. Piroxicam nanoparticles for ocular delivery: physicochemical characterization and implementation in endotoxin-induced uveitis. J Drug Target. 2007;15(6):407–16.

96. Adibkia K, Omidi Y, Siahi MR, et al. Inhibition of endotoxin-induced uveitis by methylprednisolone acetate nanosuspension in rabbits. J Ocul Pharmacol Ther. 2007;23(5):421–32.
97. De Campos AM, Sanchez A, Alonso MJ. Chitosan nanoparticles: a new vehicle for the improvement of the delivery of drugs to the ocular surface. Application to cyclosporin a. Int J Pharm. 2001;224(1–2):159–68.
98. Badawi AA, El-Laithy HM, El Qidra RK, El Mofty H, El dally M. Chitosan based nanocarriers for indomethacin ocular delivery. Arch Pharm Res. 2008;31(8):1040–9.
99. Yamaguchi M, Ueda K, Isowaki A, et al. Mucoadhesive properties of chitosan-coated ophthalmic lipid emulsion containing indomethacin in tear fluid. Biol Pharm Bull. 2009;32(7):1266–71.
100. Alonso MJ, Sanchez A. The potential of chitosan in ocular drug delivery. J Pharm Pharmacol. 2003;55(11):1451–63.
101. Granata G, Paterniti I, Geraci C, et al. Potential eye drop based on a calix[4]arene nanoassembly for curcumin delivery: enhanced drug solubility, stability, and anti-inflammatory effect. Mol Pharm. 2017;14(5):1610–22.
102. Bochot A, Fattal E. Liposomes for intravitreal drug delivery: a state of the art. J Control Release. 2012;161(2):628–34.
103. Kuppermann BD, Assil KK, Vuong C, et al. Liposome-encapsulated (S)-1-(3-hydroxy-2-phosphonylmethoxypropyl)cytosine for long-acting therapy of viral retinitis. J Infect Dis. 1996;173(1):18–23.
104. Diaz-Llopis M, Martos MJ, Espana E, et al. Liposomally-entrapped ganciclovir for the treatment of cytomegalovirus retinitis in AIDS patients. Experimental toxicity and pharmacokinetics, and clinical trial. Doc Ophthalmol. 1992;82(4):297–305.
105. Akula SK, Ma PE, Peyman GA, et al. Treatment of cytomegalovirus retinitis with intravitreal injection of liposome encapsulated ganciclovir in a patient with AIDS. Br J Ophthalmol. 1994;78(9):677–80.
106. Bochot A, Couvreur P, Fattal E. Intravitreal administration of antisense oligonucleotides: potential of liposomal delivery. Prog Retin Eye Res. 2000;19(2):131–47.
107. Zhang R, Qian J, Li X, Yuan Y. Treatment of experimental autoimmune uveoretinitis with intravitreal injection of infliximab encapsulated in liposomes. Br J Ophthalmol. 2017;101(12):1731–8.
108. Lajavardi L, Camelo S, Agnely F, et al. New formulation of vasoactive intestinal peptide using liposomes in hyaluronic acid gel for uveitis. J Control Release. 2009;139(1):22–30.
109. Lajavardi L, Bochot A, Camelo S, et al. Downregulation of endotoxin-induced uveitis by intravitreal injection of vasoactive intestinal peptide encapsulated in liposomes. Invest Ophthalmol Vis Sci. 2007;48(7):3230–8.
110. Masuda I, Matsuo T, Yasuda T, Matsuo N. Gene transfer with liposomes to the intraocular tissues by different routes of administration. Invest Ophthalmol Vis Sci. 1996;37(9):1914–20.
111. Patane MA, Schubert W, Sanford T, et al. Evaluation of ocular and general safety following repeated dosing of dexamethasone phosphate delivered by transscleral iontophoresis in rabbits. J Ocul Pharmacol Ther. 2013;29(8):760–9.
112. Olsen TW, Feng X, Wabner K, et al. Cannulation of the suprachoroidal space: a novel drug delivery methodology to the posterior segment. Am J Ophthalmol. 2006;142(5):777–87.
113. Goldstein DA, Do D, Noronha G, Kissner JM, Srivastava SK, Nguyen QD. Suprachoroidal corticosteroid administration: a novel route for local treatment of noninfectious uveitis. Transl Vis Sci Technol. 2016;5(6):14.
114. Chen M, Li X, Liu J, Han Y, Cheng L. Safety and pharmacodynamics of suprachoroidal injection of triamcinolone acetonide as a controlled ocular drug release model. J Control Release. 2015;203:109–17.
115. Yeh S. Suprachoroidally injected CLS-TA improves visual acuity and macular Edema in noninfectious uveitis: results of the phase 3 PEACHTREE study. Paper presented at American Society of Retina Specialists; 2018 July 25; Vancouver, B.C.

Index

N. A. Rao et al. (eds.), *Posterior Uveitis*, Essentials in Ophthalmology,
https://doi.org/10.1007/978-3-030-03140-4

MIX
Papier aus verantwortungsvollen Quellen
Paper from responsible sources
FSC® C105338

If you have any concerns about our products,
you can contact us on
ProductSafety@springernature.com

In case Publisher is established outside the EU,
the EU authorized representative is:
Springer Nature Customer Service Center GmbH
Europaplatz 3, 69115 Heidelberg, Germany

Printed by Libri Plureos GmbH
in Hamburg, Germany